"If you don't take care of your body, where are you going to live?"

- Jim Rohn

Written by Dr. Nivedita Lakhera, MD, Internal Medicine
Illustration by Ms. Sathvega Somasundaram & Mr. Munavar Nahas
Fed and formatted by Mr. Munavar Nahas
Proofreading by Dr. Heena Majmudar

A heartfelt shout-out to Mr. Stephen Colbert—your wit, wisdom, and humor have been a lifeline in more ways than I can express. You quite literally saved my life.

To Mr. Vidhu Vinod Chopra—your cinematic masterpiece, *12th Fail*, resonated deeply not only with me but with countless others who were profoundly moved by its raw power and message.

To My Family and Friends—you are my unwavering support, my tribe, my joy, and my strength.

And above all, to My Parents, Mr. Subhash Chandra Lakhera and Mrs. Surendra Lakhera—you are my guiding light, my faith, my happiness, my moral compass. You are my roots, my strength, and my everything. I love you so very much.

niveditalakhera.com

Dearest One,

Thank you for being here, and thank you for being you. Thank you for choosing this book and for sharing a part of your time—and therefore, your life—with me. I kiss your hand and soul in gratitude for this honor, with my humble and sincere thanks. You are amazing, worthy of everything that is good, and this book was written with that intention—to help you cultivate and augment all the goodness within you, in your mind, your heart, your brain, and every beautiful part of who you are.

Please remember, no matter who you are, where you've been, or what you've done—there is no place you cannot come back from. You are worthy. Whether you have loved or lost, hurt others or yourself, whether you have sinned or triumphed, you are worthy of beauty, redemption, healing, and new beginnings.

I hope you remind yourself that to begin is your birthright, and to simply be is your poetry. No matter who you are or where you are, I am here to hold your hand as we walk together—in rebuilding, redesigning, reliving, or simply continuing the journey of you. For as long as you have a day, another day, two days, or many days, you deserve all of your love, your compassion, and your efforts. But, like all forms of love, self-love requires action. This book is my attempt to be your soulmate and friend, helping you take one, two, or even several of those actions.

This book is part of the -Building Better You- series, a journey that begins with the understanding that what holds you back does not exist. In this series, I attempt not just to offer information, but to give you a little joy as well. In this book, *Building Better Brain*, we tend to your mind. It is volume one of the upcoming series, where we caress, care for, and cultivate the best of you and all parts of you—heart, liver, bones, muscles, immunity, and so much more. Together, we embrace the beauty and resilience within you, and all that the world has to offer, so you can shine with all your light.

My mission is to close the gap between science and your everyday life. This is me, trying to take care of you. When you hold this book, you are holding me—my strength, my love, my compassion, and my knowledge. Whether you need to rest, grieve, celebrate, or just be—I am right here, next to you.

You are an extraordinary gift from the universe, and you deserve nothing less than the best this life has to offer. Thank you for allowing me to be part of your journey. I promise to stand by you with everything I have. And if we ever falter, I ask you to find extra love and forgiveness in your heart for both of us, so we can rest, reflect, and restart when needed. Come, let's go...

Sincerely- nivedita lakhera

the best part
about being human
is that
we have the capacity
to recreate our minds
and therefore
recreate our lives,
and we start there.

no one is coming
to save us
from ourselves;
this job falls on us,
not just to save ourselves
but to excel
at being
our best selves.

and it starts
with a decision

Come, let's go.
what holds you back
does not exist.

I recognize the immense privilege of having access to clean drinking water and proper nutrition. Around 2.2 billion people worldwide lack access to safe water, while 2.4 billion people do not have reliable access to food.

All of the profits from this book's sales will be donated to the World Food Programme (WFP) and Water.org. The World Food Programme, a branch of the United Nations, provides food assistance to over 90 million people in more than 73 countries. Water.org is a global nonprofit organization committed to bringing clean water and sanitation to those who need it most.

I want to extend my deepest gratitude to anyone who, in any capacity, contributes to helping others secure basic human rights such as dignity, education, safety, clean water, and proper nutrition.

This book is dedicated to each of you. Thank you from the bottom of my heart.

# अति सर्वत्र वर्जयेत्

Extremes of anything is to be avoided.

A Sanskrit verse highlights the importance of balance—neither too little nor too much. This reflects how our body is designed: when everything is in just the right measure, we feel in harmony.

Your body is a part of nature and thrives in balance.

To maintain this balance, avoid excess desires, attachments, indulgence, and emotions, as these are the true enemies of human well-being.

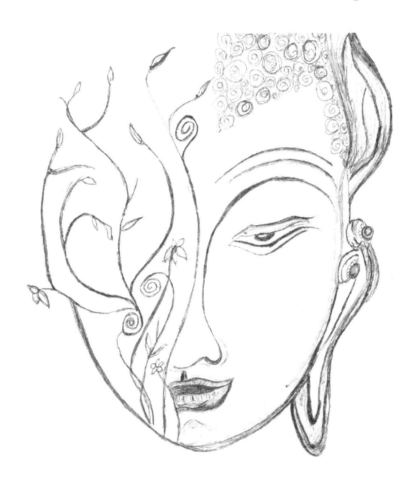

# Table of Contents

# History of Memory

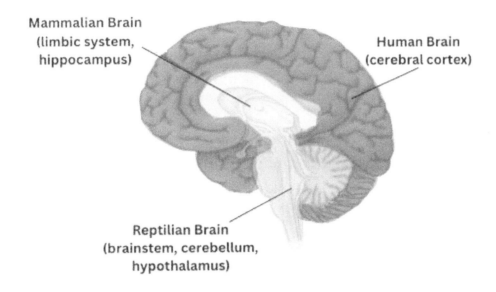

Mammalian Brain
(limbic system,
hippocampus)

Human Brain
(cerebral cortex)

Reptilian Brain
(brainstem, cerebellum,
hypothalamus)

# A Trip Down Memory Lane

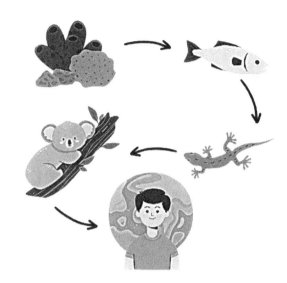

Let's start at the very beginning—about 600 million years ago—with sponges, the ultimate couch potatoes of the sea. These organisms didn't bother to develop a brain because, well, they didn't need one! Sponges are simple, filter-feeding organisms that just sit there, letting water flow through them and filtering out tiny bits of food. No need to think, no need to move—just a slow, relaxing life of endless filtering. Talk about living the dream! Sponges may not have had a brain, but they weren't completely clueless.

They possess some basic molecular machinery that would later be crucial in brain development. For instance, sponges have genes related to synapses (the junction where two neurons exchange information), even though they don't have neurons (brain cells) (Panichello et al., 2019). Think of them as the original tech support for the brain's wiring.

## Meet the Agnathans, the Original Brainiacs
Fast forward 100 million years to around 500 million years ago, where the ultimate evolution game show was underway. Contestants? The earliest fish-like creatures. Prize? The first-ever brain! Cue the dramatic drum roll because the winners of this prehistoric showdown were the Agnathans—jawless fish who had the guts (and the neurons) to develop the very first brains.
Fossils of early Agnathans have revealed the presence of primitive neural structures. These creatures showcased the earliest signs of a central nervous system that included a brain (Sheng, 2023).

Agnathans were among the earliest vertebrates to sport a brain divided into three parts: the forebrain, midbrain, and hindbrain, which handled essential tasks like sensory processing and movement. They went from being passive sea blobs to active participants in the underwater survival game.

## Ray-Finned Fish: The Brain Gets a Glow-Up

Fast forward a few million years, and we encounter ray-finned fish, which took the basic brain structure developed by the Agnathans and gave it a serious upgrade. These fish weren't just surviving; they were thriving, thanks to more complex brains that could process information, respond to their environment, and even remember things—like where the best food is. You know, the important stuff.

Ray-finned fish developed more complex brain structures, including a forebrain, midbrain, and hindbrain. These structures allowed them to process sensory information, control movement, and respond to threats—everything needed to survive in a prehistoric ocean full of hungry predators (Clark et al., 2014). Introducing epigenetics: imagine it as a dimmer switch for your genes. Just like how you can brighten or dim the lights without changing the bulb, epigenetics controls whether a gene is cranked up or toned down without altering the actual DNA. In fish, this "dimmer switch" became essential for their brains to quickly adapt to new environments—like adjusting the brightness of your phone screen depending on how sunny it is outside. So, fish brains weren't just getting new features; they were also learning to adjust to the world around them on the fly!

## The Dino Brain: More Than just a "Reptilian Brain"

Next in our evolutionary journey are the amphibians and reptiles, which took the basic fish brain and ran (or crawled) with it, developing more specialized brain regions. They beefed up their olfactory bulbs—the part of the brain that processes smells—turning themselves into prehistoric scent experts, sniffing out dinner and dodging predators! Amphibians began to develop a more defined forebrain and the early version of the limbic system—the drama department of the brain. This is the part that detects danger and triggers the fight, flight, or freeze responses (Barton & Capellini, 2011).

Reptiles took things a step further, refining their cerebral cortex, which allowed for more complex behaviors—well, to a point. But let's be real: a T-Rex wasn't about to solve a Rubik's Cube. That's because reptiles didn't evolve the complex cortex that supports higher-level thinking.

Instead, they developed the Dorsal Ventricular Ridge (DVR)—a simpler but effective brain structure. So, let's stop calling it the "reptilian brain." These ancient creatures had more going on than just basic survival instincts.
Here's where it gets really interesting: reptiles were among the first to show signs of epigenetic transmission—basically, passing down environmental hacks to their offspring like family recipes.

Environmental stressors like temperature and diet could lead to epigenetic changes in reptiles, which affected not just their own development but also that of their offspring. These changes were survival tools that helped reptiles adapt to their changing world (Kilpatrick, 2018).

**Mammals: The Brain Hits Its Stride**
Mammals took the reptilian brain and basically said, "Let's take this old-school model and give it a major upgrade!" Enter the cerebral cortex—the brain's VIP lounge where all the sophisticated thinking happens. It expanded like your Netflix watchlist during a weekend binge, especially in areas responsible for sensing the world and thinking about stuff beyond "Is this edible?" Thanks to this brain expansion, mammals were no longer just dodging predators—they were figuring out complex social behaviors, solving problems, and maybe even inventing the prehistoric version of Facebook to keep track of who was alpha in the neighborhood.

And let's not forget the brain chemistry makeover. Enter neurotransmitters—your brain's text messages—quickly delivering important info between neurons to keep everything buzzing and on track. With players like dopamine and serotonin stepping onto the scene, mammals unlocked the secret to balancing between "I'm happy" and "I need chocolate right now." These biochemical dance moves didn't just keep mammals alive; they had them thriving everywhere from the savanna to the suburbs.

## Humans: The Ultimate Brain Hack

Fast forward a few hundred million years, and we get to the human brain—the ultimate memory machine. Our ancestors weren't just memorizing which berries were safe to eat; they were mastering the arts of fire-starting, tool-making, and eventually, storytelling around the campfire. And what did that lead to? You guessed it: Snapchat filters, slime videos, and the endless parade of cat memes that dominate the internet. Who would've thought that the same brain that once struggled to remember where it buried a nut would one day create the *Gangnam Style* dance? Talk about an evolutionary plot twist!

The human brain didn't just stop at the basic mammal blueprint—it went full-on turbo mode. The prefrontal cortex, the brain's command center, became a powerhouse for decision-making, future planning, and, let's be real, overthinking everything.

But our brains aren't just running on logic. They're chemical playgrounds where neurotransmitters like dopamine drive us to seek rewards (think: pizza), serotonin tries to keep our moods steady (good luck with that), and glutamate helps us learn and remember everything from algebra to the lyrics of every Taylor Swift song.

These biochemical processes are the reason we can solve complex problems, fall in love, and, of course, argue on the internet about which Marvel movie is the best.

## The Human Brain: An Epigenetic Whiteboard

The human brain is like a massive whiteboard where life scribbles its messy notes, doodles, and occasionally, full-blown masterpieces. These epigenetic scribbles can have a huge impact on mental health, cognitive function, and even your daily behavior. Imagine your brain's epigenome as a giant, erasable whiteboard that's been getting written on by your ancestors, your experiences, and maybe even that one time you tried kombucha.

And in humans, epigenetics can be a bit of a double-edged sword. Sure, these changes can help with survival, but they can also pass down trauma. Studies have shown that trauma experienced by one generation can alter DNA methylation in their offspring, increasing their susceptibility to mental health issues like anxiety and depression. It's like inheriting your grandparents' DNA, along with a side of their trauma. This phenomenon, known as generational trauma, has been observed in various human populations, including descendants of Holocaust survivors and those affected by severe stress or famine (Kato & Ikeguchi, 2016; Hall et al., 2018). This has profound implications for mental health, highlighting the importance of understanding how environmental factors and experiences shape our genetic legacy (Benoit & Anderson, 2012).

## To remember some, you must forget some; to forget some, you must remember some!

As humans evolved, they couldn't help but wonder why they could remember every detail of their wedding day but couldn't, for the life of them, remember where they abandoned their spouse in the chaos of Target. This baffling paradox sent scientists on a wild goose chase to uncover the mysteries of memory. How do these tiny neurons manage to hold onto our life's greatest hits while conveniently misplacing the grocery list?

Turns out, memory is like a finely tuned orchestra of neurons, each one playing its part to help you recall that cringe-worthy high school dance but not the keys you set down five minutes ago. And here's the kicker—forgetting is actually a feature, not a bug. Yep, your brain has an entire system dedicated to deciding which memories to keep and which ones to toss into the "who needs this?" pile.

## Nobel Glory: Cracking the Memory Code, From Slug to Scholar

The quest to understand memory eventually caught the eye of the Nobel committee. In 2000, the Nobel Prize in Physiology or Medicine was awarded to three brainiacs—Eric Kandel, Arvid Carlsson, and Paul Greengard—who cracked the code on how our brains store memories.

Kandel's groundbreaking work with the sea slug *Aplysia* (yes, a slug won a Nobel!) showed that learning and memory are all about changes in nerve connection strength and the formation of new nerve connections.

It's like discovering that your brain can build new filing cabinets just to store all those life lessons. And let's give credit where it's due—to the slug itself.

In *Aplysia,* neurons don't just talk the talk—they stretch the stretch! These little sea slugs have neurons so long they could practically form a conga line on the ocean floor. Some of their neurons extend up to 10 cm, making them the skyscrapers of the neuron world. Researchers adore these slugs because, with neurons that big, it's like studying brain function with a magnifying glass on the Empire State Building—hard to miss and packed with useful info!

So, the next time you recall a fond memory, tip your hat to the neurons that, after billions of years of evolution, figured out how to store and recall information—and to the scientists who finally decoded their secrets. And of course, don't forget to give a shoutout to that legendary slug!

While Kandel was busy making slugs famous, Arvid Carlsson and Paul Greengard were hard at work decoding how neurotransmitters—those brain chemicals that send little text messages between neurons—like dopamine, influence brain signaling and memory. Their discoveries laid the groundwork for understanding not just memory, but a whole host of neurological conditions.

So, the next time you recall a fond memory, tip your hat to the neurons that, after billions of years of evolution, figured out how to store and recall information—and to the scientists who finally decoded their secrets. And, of course, don't forget to give a shoutout to that legendary slug!

Memory might have kicked off as a simple survival mechanism—like, "Hey don't eat that berry again"—but it has since leveled up into the complex cognitive tool that makes us, well, us. Whether you're trying to remember where you left your spouse or recalling the name of that scientist who won a Nobel Prize for studying slugs (gotcha! It's Eric Kandel, by the way), memory is one of our brain's most impressive party tricks. Who knew that one of our most remarkable evolutionary achievements started with a bunch of neurons just trying to keep it together in a rough-and-tumble world? It's like the brain went from surviving on ramen noodles to cooking up gourmet meals—with a side of existential crises, of course.

# Humans, Brunch, xoxo-
## Best Part of Evolution

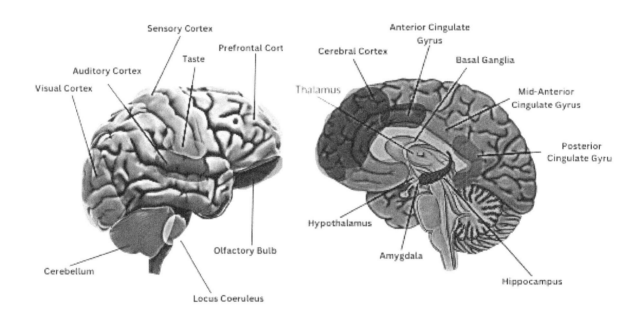

# The Brunch, Best Friends & Colbert

Niv wakes up with butterflies in her stomach because today's not just any day—she's about to have brunch with her besties, Mona (aka Jasdeep Virdi), Gautami Agastya, and Kavitha Jayachandran. And she's got some news that's going to blow their minds. As she finally makes her way into their favorite café, Appakadai, nestled in the heart of Mountain House, California, she's practically floating on air. Why? Because she was just invited to be on *The Stephen Colbert Show*! Yes, that Stephen Colbert. Niv has been head-over-heels, totally in love with him since forever, and now she's going to meet him! Emotions are running high, and this brunch is about to go down in history.

### Visual Cortex: Capturing the Scene

Niv's visual cortex, the part of her brain responsible for processing visual information, kicks into high gear as she finally spots her friends waving (and definitely rolling their eyes at her lateness) from their usual table at Appakadai. The brain's equivalent of a camera, the visual cortex, snaps mental pictures of her friends' smiling faces, the steaming plates of appam, and the aromatic cups of South Indian coffee, ensuring these images are locked in for later.

### Olfactory Bulb and Orbitofrontal Cortex: Savoring the Smells

As soon as Niv enters Appakadai, the warm, slightly fermented aroma of appam and the rich scent of South Indian coffee hit her like a wave of nostalgia and comfort. Her olfactory bulb, which processes smells, sends this sensory data directly to the orbitofrontal cortex, where her brain decides, "This smells like happiness," tagging these scents with emotional significance (Simonini, 2024). And here's something fun and diva-worthy: Unlike all the other senses that need the thalamus to relay information to the brain, olfaction takes the VIP route! It bypasses the thalamus entirely and heads straight to the brain's higher centers. Yes, your sense of smell doesn't wait in line—it goes straight to the head of the party!

**Auditory Cortex: The Soundtrack of Joy and Banter**

When Niv finally sits down, her friends are already buzzing with curiosity.

"Alright, Niv, what is it this time? Another Colbert marathon?" Mona teases, her eyes twinkling with mischief, barely able to contain a smirk.

Gautami, not missing a beat, adds, "Let me guess, you're finally getting that restraining order lifted?"

Niv bursts out laughing but quickly shakes her head. "No, you guys, this is serious! I'm going to be on *The Stephen Colbert Show!*"

The table erupts into gasps and squeals, but it doesn't stop the teasing. Kavitha, grinning widely, says, "Oh my God, Niv, he's really going to meet his biggest fan! The man who 'saved your life'!"

Mona, raising an eyebrow, jumps in, "Niv, if he saved your life, does that make him your 'Colbert Knight in Shining Armor?'"

Niv rolls her eyes but can't help but smile. "You know it's true," she says, her tone half-joking, half-serious. "As I cried through the stroke and divorce, Colbert was my lifeline. His show was the only thing that kept me going. Remember 'The Word' segment? It gave me laughter, smiles, and for some reason, hope when everything else felt like it was falling apart."

Kavitha chimes in again, "Ahem—that's all? Are you sure you're not missing any other details?"

Mona adds with a wicked grin, "Yeah, Niv. Don't forget that Colbert also taught you how to properly use sarcasm as a defense mechanism. I mean, he didn't just save your life, he also helped you weaponize that dry wit!"

"Ha ha ha! Also, he's handsome, alright!" Niv replied with a grin.

Gautami smirks, "Well, Niv, you'd better tell him that when you meet him. Just maybe don't lead with 'You saved my life, Stephen!' You don't want to scare the poor guy!"

Mona can't resist adding, "Yeah, Niv, save the 'I love you, Stephen!' for after the commercial break. You want him to finish the interview, not sprint off the set!"

The whole table bursts into laughter again, and Niv's auditory cortex is on overdrive, capturing every word, laugh, and teasing remark, making sure this banter-filled announcement is stored in her memory as clearly as the day she met her best friends (Gopaldas, 2024).

**Somatosensory Cortex: Feeling the Comfort**

As her friends continue to tease her ("Do you think you'll get to sit at the desk with him?"), Niv wraps her hands around her cup of South Indian coffee, the warmth grounding her in the moment. This feeling is processed by her somatosensory cortex, which is responsible for processing touch and physical sensations. The cozy comfort of the warm coffee cup, coupled with the teasing affection of her friends, adds another layer to the memory, making it something she can physically feel as well as remember (Montgomery, 2024).

**Gustatory Cortex: Tasting the Moment**

As Niv takes a bite of her appam, the gustatory cortex—the part of her brain that processes taste—comes alive. The savory, coconutty flavor of the dish is the perfect accompaniment to the excitement bubbling at the table. It ensures that the taste is remembered just as vividly as the sight and sound of this special brunch. For Niv, this isn't just food; it's the taste of joy, friendship, and dreams coming true (Simonini, 2024).

**Thalamus: The Brain's Relay Station**

As all these sensory inputs are being processed, the thalamus—the brain's central relay station—works behind the scenes, directing each piece of information to the appropriate brain regions. It's like an air traffic controller, making sure that every detail, from the smells to the sounds to the tastes, gets to where it needs to go in the brain (Sun, 2024). Of course, not every sensation takes the thalamus route— smell is too fabulous for that! It skips the thalamus entirely and goes straight to the brain for instant attention.

**Amygdala: Tagging the Emotions**

The amygdala, known for its role in processing emotions, steps in to tag this brunch with an emotional highlight marker. It's the part of Niv's brain that says, "This is important! Let's remember how happy this moment feels," ensuring that the emotional significance of her big news is attached to the memory (Sun, 2024).

**Locus Coeruleus: Enhancing Attention**

The locus coeruleus, a small but mighty nucleus in the brainstem, releases norepinephrine to enhance Niv's attention and focus on the moment. It's like the brain's way of saying, "Pay attention! This is a memory you're going to want to keep!" (Bennett, 2024).

**Hippocampus: Storing the Experience**

The hippocampus, the brain's main memory center, takes all this sensory information and emotional significance and begins the process of turning this brunch into a long-term memory. It's the part of the brain responsible for making sure Niv can look back on this moment days, months, and years from now and remember every detail, including the jokes, the teasing, and the shared excitement (Montgomery, 2024).

**Cerebellum: Coordinating the Experience**

As Niv toasts to friendship and her upcoming adventure with Colbert, the cerebellum—known for its role in coordinating movement—helps her keep her balance and composure. But beyond that, it also plays a role in enhancing cognitive functions, subtly helping Niv integrate all these sensory experiences into a cohesive memory (Bennett, 2024).

**Neocortex: The Final Storage**

When Niv goes to bed that night, her hippocampus replays the entire brunch, backward, and transfers those memories to the neocortex for long-term storage. The neocortex, responsible for higher-order brain functions like reasoning and sensory perception, ensures that every detail of this special day, from the friendly banter to the thrilling news, is stored safely for future recall (Carbone, 2024).

So, lovely people, apart from the truthiness of this story, this is how memory is formed. Any dysfunction in that pathway spells trouble for memory formation. Now that you've learned everything there is to know about the brain and memory, you can close the book and go have your own brunch. Just kidding! We're just getting started—hold onto your horses! Woo hoo! Let's make some new memories through this book. Come on, let's go! ☺

# The Divine Forces in Brain Health

**Brahma, Vishnu, Mahesh, and Shakti: The Divine Forces in Brain Health**

The intricate interplay of biological processes within the human brain can be likened to the cosmic roles of Brahma, Vishnu, Mahesh (Shiva), and Shakti. Each of these forces symbolizes critical biological processes that contribute to brain health and functionality.

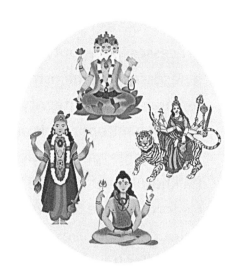

**Brahma: The Creator—Neural Stem Cells, Neurons, and the Miracle of Creation**

Brahma, as the creator, parallels the role of neural stem cells in the brain, which are responsible for generating new neurons throughout life. Recent studies indicate that these stem cells are not only active during early development but also continue to produce neurons in adulthood, albeit at a reduced rate and with increased selectivity (Milder, 1992). This process is crucial for neurogenesis, essential for learning and memory (Onishi et al., 2021). The limited production of neurons in adults can be viewed as a refined approach to brain development, akin to Brahma's careful crafting of the universe (Eshraghi et al., 2021).

**Vishnu: The Preserver—Maintaining Balance in the Brain**

Vishnu's role as the preserver is mirrored in the brain's antioxidant and anti-inflammatory systems, which protect against oxidative stress. Oxidative stress arises from normal metabolic processes and can lead to neuronal damage if not properly managed (Xie et al., 2022). Antioxidants act as protectors, neutralizing free radicals and preventing cellular damage (Li et al., 2022). Furthermore, anti-inflammatory responses in the brain help maintain homeostasis, ensuring that inflammation does not escalate into neurodegenerative conditions (Schmid et al., 2022). This preservation of brain health is vital for maintaining cognitive function and overall well-being.

## Mahesh (Shiva): The Destroyer—Apoptosis, Autophagy, and the Art of Letting Go

Shiva's role as the destroyer is essential for brain health, particularly through processes like apoptosis and autophagy. Apoptosis, or programmed cell death, is a necessary mechanism for eliminating dysfunctional neurons, thereby maintaining the integrity of neural networks (Han et al., 2021). Autophagy, including mitophagy, is another critical process that removes damaged cellular components, particularly mitochondria, which are vital for energy production (Sukhorukov et al., 2021). Recent research emphasizes that mitophagy not only clears defective mitochondria but also plays a protective role in neurodegenerative diseases by preventing the accumulation of damaged organelles (Cen et al., 2021). This balance of creation and destruction is crucial for a healthy brain, ensuring that only the most functional cells persist (Doxaki & Palikaras, 2021).

## Shakti: The Goddess of Power—Mitochondria, the Powerhouses of Life

Shakti represents the mitochondria, the energy-producing organelles within cells. Mitochondria are essential for neuronal function, providing the ATP necessary for various cellular processes (Liu, 2024). They also possess their own DNA, inherited maternally, highlighting their unique role in cellular energy dynamics (Okarmus, 2024). Mitochondria are not merely energy producers; they are involved in signaling pathways that regulate cell survival and apoptosis (Zheng, 2023). The process of mitochondrial biogenesis, where new mitochondria are formed, is vital for meeting the energy demands of neurons, particularly during periods of high activity (Gao et al., 2022). Moreover, the interplay between mitochondrial health and mitophagy ensures that energy production remains efficient, preventing toxic buildup that could lead to neuronal death (Liu et al., 2021).

**The Cosmic Symphony in Your Brain**

In summary, the divine forces of Brahma, Vishnu, Mahesh, and Shakti symbolize the essential processes of creation, preservation, destruction, and energy management within the brain. Neural stem cells continuously generate new neurons, antioxidants and anti-inflammatory systems maintain balance, apoptosis and autophagy clear out dysfunctional cells, and mitochondria provide the necessary energy for all these processes. This harmonious interplay ensures that the brain remains a vibrant and functional organ, capable of adapting and thriving throughout life.

# Blood-Brain Barrier:

No Toxins Allowed-

Strict Dress Code Enforced

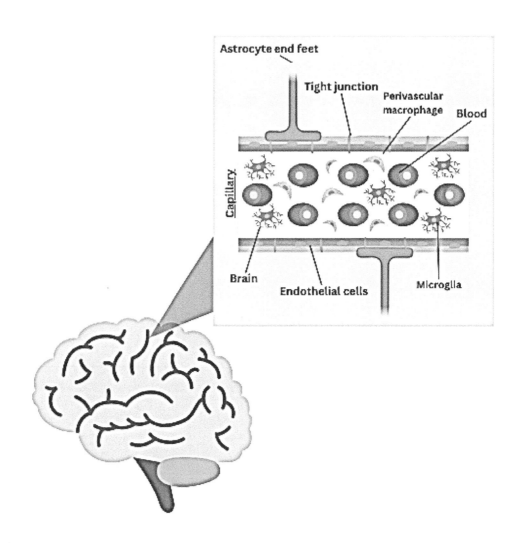

# Tight Junctions, Tighter Rules: BBB

Once upon a time, in a distant kingdom called Cerebria, there was a great castle named Brainfort, home to the most important ruler in all the land: King Brainus. His castle was the very heart of the kingdom, where every important decision was made, from controlling the kingdom's weather to helping the squirrels store nuts for the winter. Naturally, such a critical place required the best protection, and it had just that: the **Blood-Brain Barrier** (Zlokovic, 2008).

The Blood-Brain Barrier, a highly specialized security force, was no ordinary barrier. It was like a high-tech filtration system, allowing only the most essential nutrients like glucose, ketones, oxygen, and amino acids to enter the castle, while keeping out harmful invaders such as toxins, pathogens, and other undesirables (Greene et al., 2020). This tight-knit security system was managed by Captain Endo, the leader of the endothelial cells, who were responsible for creating the barrier. These cells formed an impenetrable wall around Brainfort, held together by tight junctions (Sweeney et al., 2019).

Endo didn't work alone, though. He had a loyal squad of cells backing him up: Astrocyte Annie, Pericyte Percy, and the stalwart Extracellular Eddie, all working together to ensure the integrity of the Blood-Brain Barrier (Sweeney et al., 2019; Profaci et al., 2020). Their job was crucial, ensuring that Brainfort remained safe and secure so King Brainus could function properly, storing and retrieving memories without distractions. Without this protection, the king would have trouble making decisions or even remembering his own royal duties (Nation et al., 2019).

One day, as the castle's guards went about their regular patrols, trouble began to stir from the distant Kingdom of Gut. The Gut Kingdom, while far away, had a strong influence on Brainfort. When Gut was happy and balanced, Brainfort operated smoothly. But when Gut became unruly, especially when the people of Gut neglected their fermented foods and fiber-rich diets, the situation could turn grim very quickly (Kim, 2024; Loh, 2024).

On this particular day, Gut was in chaos. The people had stopped eating their sauerkraut, yogurt, and fiber-rich foods, leading to unrest. Inflammatory messages began to pour out of Gut, making their way toward the blood-brain barrier. Captain Endo and his team were immediately on high alert.

"Trouble is brewing!" shouted Endo. "The Gut Kingdom is sending inflammatory signals our way. We must remain vigilant!"

But just as the Blood-Brain Barrier guards prepared for battle, a new threat appeared on the horizon. Chronic Stress, a notorious troublemaker, arrived at Brainfort's gates. Chronic Stress was known for his sneaky tactics, weakening the Blood-Brain Barrier and letting in harmful elements like neuroinflammation and even toxins. Chronic Stress gleefully poked holes in the once-impenetrable barrier (Shi, 2022).

"Time to cause some chaos!" cackled Chronic Stress as he slipped through the cracks he had created in the Blood-Brain Barrier. Once inside, Chronic Stress invited his terrible friends—Neuroinflammation and Memory Loss—into Brainfort. Soon, the once peaceful castle was in disarray. King Brainus found it hard to think clearly, and his memory of important matters started to slip. He couldn't remember where he had placed his crown, let alone how to run the kingdom!

The situation worsened when High Blood Sugar, an even more dangerous villain, joined forces with Chronic Stress. High Blood Sugar, emboldened by a lack of proper diet and exercise, wreaked havoc on Brainfort. He weakened the blood-brain barrier even further, letting in amyloid-beta peptides, which contributed to a faster decline in cognitive function (Cai et al., 2021). It was like watching the once-great walls of Brainfort crumble under the pressure (Sakib, 2023; Feng, 2024).

"It's a disaster!" shouted Endo. "The Blood-Brain Barrier is collapsing, and Brainfort is being overrun!"

Just as all seemed lost, a hero appeared. From the peaceful skies above, **Melatonin**, the guardian of restful sleep, arrived to save the day. Melatonin was known for her remarkable ability to calm chaos and restore balance. She was famous for protecting the integrity of the Blood-Brain Barrier, especially when it was under attack by the likes of Chronic Stress and High Blood Sugar (Wang et al., 2021).

With a wave of her glowing staff, Melatonin cast her anti-inflammatory and antioxidant spells, strengthening the blood-brain barrier and restoring order to Brainfort. She worked swiftly, sealing up the holes in the barrier and ensuring that the tight junctions between endothelial cells were reinforced. Her magic suppressed harmful agents like matrix metalloproteinase-9, which had been tearing down the barrier's walls (Wang et al., 2021; Raghavan et al., 2022).

As Melatonin worked, Brainfort began to recover. The harmful elements were pushed back, and King Brainus regained his clarity of thought. He remembered where he had placed his crown and began to restore order in the kingdom. But Melatonin wasn't finished yet. She reminded everyone in the kingdom of the importance of maintaining a healthy lifestyle to keep the blood-brain barrier strong.

"Sleep well, eat plenty of fermented foods, and exercise regularly," Melatonin advised. "If you do not, you will only make it easier for Chronic Stress, High Blood Sugar, and their friends to sneak in and cause more trouble."

With Brainfort restored and the blood-brain barrier fortified, King Brainus declared a kingdom-wide celebration. From that day forward, the people of Cerebria vowed to prioritize their health, following a high-polyphenol Mediterranean diet full of fruits, vegetables, and healthy fats, while also making sure to exercise regularly (Kaplan et al., 2022; Smith et al., 2010).

Thanks to Melatonin and the efforts of Captain Endo and his squad, the kingdom of Cerebria lived happily, and cognitively, ever after.

# Neurotransmitters, Melatonin & Nitric Oxide

## Tiny Chemicals, Big Attitudes- Brain's Tiny Overlords

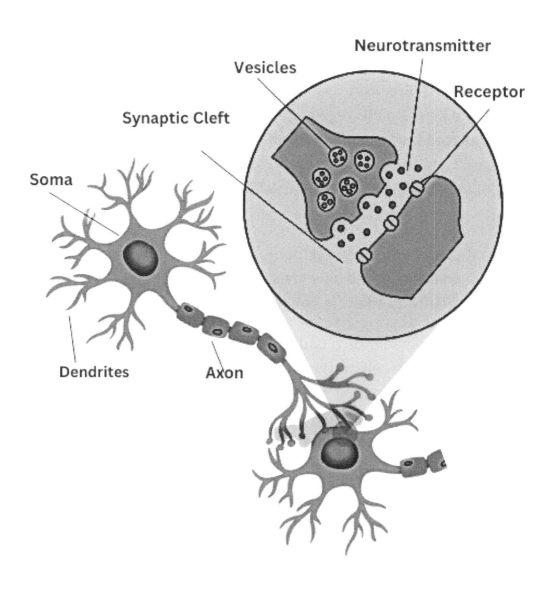

# Neurotransmitters Assemble: Epic Saga of Brain Cell Creation

In the deep recesses of the brain, where thought, memory, and mood come to life, a grand meeting of the mind's most important players was taking place. This wasn't just any meeting—it was a gathering of the molecular powerhouses and neurotransmitters that drive neurogenesis, the process of creating new neurons. At the head of the room stood Brain-Derived Neurotrophic Factor (BDNF), the wise old leader. "Alright everyone, listen up!" BDNF called out, tapping a neuron-shaped gavel on the table. "We've got a lot of work to do. The brain needs new neurons, and I'm counting on each of you to play your part!"

First to stand was Wnt, the elegant orchestrator of cellular development. "We've got this covered. I'll ensure that all the neural progenitor cells are in order," Wnt said, a bit haughtily. "By activating beta-catenin, I'll regulate the proliferation and differentiation of neural stem cells (NSCs). Everything will be perfectly timed, just as always."

Notch, always cautious, nodded in agreement but chimed in, "I'll keep those progenitors from rushing into becoming neurons too quickly. We need a steady supply, after all. Can't have everyone differentiating all at once."

From the back of the room, Sonic Hedgehog (Shh) made his entrance, rolling in like a rock star. "Don't worry folks, I've got the proliferation side of things locked down," Shh said with a smirk. "By binding to my trusty receptor Patched and activating Smoothened, I'll get those NSCs multiplying in no time."

As the molecular players discussed the groundwork, the door burst open. The neurotransmitters—arguably the most colorful group—had arrived, full of energy (and some with a bit too much).

Glutamate, the overachiever, barged in first. "Alright, everyone, let's get moving!" he said, brimming with excitement. "I'm driving this neurogenesis train by activating N-Methyl-D-Aspartate (NMDA) receptors, bringing in that sweet calcium influx!" (Crispino et al., 2020). Glutamate waved a hand, triggering a cascade of calcium signals through the room. "More neurons, more action!" he added, almost bouncing off the walls.

From the corner, in a calm and composed manner, Gamma-Aminobutyric Acid (GABA)—the Zen master—slowly rose and raised a hand to settle things down. "Balance, my dear Glutamate," GABA said, his voice a soothing contrast to Glutamate's intensity. "While you're promoting proliferation with all that excitement, remember that I'm here to ensure these newborn neurons mature properly." He gestured towards the growing neurons, stabilizing their progress with GABA_A receptor activation. "I help guide them through depolarization early on, but I'll take care of their inhibition when the time comes" (Gustorff et al., 2021).

Glutamate rolled his eyes but didn't argue—GABA's wisdom was undeniable. Dopamine swaggered into the room next, flipping a coin and smirking at his colleagues. "I bring balance to neurogenesis, especially in times of stress," he said with a grin. "With my D1 receptors, I'll stimulate gene expression for new neurons, but if things get too crazy, I'll let the D2 receptors step in and cool things down" (Winner et al., 2023; Jayakumar et al., 2022). Dopamine, ever the gambler, liked to keep the brain's neurogenic potential in check, only stepping in when necessary.

Before Dopamine could finish his smooth speech, Serotonin—the mood maestro—took the stage. "Ah, dopamine, always the balancing act, aren't you?" Serotonin said, smiling warmly. "But I, my friends, am the one who really sets the tone for neurogenesis, especially when things are tough." Serotonin walked over to a group of neurons, gently activating his 5-HT1A and 5-HT7 receptors. "With my help, I'll not only promote neurogenesis but also enhance the survival of these neurons by boosting BDNF levels" (Jayakumar et al., 2022). The neurons thrived under Serotonin's care, growing stronger and more resilient.

Suddenly, Acetylcholine—the brain's architect—joined the discussion. "Now that we've got these new neurons, I'll make sure they're well-integrated into the brain's memory circuits," Acetylcholine said, busy sketching out neural blueprints. "Through muscarinic receptors, I'll make sure everything fits into the hippocampus like a finely crafted puzzle. After all, without memory and learning, what good is neurogenesis?" (Li et al., 2024).

In the background, Norepinephrine—the ever-stressed stress manager—was scribbling notes frantically. "Alright, everyone, don't forget the balance!" Norepinephrine exclaimed. "Too much stress can shut down neurogenesis, but under the right circumstances—like with antidepressants —I can actually stimulate the birth of new neurons" (Weselek et al., 2020). Norepinephrine paced nervously, reminding everyone of the fine line they walked between helping and harming neurogenesis.

As the neurotransmitters and molecular managers debated and collaborated, the door cracked open once more, and Endocannabinoids sauntered in. "No worries, everyone. I'm here to modulate things and keep it all chill," Endocannabinoids said, leaning against the wall, clearly not in a rush. "I'll enhance synaptic plasticity and make sure those newborn neurons survive. Just relax and let me do my thing" (Weselek et al., 2020).

As the meeting progressed, it became clear that every single molecule and neurotransmitter had a crucial role to play. From the orchestrating growth factors like BDNF and Fibroblast Growth Factor-2 (FGF-2), which laid the groundwork for proliferation, to the neurotransmitters like Glutamate and GABA that drove the neural activity, each piece of the puzzle fit together perfectly. The molecular players ensured that neurons were born, while the neurotransmitters made sure they matured, integrated, and functioned smoothly.

**Neurons on Overdrive: When Two Hyperactive Neurotransmitters Throw a Wrench in Brain Gains!**

Meanwhile Cortisol and Norepinephrine (NE) crash a meeting led by Brain-Derived Neurotrophic Factor (BDNF). When cortisol levels rise, it's like your brain ringing the "stress alarm," activating the hypothalamic-pituitary-adrenal (HPA) axis, which kicks off a stress assembly line. The hypothalamus, like a frazzled project manager, releases corticotropin-releasing hormone (CRH), screaming, "We've got a situation here!" CRH rushes to the pituitary gland, which is like a frazzled intern, saying, "Oh no, now I have to release adrenocorticotropic hormone (ACTH)!" ACTH, in turn, knocks on the door of the adrenal glands, which are like the overworked, caffeine-fueled supervisors, pumping out cortisol like there's no tomorrow.

Once cortisol enters the scene, it's ready to cause chaos. Cortisol binds to glucocorticoid receptors (GRs) in the hippocampus, the part of your brain that handles memory. It's like a grumpy city inspector showing up at a construction site, immediately shouting, "Shut it down! No more building neurons here!" This triggers a series of unfortunate events, downregulating BDNF—the brain's neuron cheerleader who normally says, "Hey, let's make some new neurons!" But now BDNF's voice is muffled, and without it, the brain struggles to grow and maintain those shiny new neurons, especially in the hippocampus (Dupre et al., 2021).

Meanwhile, norepinephrine (NE)—the brain's equivalent of a hyperactive security guard—gets called in by the sympathetic nervous system during stress. NE binds to adrenergic receptors in the brain and amps up the alertness and fight-or-flight response. It's like turning up the volume in an already chaotic situation. Sure, this is great if you're running from a bear, but for your neurons, it's like throwing gasoline on a bonfire.

NE ramps up excitatory signaling, great for short-term survival, but bad news for long-term neuron health. It also unleashes a wave of inflammation that damages neurons and throws a wrench into neurogenesis (Caceres, 2023).

As if that wasn't enough, cortisol and norepinephrine also summon the inflammatory cavalry, calling in pro-inflammatory cytokines like interleukin-6 (IL-6) and tumor necrosis factor-alpha (TNF-α), which are basically the wrecking crew of the brain. They induce apoptosis, or programmed cell death, in neural progenitor cells—the rookie neurons in training. These poor cells don't stand a chance, and the brain's ability to generate new neurons is further reduced (Borsini et al., 2020).

Cortisol, still acting like that grumpy city inspector, keeps slapping "STOP WORK" signs on neurogenesis, redirecting resources to short-term stress responses like "DON'T DIE RIGHT NOW" instead of long-term investments like memory and learning. The combination of cortisol and norepinephrine creates an environment that's a neurogenesis wasteland—full of inflammation, oxidative stress, and neuron death (Caceres, 2023).

While cortisol and norepinephrine might help you dodge a bear in the woods, over time, they turn your brain into an underfunded city of abandoned neuron projects. Chronic stress leads to reduced neurogenesis, impaired cognitive function, and a brain that's more vulnerable to neurodegenerative issues (Beckner et al., 2021). The suppression of BDNF, combined with oxidative stress and chronic inflammation, leaves you with the perfect storm for depression, anxiety, and cognitive decline (Dupre et al., 2021; Borsini et al., 2020). It's like your brain's infrastructure is crumbling under the weight of all that stress without any new neurons to help rebuild it.

Luckily, you can fight back with lifestyle interventions:

1. **Yoga:** Studies show yoga lowers cortisol and improves well-being. Prenatal yoga, for instance, reduced cortisol levels and improved mental health in pregnant women (Danti et al., 2020), while structured yoga programs helped reduce stress in healthcare workers during the pandemic (Misra et al., 2023).

2. **Meditation:** Mindfulness and meditation significantly decrease cortisol levels. Practicing heartfulness meditation has been linked to reduced

anxiety and stress, promoting a healthier brain environment for neurogenesis (Miyoshi et al., 2022; Thakur, 2023).

3. **Diet:** Foods rich in omega-3s (like fatty fish and flaxseeds) and antioxidants (fruits and veggies) help combat oxidative stress and lower cortisol levels (Wan, 2023). Blueberries are stress-fighting ninjas, packed with antioxidants that calm cortisol (Lau et al., 2020). Leafy greens like spinach? Full of magnesium that tells cortisol to take a hike. And don't forget ashwagandha and turmeric—herbs that lower stress and boost neurogenesis (Chandrasekhar et al., 2022). Talk about nature's happy pills! Adaptogenic herbs like ashwagandha and rhodiola roseaalso reduce cortisol (Janssen, 2022).

4. **Exercise:** Regular exercise boosts BDNF and reduces cortisol, promoting neuron growth and improving cognitive function (Keller et al., 2021).

5. **Adequate Sleep**: Sleep reduces cortisol and helps the brain repair itself (Caceres, 2023). In summary, while cortisol and norepinephrine are essential in short bursts, prolonged exposure leads to significant damage in neurogenesis, particularly in the hippocampus. Incorporating yoga, meditation, proper diet, exercise, and sleep can help mitigate these effects and protect your brain's capacity to generate new neurons (Keller et al., 2021; Dhar et al., 2021; Danti et al., 2020).

6. **Classical Music:** Bach to Calm: Picture this: you're stuck in traffic, cortisol's rising like bread in an oven, but you hit play on some Mozart. Boom! Cortisol levels drop like a bad Wi-Fi connection. Studies (Chanda & Levitin, 2021) found classical music helps reduce cortisol, especially the heart-soothing symphonies of Bach and Tchaikovsky. Who knew defeating stress was as simple as a playlist?

7. **Grounding and Humming**: Nature's Chill Pill: Want to zap stress? Kick off your shoes and touch the Earth. Grounding (Chevalier et al., 2020) helps

absorb calming electrons from the ground, reducing cortisol. Pair it with humming—a vagus-nerve-activating trick—and you've got a double dose of relaxation. Next time you're stressed, just hum your way to peace, literally.

8. **Essential Oils:** Smells Like Victory: Lavender, rosemary, and chamomile aren't just for fancy spas—they're cortisol-busters. Lavender's relaxing scent reduces stress (Koulivand et al., 2021), while rosemary fights brain fog, and chamomile is your herbal therapist. One whiff and those stress hormones are running for the hills!V

9. **Vitamins D3, K2, and B12**: The Sunshine Trio : Vitamin D3 is like sunshine in a pill—lowering cortisol and improving mood (Grudet et al., 2020). K2 is D3's sidekick, helping calcium go where it belongs (arteries, begone!), while B12 keeps your nerves cool under pressure. It's like a multivitamin spa day for your brain!

# Dopamine: Turning Mundane Tasks into Epic Adventures (Like Doing Laundry!)

Dopamine is like your brain's personal hype-man, constantly saying, "You got this!" whenever you do something remotely rewarding—whether it's reading this book or finding the TV remote without getting up. This "feel-good" neurotransmitter is produced mainly in the *ventral tegmental area* (VTA) and the *substantia nigra*—two fancy parts of the brain that sound like exclusive spa resorts but are actually key to making sure you feel motivated enough to get out of bed. Plus, around 50% of dopamine is actually produced in your gut (Bagarolo et al., 2023). So, yes, when your stomach tells you to grab that extra slice of pizza, it's not just hunger—it's your gut pulling some dopamine strings too!

Back in the 1950s, scientists stumbled upon dopamine while poking around the brain's reward system. Swedish scientist Arvid Carlsson was the first to uncover that dopamine wasn't just a boring precursor to other neurotransmitters but an all-star player in the brain's pleasure circuit. Imagine his surprise when he realized dopamine wasn't just the opening act but the main headliner (Carlsson et al., 1958). He might as well have shouted, "Dopamine, you're the Beyoncé of neurotransmitters!" His groundbreaking work earned him the Nobel Prize in Physiology or Medicine in 2000, for showing that dopamine wasn't just a backstage roadie but the lead singer of the neurotransmitter band, especially in its role related to motor control and Parkinson's disease. So basically, Carlsson got the Nobel Prize for recognizing dopamine as the rock star it truly is!

Dopamine gets synthesized from the amino acid *tyrosine* (found in chicken, tofu, and, apparently, happiness). First, *tyrosine hydroxylase* converts it into *L-DOPA*—think of it like turning raw dough into pizza. Then *DOPA decarboxylase* steps in to complete the process and voilà—dopamine, the brain's "happy sauce," is ready (Xiao et al., 2020). Interestingly, about 50% of dopamine is also produced in the gastrointestinal tract, indicating that our gut plays a significant role in dopamine production and may influence our cravings (Bagarolo et al., 2023).

**Pleasure and Reward Manager**: Dopamine is primarily responsible for feelings of pleasure and reward, and its levels can be influenced by a variety of factors. Chronic stress is like dopamine's kryptonite, draining it and disrupting its balance in the mesolimbic pathway, which leads to reduced motivation and reward-seeking behavior (Baik, 2020). Poor dietary habits also don't help—low levels of tyrosine, the amino acid precursor to dopamine, can hinder its synthesis and deplete your feel-good reserves (Wang et al., 2021). Substance abuse, especially drugs like cocaine or amphetamines, may spike dopamine levels initially, but the eventual crash is brutal, leading to long-term deficits in dopamine signaling (Sagheddu et al., 2020; Wise & Jordan, 2021).

**Memory Master:** Dopamine is like the brain's personal assistant, making sure your memories don't fall into the black hole where your high school locker combination lives. It plays a key role in memory consolidation, keeping your brain adaptable and flexible when learning new things (Frick et al., 2021). However, too much or too little dopamine, and you might end up forgetting where you even got this book from (Guarnieri et al., 2016).

**Movement Maestro:** Dopamine isn't just important for memory and reward; it's also the brain's "Movement Manager." When dopamine levels drop, the body can slow down, turning into a sluggish version of itself, which is exactly what happens in Parkinson's disease when dopaminergic neurons are lost (Ko et al., 2019; Wang et al., 2021). This leads to cognitive and motor impairments, making dopamine a crucial factor in keeping your movements coordinated and smooth.

**Sleep and Social Life:** Sleep deprivation? Yep, that'll mess with your dopamine, too. It disrupts the brain's natural cycles of neurotransmitter release, leading to impaired memory consolidation and other cognitive processes that depend on healthy dopamine levels (Isotalus et al., 2020). Even your social life impacts your dopamine. Positive social interactions stimulate dopamine release, which enhances mood and motivation. On the flip side, social isolation can result in decreased dopamine, making you feel low and unmotivated (Baik, 2020).

**Stress Saboteur:** Chronic stress is dopamine's ultimate energy drain. It's like that app running in the background, slowly killing your phone's battery. Stress reduces dopamine in the mesolimbic pathway, leaving you feeling sluggish and uninterested in rewards (Baik, 2020). This is why long-term stress can feel so debilitating—it messes with your brain's ability to feel good about achieving anything.

**Reward Junkie:** But dopamine is also the brain's reward junkie. It links your motor actions to rewards, which is why you feel like a superhero after a good workout (Kempadoo et al., 2016). However, too much pleasure-seeking can lead to compulsive behavior, much like binge-watching "just one more episode" over and over (Kramar et al., 2014).

**Dopamine's Best Friends:** Fortunately, there are ways to keep your dopamine happy, and you don't need to move to Italy to do it! Regular exercise, omega-3s, and antioxidants are dopamine's best friends (Shimojo et al., 2019). Additionally, eating foods rich in tyrosine, like soy products, nuts, and legumes, helps boost dopamine production. Chickpeas aren't just for hummus—they're brain fuel! Maintaining a balanced lifestyle, rich in nutrients and social connections, is crucial for keeping dopamine levels in check and ensuring optimal brain function (Baik, 2020).

**The Crash:** When dopamine levels drop, the party ends—movement becomes sluggish, rewards lose their appeal, and motivation hits rock bottom. With low dopamine, even the most exciting activities feel dull. Without sufficient dopamine, memory, movement, and mood all start to suffer. In cases of extreme dopamine depletion, like in Parkinson's disease, the cognitive and motor impairments can be severe (Wang et al., 2021).

**The Dopamine Quest: A Fairytale of Brainy Bliss**

Once upon a time, in a land where everyone was a little grumpy, there lived a Brain named Doppi. Doppi ruled over the kingdom of Feel-Good with his mighty chemical sword: dopamine. But alas, the dopamine supply was running low, and the villagers were turning into zombies, yawning through their days, and binge-watching shows with no joy.

The wise Brain Council gathered and sent Doppi on a heroic quest to restore dopamine to the kingdom. Armed with nothing but a banana, a tub of hummus, a pair of dancing shoes, a steaming cup of coffee, dark chocolate, and a checklist of lifestyle interventions, Doppi set off on his adventure.

**1. The Enchanted Banana Forest**

Doppi's first destination was the legendary Banana Forest. Here, magic bananas hung from every tree, said to be full of L-tyrosine, a key ingredient in crafting dopamine. Doppi learned that bananas contain around 14 mg of L-tyrosine per fruit, alongside vitamin B6, which aids dopamine production. The wise herbalist Darcey had once mentioned the power of tyrosine-rich foods, and Doppi knew this was the perfect place to start his journey (Darcey et al., 2022). But it wasn't just bananas. Doppi also discovered chicken, cheese (with 500 mg of L-tyrosine per 100 grams), almonds (500 mg per 100 grams), walnuts, and a hidden hummus well, all full of L-tyrosine and omega-3 fatty acids, essential for brain function and dopamine production (Fernstrom et al., 2007).

He munched on sprouted or fermented whole grains that can crank out bioactive tyrosine derivatives, giving dopamine production an extra boost (Canlı et al., 2021). So yes, sourdough bread rocks.

He packed less fat for his journey because he knew, eating too much fat, especially bad stuff like palmitic acid, can turn his brain's dopamine transporter (DAT) into a lazy couch potato. Normally, DAT is supposed to clean up dopamine from your brain's synapses, but when one eats a high-fat diet, DAT's productivity drops (Fordahl & Jones, 2017). This leaves dopamine hanging around too long, overstimulating the brain, which initially feels great—like you're winning at life—but eventually makes you crave more junk food to get the same dopamine hit (Carlin et al., 2013). Add some brain inflammation to the mix, courtesy of saturated fats, and dopamine neurons start throwing in the towel (Hryhorczuk et al., 2015). So, in short, too much fat turns the brain into a dopamine drama queen.

He also packed salt lightly because he knew a high-salt diet increases dopamine levels, thanks to kidneys suddenly deciding they're dopamine producers now (Yang et al., 2015). At first, Doppi's like, "Cool, more dopamine!" But soon, he knows he will get overwhelmed—salt overload leaves dopamine hanging out too long in his brain, and will be wondering why he can't stop inhaling chips (Carlin et al., 2013).

## 2. The Dance Battle with the Cardio Troll

On his path, Doppi encountered the fearsome Cardio Troll, a towering creature who only allowed passage through a dance-off. Doppi, unafraid, put on his dancing shoes and challenged the troll. With every step, Doppi's heart raced, and his brain lit up with dopamine magic. He moonwalked, twirled, and before long, he had outdanced the troll. The dopamine rush from all the exercise left Doppi feeling lighter than ever (Meeusen et al., 1995).

## 3. The Coffee Springs and Dark Chocolate Falls

Doppi's journey then led him to the Coffee Springs, where the air was filled with the rich aroma of freshly brewed coffee. Doppi took a deep sip and felt an instant surge of energy. The magic of coffee was more than just its warmth—it contained bioactive compounds like caffeine, which blocked adenosine receptors, allowing dopamine to flow more freely. Coffee wasn't just a morning hero—it was dopamine's wingman, especially in protecting against Parkinson's disease. Caffeine helped block the brain's "slow down" signals, giving dopamine room to work and preventing the depletion of dopamine that occurs in Parkinson's (Saarinen, 2024; Köhn et al., 2022; Wang et al., 2023).

Doppi also learned the secret to preserving coffee's brain-loving benefits: go for light-roasted, organic coffee. Light roasting keeps the brain-protecting polyphenols intact, and choosing organic, single-origin beans avoided pesticides and packed more polyphenols into each sip (Wu et al., 2022; Wang et al., 2022; Ludwig et al., 2014). As a finishing touch, Doppi added a twist of lemon to his brew. The vitamin C from the lemon supercharged the antioxidants in coffee, making them even more powerful for brain health, while also adding a refreshing flavor that pleased both the brain and the belly (Huang, 2024; Marie, 2024). Nearby, Doppi discovered the Dark Chocolate Falls, where streams of 70-90% dark chocolate flowed freely. Rich in L-tyrosine and phenylethylamine, dark chocolate increased dopamine levels, with about 70-90 mg of L-tyrosine per 100 grams, giving Doppi another boost (Quintana et al., 2020).

## 4. The Musical Muse

Deep in the forest, Doppi heard the sweet sounds of the Musical Muse playing her magical flute. Entranced by the melody, he sat and listened as the music danced through the air. His brain flooded with dopamine, bringing a sense of euphoria that was even stronger than when he had won the dance battle (Salimpoor et al., 2011).

## 5. The Sleepy Sorcerer

Doppi's journey led him to the lair of the Sleepy Sorcerer, a powerful being who caused insomnia in all who dared approach him. But Doppi knew the sorcerer's weakness: the importance of sleep. Armed with this knowledge, he cast the "Sleep Tight" spell, allowing the sorcerer to fall into a deep slumber. With a full night's rest, Doppi's dopamine reserves were replenished (Volkow et al., 2012).

## 6. The Morning Ritual: Making the Bed

Before continuing his quest each day, Doppi started each morning with a simple task: making his bed. As he straightened the sheets and fluffed the pillows, Doppi felt a small yet satisfying boost in his mood. This small accomplishment was enough to set a positive tone for the day, and he could feel the dopamine spark in his brain, preparing him for the challenges ahead (Murayama et al., 2010).

## 7. The Sunlight Mountain: The Power of Blue Light

Doppi's path led him to the great Sunlight Mountain, where the sun's rays warmed his skin and energized his soul. It was the blue light from the morning sun that was particularly powerful, interacting with his brain and promoting dopamine production (Lambert et al., 2002; Vandewalle et al., 2020). Doppi knew that blue light, especially in the early hours, was key to activating the dopamine pathways in his brain.

## 8. The Salmon River and Avocado Hills

As Doppi ventured further, he arrived at the Salmon River, where the fish swam upstream, bringing omega-3 fatty acids essential for brain health. Doppi learned that omega-3s, found abundantly in salmon and mackerel, not only supported brain cell membranes but also helped in dopamine synthesis and protection. These fatty acids facilitated the release of dopamine and enhanced receptor sensitivity, allowing dopamine to work more effectively. Omega-3s also protected neurons from oxidative stress, which could otherwise damage dopamine-producing cells (Quinn et al., 2017; Shimojo et al., 2019).

Across the river stood the Avocado Hills, offering Doppi creamy fruits rich in healthy fats and B vitamins like folate, which supported dopamine synthesis. The avocado trees provided about 19 mg of folate per 100 grams, just what Doppi needed for a balanced brain.

## 9. The Meditation Meadow

While traversing a meadow, Doppi stumbled upon a group of monks practicing mindfulness meditation. Curious, he joined them in their serene practice. As Doppi focused on his breath, he felt his mind clear and his dopamine levels rise. The meditation calmed his thoughts, and Doppi realized the profound effect that mindfulness had on his brain's chemistry, much like Yoga Nidra had done for the people of Neurolia (Datta et al., 2022).

## 10. The Dopamine Salad and Tea

In Doppi's dopamine-boosting journey, things get chaotic—imagine him diving headfirst into a bowl of broccoli like he's found the secret to eternal brain power. Sulforaphane, the unsung hero lurking in cruciferous veggies like broccoli, Brussels sprouts, kale, cauliflower, and radishes, acts like the brain's very own cleanup crew. It rolls in, activates the Nrf2 pathway, and sends out a team of detox enzymes and antioxidant bodyguards to fend off oxidative stress (Davuljigari et al., 2021; Bose et al., 2020).

Sulforaphane doesn't stop there—it also takes care of inflammation, lowering levels of pesky inflammatory markers like TNF-$\alpha$ and IL-1$\beta$, which would otherwise mess with dopamine production. Thanks to this, tyrosine hydroxylase (the enzyme responsible for converting L-tyrosine into dopamine) gets to work smoothly, cranking out dopamine like it's on a mission (Yeger & Mokhtari, 2020). But Doppi's real nemesis? Dopamine quinone—a toxic byproduct of dopamine metabolism that loves to stir up trouble by piling on reactive oxygen species (ROS). Sulforaphane steps in here too, blocking this troublemaker and keeping Doppi's neurons from going haywire (Guerrero-Hue et al., 2020).

To really supercharge sulforaphane's effects, Doppi throws in mustard seeds and garlic like secret weapons. These bad boys dramatically increase sulforaphane's absorption, while pepper and olive oil get in on the action, making sure it's absorbed even better (Marx, 2023; Loizzo et al., 2021). Olive oil, rich in monounsaturated fats, acts like a soft cushion for Doppi's neurons, keeping them comfy and well-protected (Mansour-Gueddes & Naija, 2021).

## 11. The Celebration of Small Wins

As Doppi crossed the final bridge to his next destination, he reflected on his journey so far. With every step, he celebrated the small victories—finding his way through the forest, defeating the troll, enjoying the music, sipping coffee, and soaking up the sunlight. Each high-five he gave himself sent a fresh surge of dopamine through his brain, leaving him feeling invincible. After all, even the smallest achievements, when acknowledged, could unleash the power of dopamine (Murayama et al., 2010).

## 12. The Social Butterflies

At last, Doppi arrived in the village of the Social Butterflies, where laughter and camaraderie filled the air. As he joined in their conversations, Doppi felt an immediate uplift in his mood. The warmth of friendship and social connection had always been known to increase the flow of dopamine, and this village was living proof (Mobbs et al., 2009).

## 13. Doppi's Dynamic Duo: How Vitamin D and B12 Saved the Day (and the Dopamine)

As Doppi continued his quest, he stumbled upon a quirky duo living on the sunny side of a hill: Vitamin D and Vitamin K2, the kingdom's "sunshine warriors." These two had an odd but delightful partnership—Vitamin D would bask in the sun, soaking up rays like a lizard on vacation, while Vitamin K2 played the role of the wingman, helping Vitamin D do its job of regulating dopamine production. Molecularly, Vitamin D interacts with dopamine-producing neurons by modulating the expression of genes responsible for dopamine synthesis and release. Specifically, Vitamin D boosts the activity of tyrosine hydroxylase, the enzyme that converts L-tyrosine into L-DOPA, the precursor to dopamine. This, in turn, ramps up dopamine production (Silva et al., 2022). Meanwhile, Vitamin K2 ensures proper calcium regulation in the brain, reducing oxidative stress that can damage dopamine neurons, keeping Doppi's brain cells in prime dopamine-making condition (Daniello et al., 2021).

Not to be outdone, B Vitamins showed up like the ultimate hype crew, each one with its own flair. "I'm B6," one said, flexing its muscles, "I help convert all that L-tyrosine into dopamine, baby!" (Fenzl et al., 2020). At the cellular level, Vitamin B6 acts as a coenzyme for aromatic L-amino acid decarboxylase, the enzyme responsible for converting L-DOPA to dopamine, the final step in dopamine synthesis.

"And don't forget me, B12!" another chimed in, "I keep those nerve cells in shape, so they don't slack off when it's dopamine production time." Physiologically, B12 plays a crucial role in maintaining the myelin sheath around neurons, ensuring proper transmission of dopamine signals across synapses. This allows for smooth communication between neurons, optimizing dopamine function (Kennedy, 2022).

## 14. Dopamine Diaries: How 'Building Better Brain' Turned Neurons Into Bookworms

One day, Doppi stumbled upon a mysterious book titled "Building a Better Brain" by Dr. Nivedita Lakhera, sitting under a tree, looking all intellectual. "What's your deal?" Doppi asked, intrigued. The Book, not even looking up, replied coolly, "I boost dopamine like a pro. Every time you turn a page, your brain gets a little hit of dopamine—reward and pleasure all wrapped in one. Plot twists? That's like a dopamine birthday party!" (Soroka & Zajac, 2021). Doppi's eyebrow raised. "But why?"

"Well," said the Book, "reading engaging stories releases dopamine, making the whole experience more rewarding. It enhances motivation and keeps you hooked, especially with a good narrative (Michely et al., 2020; Westbrook et al., 2020). When you finish me, your brain throws a dopamine bash, and all you did was move from bed to couch. And don't even get me started on reading with others. That's a social dopamine explosion! Shared reading amplifies everything, making it even more fun and enriching (Noble et al., 2020; Vuong et al., 2021)." Plus, the aesthetic appeal of a well-designed book or a compelling story further fueled that dopamine fire, creating a positive loop where readers just wanted more (Zheng et al., 2022; Tang, 2022).

**Happily Ever After**- With his dopamine supply fully restored, Doppi returned to the kingdom of Feel-Good. The once-dreary villagers rejoiced, dancing, sleeping, basking in the sun, meditating, inhaling essential oils, drinking coffee, and feasting on hummus, bananas, chicken, and almonds like there was no tomorrow. The Dopamine River flowed freely once more, bringing joy, motivation, and energy.

# Acetylcholine: Keeping Your Memories from Ghosting You Since Forever

Once upon a synapse, there was a little molecule called **Acetylcholine** (ACh for short), bustling around the brain like a chatty barista serving up essential neuro-espresso. Discovered in the early 20th century, acetylcholine's rise to fame took a leap in the 1930s when it was identified as a neurotransmitter. But this isn't just your run-of-the-mill brain chemical—it's the ultimate multitasker, playing a role in memory, movement, sleep, and even immune responses.

But what is this acetylcholine, and where does it hang out? Let's take a closer look at its neighborhood.

### Acetylcholine's Home Turf

Acetylcholine is produced primarily in the basal forebrain, specifically in places like the medial septum and the nucleus basalis of Meynert. This chemical production process begins with the enzyme choline acetyltransferase, which takes choline and acetyl-CoA (imagine them as ingredients in a neurochemical recipe) and mixes them together to create acetylcholine (Juliet et al., 2023). From here, acetylcholine is sent out into the synaptic cleft like a courier with a very important message. Once released, it binds to nicotinic and muscarinic receptors, triggering a variety of responses, depending on which part of the brain it's hanging out in. Acetylcholine is also found in motor neurons, where it helps your muscles get the memo to move. Think of it as the email your brain sends to your arm when it's time to wave at someone—or when you're trying to act like you weren't just checking your reflection in a shop window. Beyond the brain, acetylcholine also plays a key role in the peripheral nervous system, particularly at the neuromuscular junction, where it's the reason you can move at all. Without acetylcholine, you'd feel as immobile as a statue.

## The Many Hats of Acetylcholine

**Memory Magician**: In the hippocampus, acetylcholine is crucial for learning and memory. It's like the magical librarian of the brain, helping you store new information and retrieve old memories (Matta et al., 2021). Without it, your brain becomes a bit like a library where all the books are in the wrong places—you might know the information is there, but good luck finding it.

**Attention Manager**: In the prefrontal cortex, acetylcholine helps you focus and pay attention. Imagine you're trying to read a book but keep getting distracted by a noisy squirrel. Acetylcholine steps in and says, "Ignore the squirrel—focus on the book!" It's essential for getting things done without wandering off into a daydream.

**Motor Maestro:** In the striatum, acetylcholine helps regulate movement by coordinating messages between neurons that control voluntary movements (Matta et al., 2021). Whether you're kicking a ball or trying to pull off an elaborate dance move, acetylcholine is your choreographer, making sure your muscles know exactly what to do.

**Sleep-Wake Cycles Supervisor:** Down in the brainstem, acetylcholine regulates arousal and the sleep-wake cycle, making sure you wake up in the morning and don't doze off during that important Zoom meeting (Hay, 2021). It's like your brain's internal alarm clock, ensuring you're alert when you need to be and drowsy when it's time to hit the pillow.

**Immune Influencer:** Acetylcholine also has surprising non-neuronal roles. Recent research has shown that it influences immune responses and inflammation by acting on α7 nicotinic receptors in immune cells (Kawashima, 2024). It's like the brain's ambassador to the immune system, ensuring communication lines are open between neurons and immune cells to keep everything running smoothly.

**The Tale of Too Little Acetylcholine: Brain on Vacation**
When acetylcholine is running low, things start to get foggy, both mentally and physically. It's like sending your brain on an unexpected vacation to a remote island with no Wi-Fi.

**Memory Malfunctions:** In the hippocampus, low acetylcholine levels are a major culprit behind cognitive decline and memory impairment, as seen in conditions like Alzheimer's disease. The basal forebrain neurons that produce acetylcholine deteriorate, leaving your memory in disarray like a broken filing system (Ali et al., 2022). Think of it as trying to recall where you parked your car in a parking lot the size of Texas—with no idea where you started.

**Motor Mishaps:** Without enough acetylcholine in the motor neurons, you could face muscle weakness, fatigue, or worse, as seen in myasthenia gravis, where the body's ability to communicate with its muscles is severely compromised (He et al., 2022).

**Attention Deficits:** Low acetylcholine in the prefrontal cortex leads to attention deficits. Imagine trying to read a book while simultaneously juggling flaming bowling pins—it's just not happening (Smith et al., 2021).

**The Tale of Too Much Acetylcholine: Brain on Espresso**
On the flip side, an excess of acetylcholine can turn your brain into an over-caffeinated mess.

**Cholinergic Crisis:** An overdose of acetylcholine can result in a cholinergic crisis, as seen in organophosphate (class of chemicals primarily used in pesticides and insecticides) poisoning, which leads to severe symptoms like muscle spasms, respiratory failure, and sometimes even death (Aroniadou-Anderjaska et al., 2023). It's like your muscles receiving way too many instructions at once, causing them to panic and throw a fit.

**Over-Excitation:** Too much acetylcholine can lead to hyper-excitation of muscles, causing spasms and cramps. Picture trying to sit still while your muscles decide to do the cha-cha against your will (Johnson et al., 2022).

**Anxiety Overload:** In the amygdala, too much acetylcholine can crank up your anxiety levels. Suddenly, you're not just wondering if your neighbor's cat is judging you—you're pretty sure it's plotting against you (Lee et al., 2022).

**The Balancing Act of Acetylcholine**: Acetylcholine is the Goldilocks of neurotransmitters—it needs to be "just right." Too little, and your brain and muscles feel like they're wading through molasses. Too much, and you're on a rollercoaster of muscle twitches, hyper-focus, and anxiety. Whether it's facilitating memory, regulating muscle contractions, or modulating immune responses, acetylcholine is a key player in the grand performance of life. But like any good story, it requires balance—too much or too little, and things quickly spiral out of control.

**The Adventures of Captain Acetylcholine and His League of Neurotransmitters**
In the mystical land of Brainovia, there lived a superhero named Captain Acetylcholine—the neurotransmitter responsible for muscle activation, memory, and learning. While our hero was known for his quick reflexes and sharp mind, he needed constant support to stay in top shape. Luckily for him, a variety of magical foods, supplements, and lifestyle practices acted like his loyal sidekicks, ensuring he could always save the day from the dastardly duo of Brain Fog and Forgetfulness.

**1. Food: The Delicious Path to Acetylcholine**
First things first, let's talk about what you're putting on your plate. Foods rich in choline are your best friends on this journey. These foods were known as the Choline Champions.

a) **Eggs:** The Original Brain Eggs-ercise- Our story begins with Eggs. Legend has it that the yolks of these delicious orbs contain high amounts of choline, the building block for acetylcholine (*Zeisel & Da Costa, 2009*). Studies have shown that dietary choline can significantly increase acetylcholine levels in the brain, enhancing cognitive function and memory (*Matera et al., 2023*). Not only did Captain Acetylcholine love his eggs scrambled, but they gave him the mental clarity of a hawk.

b) **Nuts and Seeds:** Tiny Titans of Power- Captain Acetylcholine loved snacking on Almonds and Walnuts, not just because they were tasty, but because they provided him with healthy fats and choline, which are essential for acetylcholine production (*Matera et al., 2023*). These nuts also boosted his overall brain health, making them an unsung hero in his diet.

c) **Fatty Fish:** Swimming in Smartness- Captain Acetylcholine was known to swim alongside Salmon, Mackerel, and Sardines, who were high in omega-3 fatty acids (*Karr et al., 2011*). These fatty fish helped in producing acetylcholine and also protected him from the evil forces of Inflammation, which frequently targeted Brainovia.

d) **Cruciferous Crusaders:** Broccoli, Brussels Sprouts, and Kale- As tough as Captain Acetylcholine was, he owed much of his resilience to the Cruciferous Crusaders—a group of green vegetables that boosted his powers. Rich in choline and antioxidants, these foods helped keep his neurons firing at rapid speeds (McNamara & Liu, 2015).

e) Sulforaphane (SFN) teams up with Nrf2, to help reduce oxidative stress, which is like cleaning up the brain's clutter so neurons can function properly (Li et al., 2022; Kim, 2021; Santos, 2023; Shimizu et al., 2022).

f) They also sneak up on acetylcholinesterase (AChE)—the party pooper enzyme that breaks down ACh—and gives it a little smackdown (Kim et al., 2022; Pant, 2024).  With AChE out of the way, ACh levels skyrocket, leaving more of this precious neurotransmitter floating around your synapses, ready to make you the sharpest version of yourself.

g) **The Choline Champions**—egg yolks were his go-to, loaded with choline to keep his mental muscles flexed (Zeisel & Da Costa, 2009). When he needed a snack, almonds and walnuts provided the crunchy brain fuel he craved (*Matera et al., 2023*). Even tart cherries pitched in, boosting his post-battle recovery and acetylcholine production (*Squires, 2024*). But his ultimate weapon? Sunflower Lecithin, bursting with phosphatidylcholine to ensure no brain fog villain stood a chance (*Blusztajn, 1998*). With these foods in his arsenal, Captain Acetylcholine was always a step ahead!

**2. Lifestyle Interventions: The Fun Side of Brain Health**

Now that we've covered food, let's move on to lifestyle interventions. After all, Captain Acetylcholine didn't become a superhero just by eating well—he had some fun with his daily routine.

a) **Exercise:** The Movement Mantra- Captain Acetylcholine wasn't just a fan of thinking—he loved to move. Whether it was running, cycling, or even dancing, every bit of exercise pumped his brain with oxygen and increased acetylcholine levels (*Cotman et al., 2007*). Studies show that physical activity increases levels of major cholinergic neurotransmitters, including acetylcholine, which plays a crucial role in memory and learning (*Yang et al., 2022; Zong et al., 2022*). After a solid workout, Captain Acetylcholine felt as strong as a mythical creature with abs of steel.

b) **Meditation:** Zen Mode Activated- Even a superhero needed to calm his mind occasionally. Captain Acetylcholine would sit under the mystical Bodhi tree in Brainovia and practice mindfulness meditation. Research has linked mindfulness practices to improved cognitive function and reduced stress, both of which help maintain healthy neurotransmitter levels (*Ahmad et al., 2022*). With a clear mind, no villain could outsmart him.

c) **Sleep:** The Restorative Recharge- After a long day of battling Brain Fog, Captain Acetylcholine knew the importance of sleep. When he closed his eyes for a solid 7-8 hours, his acetylcholine reserves were replenished. Sleep improved his memory and reaction time, preparing him for the battles ahead (*Walker, 2017*).

**3. Supplements:** The Cherry on Top- If Captain Acetylcholine needed a little extra oomph, he turned to supplements for support. These magical concoctions gave him an edge when ordinary food wasn't enough.

**Alpha-GPC (L-Alpha glycerylphosphorylcholine)** is renowned for its ability to elevate acetylcholine levels rapidly, thus enhancing memory and cognitive performance. Studies indicate that Alpha-GPC supplementation can significantly improve cognitive function, particularly in aging populations and those with cognitive impairments (Olaso-González et al., 2021). Its efficacy in promoting acetylcholine synthesis makes it a favored choice for individuals aiming to enhance memory retention and recall. Food sources: found in small amounts in organ meats, dairy products, eggs, and soy products.

**Huperzine A**, derived from the Chinese club moss, acts as a potent inhibitor of acetylcholinesterase, the enzyme responsible for breaking down acetylcholine. This inhibition prolongs the action of acetylcholine in the brain, thereby enhancing learning and memory capabilities (Russell-Jones, 2022). Its neuroprotective properties make it a valuable supplement for those facing cognitive challenges.

**Rosemary Oil**, particularly its active compound 1,8-cineole, has been shown to inhibit acetylcholinesterase, thereby preserving acetylcholine levels. Recent studies have demonstrated that rosemary oil can improve cognitive performance and memory, making it an effective natural supplement for enhancing mental clarity (Voltas et al., 2020).

**Brahmi** (Bacopa Monnieri) is celebrated for its cognitive-enhancing properties, particularly in memory and learning. Research indicates that Brahmi can enhance acetylcholine release and reduce anxiety, thereby supporting cognitive function (Pervaiz, 2023).

**Shankhpushpi** is recognized for its ability to enhance memory by improving acetylcholine signaling, which is essential for cognitive clarity and focus, particularly during stressful situations (Xu et al., 2022).

**Moringa** is a nutrient-dense plant that supports brain health through its neuroprotective properties and ability to enhance acetylcholine production. Its rich antioxidant profile helps reduce cognitive fatigue, making it an essential supplement for maintaining cognitive vitality (Alruwaili et al., 2023).

**Magnesium** is essential for neurotransmitter release, including acetylcholine. Adequate magnesium levels are crucial for optimal cognitive function, as deficiencies can impair memory and cognition (Asadi et al., 2022). Food sources: spinach, almonds, avocado, black beans, and pumpkin seeds.

**Phosphatidylserine** is vital for maintaining healthy brain cell membranes and supporting acetylcholine production, with evidence suggesting it enhances memory and cognitive health (Soh et al., 2020). Food sources: soybeans, white beans, mackerel, herring, and chicken liver.

**Vitamin B5 (Pantothenic Acid)** is crucial for synthesizing acetylcholine, as it aids in converting choline into this neurotransmitter. Sufficient levels of B5 are necessary for optimal cognitive function (Lee, 2024). Food sources: mushrooms, avocados, chicken, sunflower seeds, and eggs.

**Vitamin B12** supports acetylcholine production, and deficiencies can lead to cognitive decline, making it critical for maintaining brain health (Moreno-Pino et al., 2021). Food sources: beef, fish (salmon, tuna), eggs, dairy products, and supplements.

**Ginseng** acts like a brain mechanic, boosting the production of acetylcholine (ACh), the neurotransmitter critical for memory and learning (Lee et al., 2017; Lee, 2024). It also enhances choline acetyltransferase (ChAT) and vesicular acetylcholine transporter (VAChT), ensuring ACh is produced and delivered efficiently to regions like the cortex and hippocampus (Lee et al., 2017). Simply put, Ginseng keeps your cognitive gears running smoothly.

**Omega-3 fatty acids**, found in fish oil, maintain neuronal membranes and promote neurogenesis (Rokot et al., 2016; Xue et al., 2012). They also reduce inflammation, protecting the brain from cognitive decline and neurodegenerative diseases. Plus, they stimulate brain-derived neurotrophic factor (BDNF), encouraging neuron growth and enhancing learning (Rokot et al., 2016).

**Vitamin D3 and K2** work together to regulate calcium, which is crucial for neurotransmitter release (Rokot et al., 2016). D3 boosts cognitive performance, while K2 ensures calcium ends up in the right places, preventing harmful buildup. This duo also helps reduce neuroinflammation, keeping the brain healthy and functioning properly.

# Norepinephrine and the Case of Missing Focus

Once upon a time, in the bustling city of Brainopolis, there lived a neurotransmitter named Norepinephrine. Now, Norepinephrine wasn't just any ordinary chemical. It was the brain's personal alarm clock, the one responsible for keeping things running smoothly, especially when life got a bit chaotic.

Norepinephrine's daily routine involved a lot of important tasks. Whether it was making sure you stayed alert during a tedious work meeting (which honestly could have been an email) or helping you react quickly when a loud sound startled you, Norepinephrine was always there, ready to jump into action. Like a caffeine-charged superhero, it kept you on your toes (Atta & Ahmed, 2011).

Norepinephrine had a sibling, Dopamine. While Dopamine was all about rewarding you with feel-good vibes for achieving goals, Norepinephrine had a more serious job. It was made from Dopamine, courtesy of a brain enzyme that acted like a supercharged chef whipping up a neurotransmitter cocktail (Wassenberg et al., 2020). But Norepinephrine was the more intense sibling—focused, alert, and sometimes a little stressed out.

Norepinephrine loved to hang out in important areas of Brainopolis, like the prefrontal cortex. This was the part of the brain that made "adulting" possible, helping with decision-making and focus. Then there was the amygdala, the brain's personal alarm system, which sounded the bells when something felt emotionally important or threatening. Finally, there was the hippocampus, a memory vault where all your embarrassing and not-so-embarrassing moments were stored for future cringe sessions. In Brainopolis, Norepinephrine took on the role of a drill sergeant when it came to memories. It made sure you didn't forget where you left your keys or that awkward thing you said at a party five years ago. Working closely with the hippocampus and the amygdala, Norepinephrine tagged certain memories as "super important," making them harder to forget. It even had its own headquarters, the locus coeruleus, where all Norepinephrine-related matters were managed with precision and care (Colucci et al., 2021).

But Norepinephrine wasn't alone in these memory adventures. It teamed up with its pal Dopamine to help seal the deal when it came to remembering things. Together, they made sure the memory scrapbook in your brain was filled with all the standout moments (Jacobs et al., 2020).

One of Norepinephrine's favorite things to do was activate beta-adrenergic receptors. Think of this as giving the brain a shot of adrenaline, ramping up the ability to remember things. This mental boost helped solidify memories, ensuring they stayed put for years to come (Tt et al., 2020; Ravache et al., 2023). Norepinephrine was like the diligent note-taker in a meeting, frantically scribbling everything down so nothing would be forgotten (Wilmot et al., 2022; Mulvey, 2024).

But Brainopolis wasn't always a calm and organized place. When Norepinephrine levels went haywire, things could get a bit out of hand. Too much Norepinephrine could make Brainopolis feel like it was in constant emergency mode. Residents, like Amy from the Amygdala District, were always on edge. Anxiety and stress-related issues started to emerge, as Norepinephrine ramped everything up to eleven, leaving the city stuck in a state of hyper-alertness (Zhou, 2024; Yang, 2024). This hyperactivity was tied to a strange phenomenon known as the hypothalamic-pituitary-adrenal axis. When overstimulated, it caused chronic inflammation, which in turn led to mental health challenges like depression. Even Norepinephrine was having a hard time keeping up with the stress levels (Santamarina, 2024; Chang, 2024).

On the flip side, when Norepinephrine levels were too low, Brainopolis felt sluggish and foggy. It was as if the city had lost its spark. Low levels were linked to mood disorders, such as major depressive disorder, where Brainopolis struggled to regulate emotions and stay focused. It was like trying to drive through the city with the brakes on (Higuchi, 2024; Sala-Cirtog, 2024). This imbalance even messed with the brain's sleep patterns, leading to insomnia. And once sleep was disrupted, the whole city of Brainopolis started to fall apart (Gu, 2024).

Norepinephrine's deficiency also had a hand in conditions like attention-deficit/hyperactivity disorder. With low levels of Norepinephrine, Brainopolis couldn't stay focused on tasks, and residents like ADHD Andy from the Prefrontal

Cortex had trouble concentrating and staying on track (Sindhura et al., 2022). In cases of depression, Brainopolis felt heavy and weighed down, as if Norepinephrine had taken a long vacation (El-Anwar et al., 2015).

But all was not lost for Brainopolis! Norepinephrine knew how to keep things in balance. One of the best ways to ensure a steady flow of Norepinephrine was by staying active. Physical exercise was like a boost to Brainopolis's energy grid, supercharging Norepinephrine production. This gave the city renewed focus, boosted the overall mood, and made life a bit more manageable (Ipekoğlu et al., 2017). Diet played a huge role too. Foods rich in tyrosine, such as lean meats, fish, eggs, and nuts, were like fresh supplies for Norepinephrine production. It was as if these foods were delivered straight to the Brainopolis factory, ensuring it had everything needed to keep running smoothly (Waløen et al., 2016). Add in some omega-3 fatty acids and B vitamins, and Norepinephrine was feeling strong and steady (Gupta & Sharma, 2016).

But there were also enemies lurking in Brainopolis. Sugar and processed foods were notorious for sending Norepinephrine into a downward spiral. They messed with the city's balance, leading to mood swings and brain fog (Woods et al., 2014). Alcohol, when consumed too much, was also a menace—it made it harder for Norepinephrine to bounce back from stress, leaving Brainopolis in disarray (Hans, 2024). Luckily, Brainopolis had some secret allies: adaptogenic herbs like Rhodiola rosea, ashwagandha, and Panax ginseng. These herbs helped Norepinephrine handle stress better, boosting the brain's defenses and keeping things calm (Gupta & Sharma, 2016). And then there was caffeine—the trusty sidekick that gave Norepinephrine a quick boost, making you feel like you could take on the world (Watson et al., 2010). And so, Brainopolis lived on, always bustling, always adapting, with Norepinephrine leading the charge to keep everything in balance.

# The Role of GABA: The Brain's Chill Pill

Gamma-aminobutyric acid, or GABA, is like the brain's very own chill pill. It's the principal inhibitory neurotransmitter, keeping your neurons from getting too excited and making sure everything stays in balance (Drenthen et al., 2016; Hampe et al., 2018). Think of GABA as the wise friend who knows when to tell your brain, "Take it easy." GABA does this by working through two types of receptors: GABA_A, which acts fast like a calming breath, and GABA_B, which is more of a long, soothing exhale (Zhu et al., 2018; Kilb, 2011).  But GABA isn't just about slowing things down; it's also involved in learning, memory, and helping you make sense of the world around you (Puts et al., 2011). When GABA isn't doing its job right, it can lead to a host of issues, from epilepsy and anxiety to depression and autism spectrum disorder (Puts et al., 2016; Fatemi et al., 2011).

**Disorders Associated with Abnormal GABA Levels: When the Chill Pill Fails**
Low GABA has been linked to a variety of disorders. For example, individuals with autism spectrum disorder often show reduced GABA, which can mess with sensory processing and motor function (Puts et al., 2016). Mood disorders like depression and bipolar disorder are also frequently tied to low GABA levels, contributing to the emotional roller coasters that characterize these conditions (Fatemi et al., 2011). In epilepsy, a lack of GABA's calming influence can lead to runaway neuronal activity, resulting in seizures (Hawker & Silverman, 2012). Even schizophrenia has been linked to problems with GABA receptors, highlighting how crucial this neurotransmitter is for keeping the mind steady (Fatemi et al., 2013).

## Factors That Influence GABA: How to Keep the Chill Going

**Lifestyle Factors: The GABA-Friendly Life-** If you want to keep your GABA levels in check, your lifestyle is key. Regular exercise is like hitting the refresh button on your GABA system, boosting its activity and helping you stay calm and collected (Moghaddam & Qujeq, 2016). On the flip side, chronic stress and poor sleep are like the arch-nemeses of GABA, dragging its levels down and leaving you feeling more anxious and moodier than you'd like (Hampe et al., 2018; Werner & Coveñas, 2016).

**Dietary Sources: Eat Your Way to a Calmer Brain-** Your diet also has a big say in how much GABA your brain gets to play with. Foods rich in glutamate, like tomatoes, mushrooms, and some cheeses, are GABA's raw materials, helping to ramp up its production (Yasir, 2023). Fermented foods like yogurt and kimchi are like GABA's best friends, thanks to the probiotics that might boost GABA production through the gut-brain connection (Hampe et al., 2018). But beware of overdoing it on alcohol and caffeine—they're like party crashers that disrupt GABA's calming effects, leaving your brain more excitable than it should be (Zhu et al., 2018; Werner & Coveñas, 2016).

**Supplements: GABA's Boosters-** If you're looking to give your GABA levels a little extra love, certain supplements can help. Magnesium, for instance, is like a GABA booster shot, enhancing (molecular )receptor function and increasing GABA synthesis (Hampe et al., 2018; Moghaddam & Qujeq, 2016). L-theanine, found in green tea, is another GABA-friendly compound known for promoting relaxation and giving GABA a nice boost (Hampe et al., 2018; Werner & Coveñas, 2016). But keep an eye on omega-6 fatty acids—too much can mess with GABA's calming vibes, so balance is key (Hampe et al., 2018; Werner & Coveñas, 2016).

# Keep Calm and Crank Up the Serotonin: A Guide to Staying Zen

Serotonin's story begins in the 1940s, when scientists were searching for the causes of smooth muscle contractions. Maurice Rapport, Arda Green, and Irvine Page (yes, we're name-dropping) isolated a substance from blood serum that caused blood vessels to constrict. It was so shocking and serendipitous, they gave it a literal name combining "serum" and "tonic"— hence, serotonin. Little did they know, this wasn't just some random blood-born agent. 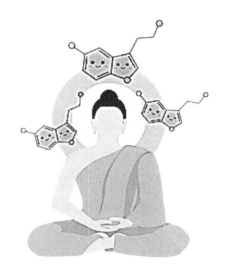 Serotonin was about to become the molecular mascot of happiness, contentment, and feeling like the world's most enthusiastic puppy when you see your favorite snack.

**The Brain's Little Prozac Factory-** While serotonin was first discovered in the bloodstream, its fame skyrocketed when scientists realized it's produced in the brain too! The brain stem, specifically the raphe nuclei, is the precious section of serotonin production. From here, serotonin likes to travel around the brain like a well-meaning grandma handing out cookies (except these cookies are neurotransmitters that regulate mood, sleep, appetite, and overall mental wellness). But serotonin doesn't just play in one venue. No, it is a world traveler. It acts on multiple parts of the brain, including:

- The cortex, where it helps you make decisions and avoids impulsive behavior (like buying that 3-foot inflatable rubber duck on sale).
- The limbic system, the emotional HQ, where it keeps your anxiety in check and gives you that warm, fuzzy feeling of "everything's going to be okay."
- The basal ganglia, involved in motor control, which serotonin helps out like a chill yoga instructor, making sure everything moves smoothly.

**The Gut Feeling: The Second Brain**

Before you think serotonin is only a brain thing, hold onto your broccoli! Most of your serotonin is actually produced in the gut. Yep, nearly 90% of serotonin is hanging out in your gastrointestinal tract, probably judging you for that third slice of pizza. This is why you get "gut feelings"—because serotonin helps regulate the contractions of your intestines and digestive process. When something's off in your tummy, it might also affect your mood. This is why scientists have lovingly dubbed the gut your "second brain." And no, it doesn't mean you're smarter if you eat more!

**Let us take a peek at what this molecule is up to**

**Memory Consolidation:** Your Brain's Filing System

One of serotonin's most important jobs was in memory consolidation. By enhancing synaptic plasticity in the hippocampus and prefrontal cortex, serotonin helped store important memories. Serotonin was produced in the brain by tryptophan hydroxylase 2 (TPH2), ensuring there was always enough to support these crucial processes (Villanueva et al., 2021).

**Why Running Makes Your Brain a Construction Site**: Serotonin takes a hammer to neurogenesis, helping create neural stem cells (NSCs) with the help of neurotrophic factors like BDNF (Arazi et al., 2022; Park et al., 2021). So, every time you lace up those running shoes, you're basically signing your brain up for a neuron renovation. It is also playing messenger in the brain-gut axis, keeping tabs on everything from your energy levels to brain development (Teng et al., 2022; Drigas & Mitsea, 2021). It's a multitasker, helping neurons grow and survive during their early years like the world's most overqualified babysitter (Janowitz, 2024).

As if that weren't enough, serotonin also manages the brain's immune cells, the microglia. These cells are like royal guards at a neuron castle, deciding which new neurons get to stay and which ones have to leave, affecting the overall health and proliferation of your brain's freshest cells (Turkin et al., 2021; D'Alessandro et al., 2021).

**The Mood Manager, Appetite & Memory Wizard:** Serotonin isn't just for keeping Neuroville's residents from tearing up during sad stories; it was their brain's project manager, ensuring that their mood remained stable, their sleep restful, and their appetites in check. Serotonin even worked with leptin, the hunger bouncer, to prevent those pesky midnight cravings (Yabut et al., 2020). Moreover, serotonin was the unsung hero of memory, consolidating short-term memories into long-term ones while the people slept, like an overnight data backup for the brain (Villanueva et al., 2021).

**The Digestion Dynamo:** While serotonin did wonders in the brain, about 90% of it was actually hard at work in the gut, ensuring that food moved smoothly through the intestines. Without serotonin, the digestive system would grind to a halt, causing discomfort and chaos (Liu et al., 2023). Friendly gut bacteria like Lactobacillus and Bifidobacterium assisted serotonin, ensuring proper digestion and regularity (Caspani et al., 2021).

**The Vascular Bouncer:** In blood vessels, serotonin plays the role of vascular bouncer, controlling blood flow by interacting with smooth muscle cells and endothelial cells. It managed vasoconstriction and vasodilation, helping to maintain healthy blood circulation (Gershon, 2022).

**The Sticky Note Expert in Platelets:** Serotonin also acted as the body's sticky note expert, stored in platelets to promote blood clotting and trigger vasoconstriction during injury, preventing excessive blood loss (Maurer-Spurej, 2022).

**The Skeleton's Personal Trainer**: Even bones depend on serotonin! Serotonin produced in the gut travels to the bones, where it plays a crucial role in regulating the activity of **osteoblasts** (cells that build bone) and **osteoclasts** (cells that break down bone). This delicate balance ensures proper bone density and skeletal strength (Pietrzak et al., 2022). Without serotonin, the regulation of these bone cells would falter, leading to weakened and fragile bones.

**The Airway Manager:** In the lungs, serotonin helped maintain proper airflow by controlling airway smooth muscle function, ensuring that the people of Neuroville could breathe easily (Andrade et al., 2020).

**The Love Regulator:** Serotonin even played a role in the realm of romance. High levels of serotonin could dampen desire, but when balanced, serotonin kept everything functioning as it should, acting like a behind-the-scenes relationship counselor (Lindberg et al., 2021).

### The Dark Side: When Serotonin Levels Go Rogue

Too much or too little serotonin, and things start to get weird. Imagine serotonin as a circus juggler, keeping everything in balance. But when levels get abnormal, it's like the juggler dropping all the balls.

- **Low serotonin**: This can lead to **depression, anxiety**, and even **memory problems**. Your brain turns into that guy at the party who forgot how to socialize.
- **High serotonin**: Known as **serotonin syndrome**, this can cause symptoms ranging from mild (shivering, diarrhea) to severe (fever, seizures). This is when serotonin becomes the overenthusiastic cheerleader who doesn't know when to stop.

### Return of Happy King: Queen Victoria's Serotonin Strategy

In the whimsical kingdom of Aetheria, King George VI sat on his throne, looking more like a sad puppy than a powerful monarch. His royal duties weighed heavy on him, and despite his best efforts to stay positive, he just couldn't shake his persistent low mood. King George was not grumpy or angry, just...sad. His subjects often found him gazing longingly out of windows, sighing dramatically as though it were a hobby.

Enter Queen Victoria, his wife, a brave, vibrant woman who had a laugh that could chase away thunderstorms and a mind sharper than a sword. Known for her unwavering optimism, she wasn't about to let her husband mope his way through life. Armed with her wit, wisdom, and a dash of science, Queen Victoria set out to boost King George's serotonin levels, because a happy king makes for a happy kingdom—and fewer unnecessary sighs.

## 1. Omega-3: Fishy Fixes for a Frowny King

The first thing Queen Victoria did was summon the royal chef and demand a steady stream of fishy delights—salmon, walnuts, and flaxseeds. Why? Because Omega-3 fatty acids, especially DHA, could turn those frowns upside down by helping King George's brain function more smoothly (Janssen & Kiliaan, 2014). "More fluid membranes, better serotonin receptors!" she declared, as George poked suspiciously at his plate of walnut-crusted salmon. To his surprise, with each bite, the fog in his mind began to lift. Queen explained- Three things let us remember-

### Membrane Fluidity

Neuronal membranes are made up of lipids, and DHA increases their **fluidity**. This flexibility allows serotonin receptors to move and signal more effectively within the membrane, ensuring that serotonin can bind to its receptors more efficiently (Janssen & Kiliaan, 2014; Tassoni et al., 2008). When your neuronal membranes are fluid, your serotonin signaling system is smoother, leading to better mood regulation.

### Serotonin Receptor Function

DHA's impact on membrane fluidity directly improves **serotonin receptor function**. A more fluid membrane means serotonin receptors can bind more easily to serotonin molecules, enhancing serotonin signaling. This improved signaling is crucial for preventing mood disorders like depression (Su et al., 2018).

## Serotonin Synthesis and Release

Omega-3s, particularly DHA, help transport **tryptophan**, the precursor to serotonin, across the blood-brain barrier. This boosts serotonin production in key areas of the brain, like the **prefrontal cortex** and **hippocampus**, which are essential for mood regulation and cognitive function (Patrick & Ames, 2015; McNamara et al., 2009). DHA also helps maintain the release of serotonin in these regions, ensuring smooth communication between neurons.

## 2. Serotonin-Boosting Feast: The Royal Menu Overhaul

Victoria, ever the wise queen, knew that George's diet could also use a boost. She introduced a royal menu filled with serotonin-boosting foods. "Alright, George, here's the plan: more turkey, eggs, cheese, and nuts—they're all rich in tryptophan, the raw material your brain needs to make serotonin," she explained as she handed him a turkey sandwich loaded with all the good stuff (Khonachah et al., 2020).

"And don't forget the complex carbs!" she added, serving up a side of whole grains like organic sorghum, ragi and sweet potatoes. "Carbs increase insulin, which helps more tryptophan get into your brain where it turns into serotonin— think of it like giving tryptophan a VIP pass to happiness" (Khonachah et al., 2020).

But that wasn't all. For a quick serotonin boost, Victoria made sure George snacked on bananas, pineapples, and tomatoes—all pre-loaded with serotonin for a fast-acting mood lift (Tang et al., 2020).

After one particularly delicious breakfast of eggs, whole grain toast, and a banana, George sighed—not out of sadness, but out of contentment. "I have to admit, Victoria, this happy brain diet is working."

## 3. Meditation: The Art of Doing Nothing (Successfully)

They sat in the royal garden, where George spent a good amount of time fidgeting before finally finding some peace. As they practiced daily, his stress melted away, and to everyone's astonishment, his sighs became less frequent (Kaushik et al., 2020). "I'm doing nothing—and it's working!" he marveled.

## 4. Grounding: Walking Barefoot Isn't Just for Hippies

Queen Victoria led King George on barefoot walks through the castle meadows, claiming grounding would connect him with Earth's electrons, reduce stress, and promote serotonin production (Choy, 2023). Though initially reluctant, George eventually admitted it improved his mood and gave him an excuse to avoid doing taxes (yes Kings in my book have to pay taxes, unlike in real life)

## 5. Magnesium and Sunshine: Nature's Happy Pills

Queen Victoria was a woman of action, so she made sure George was getting plenty of magnesium-rich foods like spinach, pumpkin seeds, quinoa and almonds. After all, magnesium was key to serotonin production (Gao et al., 2023). Magnesium helps the enzyme, tryptophan hydroxylase turn tryptophan into 5-hydroxytryptophan, then hands the wrench to aromatic L-amino acid decarboxylase to finish the job and turn 5-hydroxytryptophan into serotonin. Without magnesium, these enzymes are like workers without their tools—slow, confused, and not getting much done (Khonachah et al., 2020). So, to keep the serotonin factory cranking out happiness, magnesium is a must!

## 6. Yoga: Stretching Your Way to Happiness

To keep the serotonin flowing, Queen Victoria introduced George to yoga. "Think of it as royal stretching," she suggested. They twisted and stretched into various poses, and although George wasn't thrilled about bending himself like a pretzel, he couldn't argue with the results. Each yoga session left him feeling calmer and lighter (Metri et al., 2023). "Maybe being flexible isn't so bad," he muttered, while stuck in a downward.

## 7. The Royal Workout: Exercise for a Happy Brain

One morning, Queen Victoria marched into the throne room with a pair of walking shoes. "George, it's time to get moving!" she declared. The King, as usual, sighed, but this time Victoria had a secret weapon: science.

"When you exercise, you increase the availability of tryptophan in your brain, which then turns into serotonin," she explained (Khonachah et al., 2020). After some initial grumbling, King George agreed to daily walks, and soon realized something remarkable—exercise raises tryptophan levels in the blood by sending its rivals, the branched-chain amino acids (BCAAs), on a mission to fuel his muscles. With the BCAAs preoccupied, tryptophan waltzes across the blood-brain barrier like it's got VIP access to the serotonin party.

But that's not all. Exercise also triggers the release of free fatty acids (FFAs) into the bloodstream, which displace tryptophan from its binding protein, albumin. This increases the amount of free tryptophan circulating in the blood, giving it an even greater chance to cross into the brain (Chaouloff, 1997). With BCAAs off fueling muscles and free fatty acids freeing up more tryptophan, it's like a royal escort guiding tryptophan straight to the brain. Once there, tryptophan transforms into serotonin, leaving you both happy and sore—so it's a win-win (Fernstrom & Wurtman, 1971; Chaouloff, 1997). And the King agreed!!

## 8. Sunlight: Nature's Mood Booster

Not content with just exercise, Victoria knew that sunlight was essential for serotonin production. "Fifteen to thirty minutes in the sun can trigger serotonin production and regulate your sleep-wake cycle," she explained as she practically dragged George into the sunlight (Shelke, 2024). At first, he was reluctant, but after a few days of sunbathing in the royal gardens, King George admitted that sunlight really did brighten his mood—literally and figuratively.

## 9. Bedtime Carbs: A Sleep and Mood Hack

One night, Queen Victoria handed King George cottage cheese and a banana. "Carbs before bed boost serotonin!" she explained. "When you eat complex carbs—especially quinoa, oats, and sweet potatoes—insulin clears most amino acids from the bloodstream by moving them into your muscles, but it leaves tryptophan behind. With less competition, tryptophan easily enters the brain, where it turns into serotonin—and later, melatonin for better sleep" (Khonachah et al., 2020; Ogawa et al., 2023).

## 10. The Sauerkraut King

King George soon earned the title "The Sauerkraut King," much to his dismay. Queen Victoria had introduced him to the magic of gut bacteria, specifically Lactobacillus and Bifidobacterium, found in fermented foods like sauerkraut and yogurt (Liu et al., 2023). These tiny serotonin producers were the key to his newfound happiness.

Despite his initial reluctance, George couldn't argue with the results. His diet of yogurt, sauerkraut, garlic, and bananas, lifted his mood with every meal (Ghafouri-Taleghani et al., 2023).

## 11. Blue Light: The Royal Wake-Up Call

One sunny morning, Queen Victoria declared, "George, the secret to your happiness is the sun." Skeptical, George asked, "The sun cheers me up?"

"Trust me, Blue light from the sun activates photoreceptors in your eyes, particularly melanopsin, which signals the brain to boost serotonin production. It also regulates your sleep-wake cycle by converting serotonin into melatonin later" she said(Shelke, 2024).

"I guess I'm solar-powered now," he muttered, secretly enjoying it (Green et al., 2015; Abdel-Rahman et al., 2020). A few days later, George even stepped into the sun voluntarily, though he still grumbled, "Well, it's better than meetings."

## 12. Red Light: Mood by Moonlight

One evening, Queen Victoria took King George for a sunset walk. "The red light boosts your mood and energy by helping your cells produce more serotonin," she explained (Kolbabova et al., 2015; Hernández-Mendoza et al., 2020). "So, the sunset's magic?" George asked, half-smiling.

"Not magic, just science," she laughed. After some reluctance, George felt his stress melt away, the red glow calming him like a blanket of serotonin. "I feel… relaxed," he marveled. "Just science, dear," Victoria smiled.

## 13. Vitamin D And Sunshine: Secret Weapon for the Gloomy King

One sunny morning, Victoria nudged George out of bed and handed him his daily vitamin D supplement. George sighed. "Okay, explain to me again how this tiny pill is supposed to boost my mood and help me sleep?"

Victoria smiled. "Glad you asked! So, when you take vitamin D in the morning, it enters your bloodstream and gets converted into **calcitriol**, which is the active form of vitamin D. This **calcitriol** then finds these special **vitamin D receptors (VDR)** that are hanging out in various tissues, including your brain."

George, now slightly intrigued, asked, "And what do these receptors do?"

"Ah," Victoria continued, "once calcitriol binds to those receptors, the whole complex goes into the **nucleus** of your cells. There, it attaches itself to specific spots on your DNA—these spots are called **vitamin D response elements (VDREs)**—and starts turning certain genes on or off (Carlberg & Campbell, 2013)."

George raised an eyebrow. "Genes, huh? So this little pill messes with my DNA?"

Victoria laughed. "In a good way! One of the genes it activates produces the enzyme **tryptophan hydroxylase 2 (TPH2)**. Now, TPH2 is a big deal—it's responsible for turning **tryptophan** into **5-HTP**, which is the precursor to **serotonin**. So, more TPH2 means more serotonin, and you're in a better mood throughout the day (Mizwicki et al., 2020)."

"Okay, so that's how it boosts my mood," George said, starting to catch on. "But what about sleep?"

"Well," Victoria continued, "as the day goes on and light exposure decreases, your body's **circadian rhythm** kicks in. This activates an enzyme called **N-**

**acetyltransferase** in your pineal gland. N-acetyltransferase converts serotonin into **N-acetylserotonin**, which then turns into **melatonin**—the hormone that helps you sleep (Srinivasan et al., 2012). Without enough serotonin from earlier in the day, you won't have enough melatonin at night to help you wind down."

"Ah, I see. So, taking vitamin D in the morning ensures I have plenty of serotonin to turn into melatonin later," George said. "Exactly!" Victoria nodded. "Plus, vitamin D influences genes that control your body's **circadian clock**, like **CLOCK**and **BMAL1**. This helps regulate your natural sleep-wake cycle, making sure you're alert during the day and sleepy at night (Xu et al., 2020). It's all about keeping your brain on schedule!"

As George finished his breakfast, he paused before taking his vitamin D pill. "Hey, Victoria, what if I just took this at night? Wouldn't it still work?" Victoria laughed. "Oh, George, you could take it at night, but things might not go as smoothly. Let me explain."

"Vitamin D helps regulate your **circadian rhythm**—your body's internal clock that tells you when to be awake and when to sleep. When you take it in the morning, it activates certain genes like **CLOCK** and **BMAL1** that help keep you alert during the day and ready for sleep at night (Xu et al., 2020). But if you take it at night, you're sending mixed signals to your body. It could throw off your **sleep-wake cycle**, keeping you feeling more alert when you should be winding down (Srinivasan et al., 2012)."

George raised an eyebrow. "So, if I take it at night, I'll be wide awake when I'm supposed to be falling asleep?"

"Exactly," Victoria nodded. "Plus, when you take vitamin D in the morning, it's busy helping your body produce **serotonin**, which later turns into **melatonin** for sleep. Taking it at night could mess with that timing, and you might not get the right boost in **serotonin** during the day when you need it most (Mizwicki et al., 2020)."

"So I could end up messing up both my daytime mood and my nighttime sleep?" George said, looking a bit more concerned.

"Yep," Victoria replied. "Your body's clock depends on cues like sunlight and morning vitamin D to know when it's daytime. Taking it at night could confuse your body, and you don't want that. It's like trying to start a car after the race has already ended!"

"Alright, you've convinced me," George sighed. "Morning vitamin D it is."

George, still skeptical, asked, "But what about just standing in the sun? Doesn't that boost serotonin too? Do I really need the vitamin D?"

"Well, yes," Victoria explained, "sunlight on its own can help. When light enters your eyes, it activates a special pathway—the **retinohypothalamic pathway**—which sends a signal to your brain's **suprachiasmatic nucleus (SCN)**. This little brain region tells your body to stop making **melatonin** and ramp up **serotonin** instead (Lambert et al., 2002). So, sunlight can directly boost serotonin production."

"So, sunlight alone should be enough then, right?" George asked, clearly hoping to skip the supplements.

Victoria laughed. "Not quite. Sunlight helps increase serotonin directly, but without enough **vitamin D**, you're not making the raw material needed to produce serotonin efficiently. And don't forget, at night, vitamin D helps convert that serotonin into **melatonin** for good sleep. So really, you need both the sunlight and your vitamin D supplement to keep the whole system running smoothly."

George finally stood up, stretching. "Alright, alright. I'll take my vitamin D and go for a walk in the sun. Happy now?" Victoria smiled. "Your brain will be! You'll feel better during the day, and sleep better at night. Now, let's get moving!"

# The Tale of Melatonin: Robin Hood of the Body

Once upon a time, in the grand kingdom of the Body, there was a brave hero named Melatonin. Discovered in 1958 by a wise sage named Lerner, Melatonin wasn't just any ordinary figure. Oh no! This noble molecule, born from the pineal gland deep in the realm of the Brain, had a mission: to bring balance, peace, and restful slumber to the entire kingdom (Lerner et al., 1958).

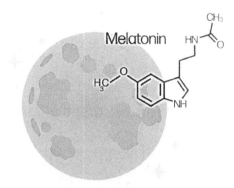

Now, Melatonin wasn't always busy in the Brain.
He had many secret roles across the kingdom. By night, he played his most famous part—the "Sandman's Secret Sauce"—singing sweet lullabies that coaxed the kingdom into a peaceful, restorative sleep. Without his nightly concert, the kingdom would fall into chaos, with villagers staying awake far too late and scrolling through glowing screens (Reiter et al., 2014).

But by day, Melatonin was like the Robin Hood of the Body. He traveled across the land, righting wrongs and defending the innocent. In the Gut, he acted as a mighty shield, protecting the people from the fiery attacks of acid reflux and ulcers, calming inflammation, and ensuring smooth digestion (Bubenik, 2002). The Gut's soldiers trusted him with their very lives.

In the Heart, Melatonin donned his superhero cape, reducing oxidative stress and lowering blood pressure like a master archer hitting his mark every time. His efforts reduced the risk of heart disease, making him a cherished hero in the Cardiovascular Forest (Reiter et al., 2014).

Not content with just defending the Gut and Heart, Melatonin rode to the land of the Skin, where he became the brave warrior who fought against the Sun Dragon's UV rays. By enhancing DNA repair and reducing inflammation, he kept the Skin young and vibrant, preventing it from aging prematurely (Slominski et al., 2012).

But Melatonin's valor did not stop there. In the Immune System's Castle, he commanded an army of T-cells and natural killer cells, the kingdom's finest soldiers. Together, they fought off invaders like infections and tumors, ensuring the safety of the realm (Srinivasan et al., 2012).

Over in the Fertility Gardens, Melatonin was a wise and gentle steward. For women, he protected eggs from the ravages of oxidative stress and regulated the cycles of the moon. For men, he ensured that sperm were healthy and strong, safeguarding future generations (Reiter et al., 2014).

And in the mysterious land of the Bones, Melatonin trained the osteoblasts, those mighty builders who maintained the kingdom's strength by forming strong, healthy bones. He also reduced the mischief caused by osteoclasts, who tried to weaken bone density as the kingdom aged (Cardinali et al., 2013).

One of Melatonin's most critical missions was in the Brain's deepest chambers. There, he was the loyal friend who dimmed the lights and whispered, "It's bedtime," every night, helping the kingdom drift into sleep (Ferracioli-Oda et al., 2018). In the peace of night, he ensured that the brain could clean up its own messes—like a janitor making sure all the metabolic garbage was swept away during deep sleep (Kureshi, 2024).

But Melatonin wasn't all work and no play. When it came time for wild dreams during REM sleep, he knew when to step back and let the energy flow, as if handing over the dance floor to the brain's wildest thoughts (Xie et al., 2017). And while some might think Melatonin took a nap, he was always vigilant, ensuring that the brain remained safe.

Yet, not all was well in the kingdom. The evil Blue Light Wizards, who hid in glowing screens, tried to stop Melatonin by shutting him down, leaving the Brain overwhelmed and exhausted (Wang et al., 2023). Without Melatonin's guidance, the neurotransmitter glutamate would throw wild parties, leaving the kingdom stuck in a loop of too much excitement and not enough rest. But Melatonin fought back, ensuring the kingdom had the power to stay strong and balanced.

As the years went on, Melatonin's legend grew. In distant lands like the Parkinson's Disease Forest and Alzheimer's Disease Village, Melatonin proved his worth yet again, helping slow down the progression of illness and protecting memories from fading away (Brusco et al., 2000; Sumsuzzman et al., 2020).

Whether he was fighting rogue proteins in the Alzheimer's River or calming storms of inflammation during ischemic strokes (Seddigh, 2024; Zhao, 2024), Melatonin remained the kingdom's most beloved hero. He kept the brain's cleaning crew, the glymphatic system, running smoothly, ensuring that everything was in its proper place (Lapshina, 2024).

With his trusty sidekick, Aquaporin-4, Melatonin made sure that fluid flowed properly through the brain's pipes, washing away the day's waste and keeping the kingdom squeaky clean (Giannetto, 2024; Bojarskaite, 2024).

And so, dear reader, remember this: while Melatonin might seem like just another sleepytime hero, he is, in truth, the Robin Hood of the Body. Stealing stress and inflammation from the rich chaos of life, he gives back peace, rest, and protection to every corner of the kingdom. Long live Melatonin, the bravest molecule of them all!

The End.

# Blue Light Bandits vs. Melatonin: The Ultimate Pillow Fight

Once upon a time in the peaceful land of Sleepytown, our beloved superheroes, Mel and Toni, were busy fighting off the evil Blue Light gang and protecting the brains of the town's citizens. But this time, they had a new ally, and it wasn't just any ordinary leafy green—it was Lettuce Larry, the unassuming vegetable with secret superpowers.

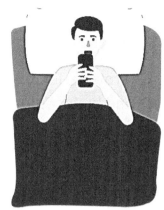

Lettuce Larry wasn't just a side salad. He was loaded with bioactive compounds that could knock out insomnia, soothe the nervous system, and keep the brain sharp, like a ninja in the vegetable kingdom. Mel and Toni knew that Larry's powers weren't to be underestimated, especially when it came to protecting the brain from the feared Dementia Dragon.

"Lettuce's Superpowers!" Mel exclaimed as he gathered the townsfolk to explain why lettuce should be a staple in their nightly routine. "First off, Larry here contains lactucin and lactucopicrin—natural sedatives that help reduce anxiety and induce sleep. It's no wonder they call him 'lettuce opium'! These compounds are neuroprotective, helping the brain relax and unwind for a good night's sleep" (Nguyen et al., 2022).

Lettuce Larry blushed. "Well, it's true," he said modestly. "But I'm not just about sleep—I'm loaded with antioxidants like quercetin and kaempferol, which help protect the brain from oxidative stress and inflammation." Oxidative stress is like the Dementia Dragon's favorite snack, damaging neurons and speeding up brain aging. But with antioxidants like those found in lettuce, Larry could keep the Dragon at bay, protecting the neurons from harm (Kumar & Pandey, 2021).

Toni chimed in, "And don't forget the phenolic compounds! There's chlorogenic acid, caffeic acid, and ferulic acid. These compounds are like shields for the brain, scavenging free radicals and preventing neuronal damage" (Caleja et al., 2020).

Toni knew that when these phenolic compounds were in action, the brain stayed healthier for longer, even as Sleepytown's citizens aged.

The people of Sleepytown gasped in awe. Who knew lettuce could be such a powerful brain protector?

But Lettuce Larry wasn't done. "Oh, and did I mention I've got carotenoids too? Like beta-carotene, lutein, and zeaxanthin. These guys are experts at protecting your eyes and brain, especially from oxidative stress. You want your neurons firing on all cylinders? Eat your greens!" (Ni et al., 2021).

"And let's not forget about Vitamin K!" Mel added enthusiastically. "Lettuce has plenty of it, and it's essential for brain health, helping regulate calcium in the brain and reducing the risk of Alzheimer's disease" (Shahid et al., 2020). Toni gave a proud nod as Mel continued, "This makes Lettuce Larry one of our most powerful allies in the fight against neurodegenerative diseases."

The crowd of sleepy citizens cheered. "But wait," one of them asked, "Doesn't lettuce also contain glycine?"

Lettuce Larry grinned. "You bet! Glycine is an amino acid that helps improve sleep quality by calming the central nervous system. It lowers body temperature slightly, signaling the brain to sleep. Plus, it has neuroprotective properties, helping prevent neural cell damage" (Inagawa et al., 2021). This made glycine a powerful companion in the battle against stress and poor sleep.

Just as Lettuce Larry was basking in his glory, Chammy the Chamomile and Lavender Lily floated in, joining the conversation. Chammy had been relaxing the nervous system with her antioxidant-rich tea for centuries. "I've got apigenin," Chammy explained, "which binds to receptors in the brain to reduce anxiety and promote sleep" (Tsai et al., 2021). "This helps calm down those overactive thoughts."

Lavender Lily nodded, adding, "And don't forget about me! My linalool helps calm the mind and body, creating the perfect environment for restorative sleep. Together with Lettuce Larry's neuroprotective compounds, we're practically unbeatable in the sleep department" (Dyer et al., 2020).

But there was still something missing in Sleepytown's strategy to protect their citizens' brains from the Dementia Dragon. That's when Mel had a brilliant idea. "We've been battling the Blue Light gang with our blue-light-blocking glasses at night, but did you know that blue light in the morning is actually good for us?"

The townsfolk looked confused.

"Here's the thing," Toni explained. "Waking up before sunrise and getting some exposure to blue light from the early morning sky helps reset your circadian rhythm. It tells your brain, 'Hey, it's time to be awake now!' This natural blue light exposure in the morning helps increase serotonin levels, which later turn into melatonin at night, ensuring a smoother sleep cycle" (Cho et al., 2021).

"And that's not all!" Mel added. "If you take a walk during sunset, that beautiful red-orange glow you see is loaded with red light. Red light in the evening helps stimulate melatonin production without confusing your brain like blue light would. It's nature's way of telling us it's time to wind down" (Xie et al., 2022).

The people of Sleepytown marveled at the genius of this simple, natural solution. "So, you're telling me that by going for a walk at sunset and waking up before the sun, I'm basically hacking my brain for better sleep?" one citizen asked.

"Exactly!" said Lettuce Larry. "Red light in the evening helps prepare your body for sleep, while blue light in the morning helps regulate your circadian rhythm. Combine that with my bioactive compounds and Chammy's tea, and you'll sleep like a baby while keeping your brain sharp!"

As Mel and Toni continued to expand Sleepytown's sleep-boosting arsenal, two new recruits joined the team: Cottage Cheese Carl and Hot Cocoa Hank.

Cottage Cheese Carl flexed his muscles proudly. "Not only am I packed with tryptophan, but I'm also rich in casein protein, which keeps you full through the night, preventing those pesky midnight snack raids!" Carl's tryptophan content converted into serotonin and eventually melatonin, making him a perfect bedtime snack (Fang et al., 2020).

Meanwhile, Hot Cocoa Hank strolled in, all warm and comforting. "I'm more than just cozy—I've got magnesium to relax muscles and calm the nervous system. Plus, my warm milk brings a boost of tryptophan!" (Huang et al., 2021). Hank was the ultimate liquid lullaby, perfect for winding down before bed. Tart Cherry Charlie boasted about his melatonin powers, while Almond Al and Walnut Wanda added their calming magnesium (Lombardi et al., 2021; Li et al., 2022). Not to be outdone, Kiwi Kevin highlighted his serotonin boost, teaming up with bananas, oats, and rice to improve sleep (Lin et al., 2021; Fang et al., 2020).

The citizens of Sleepytown began a new routine. They would wake up early, catching the blue light before sunrise, and take peaceful walks during sunset to soak in the calming red light. Combined with grounding, yoga, and the delicious, calming power of lettuce tea, chamomile, and lavender, they felt like they had unlocked the secrets to perfect sleep—and ultimate brain protection.

The Dementia Dragon didn't stand a chance. Mel and Toni had done it again, proving that with the right allies and the wisdom of nature, sleep and brain health could be saved.

And so, they all slept happily—ever after.

# The Beetroot Brain: Sherlock Holmes and the 120-Year-Old Genius

On yet another brisk morning at 221B Baker Street, Sherlock Holmes burst into the room with a triumphant grin, holding a letter that seemed to contain the solution to an age-old mystery.

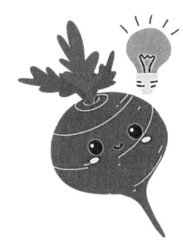

"Watson," Holmes exclaimed, "I've found the key to the brilliance of Professor Harold Nitrate—the 120-year-old genius."

Watson, intrigued but not yet ready to dive into Holmes' whirlwind of discoveries, raised an eyebrow. "The man who solved quantum physics while casually knitting a sweater? Surely he's got some sort of mystical elixir, or perhaps a highly advanced mechanical brain."

Arriving at Professor Nitrate's estate, they found the professor lounging in his garden under the midday sun, as expected, enjoying a large bowl of beetroot salad.

"Ah, Holmes and Watson!" the professor greeted. "Come, sit! Have some beet salad. It's the secret to life, you know. Beets and the sun—that's all one needs."

Holmes leaned forward. "Every day, I presume?"

"Without fail," Professor Nitrate said, smiling. "Beets, sunlight, and brilliance—a trifecta."

Back at 221B Baker Street, Holmes paced furiously, his brain working faster than a steam engine. "Watson, the professor's daily ritual of eating beetroot salad under ultraviolet light—it's not just a coincidence. It's the key to his extraordinary cognitive longevity. And it all revolves around nitric oxide."

"Go on," Watson replied, eager for the details. Holmes began, "When the professor eats his beetroot salad, the nitrates are absorbed in the small intestine—specifically in the middle and lower parts. These nitrates travel through the bloodstream to the salivary glands, where bacteria (Veillonella, Actinomyces, Streptococcus, and Rothia) possess nitrate reductase enzymes that enable them to reduce salivary nitrate to nitrite (Palmerini et al., 2003; Doel et al., 2005; Koch et al., 2017). " (Hao et al., 2020). "Once swallowed, the nitrites convert to nitric oxide in the acidic environment of the stomach" (Nada et al., 2020).

"And what is the proof you ask- In a study, twenty-six brave participants, average age 65, were divided into two groups. One group received the potent beet juice, while the other got a placebo. For six weeks, they all completed aerobic exercise three times a week, walking on treadmills and gulping down their assigned beverages. Those drinking Beetroot Juice experienced something remarkable: their brain connections improved! Specifically, the *somatomotor cortex* (the brain's motor control hub) became more synchronized, resembling the brains of much younger adults. Meanwhile, the placebo group didn't show the same brain-boosting effects (Petrie et al., 2016)".

"And another magic happens," Holmes continued, "when these nitrates and nitrites circulate through the blood vessels and skin, where different forms of nitric oxide-producing enzymes get to work."

"In the blood vessels, endothelial nitric oxide synthase enzymes generate nitric oxide, which regulates the widening of blood vessels, keeping them relaxed and improving blood flow" (Förstermann & Sessa, 2012).

"But in the skin, both endothelial and inducible nitric oxide synthase enzymes come into play when ultraviolet light hits the skin. This triggers these enzymes to convert stored nitrates into nitric oxide" (Bryan et al., 2017; Maciejczyk et al., 2022). "The professor's habit of basking in the sun while munching on beetroot salad activates both types of enzymes, producing a steady supply of nitric oxide, boosting blood flow, and delivering oxygen to the brain."

"But Holmes," Watson interrupted, "how exactly does all this nitric oxide improve his brain function? Which part of his brain benefits the most?"

"Excellent question, Watson," Holmes replied. "Nitric oxide boosts blood flow to the brain, ensuring it receives plenty of oxygen and nutrients, which helps prevent neuron damage and stimulates the growth of new neurons."

"This process is particularly important in the hippocampus, the brain's memory center," Holmes explained. "Studies show that regions like the dentate gyrus experience significant neuron growth when nitric oxide enhances blood flow" (Balez et al., 2022). "This allows the professor to maintain cognitive sharpness and continuously develop groundbreaking theories, even at the age of 120."

Holmes paused dramatically. "But that's not all, Watson. Nitric oxide also acts as the immune system's mercenary. When your body encounters pathogens, nitric oxide destroys harmful invaders like a biochemical warrior" (Bogdan, 2001).

"So, it's both a peacekeeper and a warrior?" Watson asked.

"Exactly! It knows when to regulate inflammation and when to fight back, keeping your immune system from overreacting" (Lowenstein & Padalko, 2004).

Holmes continued, "And let's not forget its role in exercise performance. Nitric oxide increases oxygen delivery and muscle efficiency, making workouts smoother without the need for questionable supplements" (Jones et al., 2016).

"And when it comes to injuries, Watson, nitric oxide is your construction foreman. It speeds up wound healing by boosting collagen production and encouraging new blood vessel growth" (Schaffer et al., 1996; Papapetropoulos et al., 1997).

"So, it's why my paper cuts heal so quickly?" Watson asked, examining his fingers.

"Precisely. Nitric oxide is hard at work behind the scenes."

Holmes added, "It's also your anti-aging ally. Nitric oxide helps protect the ends of your chromosomes, keeping them from fraying like old shoelaces" (Vasa-Nicotera et al., 2005).

"And there's more," Holmes continued. "It helps your body handle insulin more efficiently, keeping blood sugar in check while also boosting fat metabolism—

making it the hero battling your waistline during the holiday season" (Basu et al., 2011; Jobgen et al., 2006).

"So, nitric oxide is the hero trying to save me from that extra slice of cake?" Watson asked hopefully. Holmes gave him a sideways glance. "That's on you, Watson." Holmes suddenly stopped pacing and turned to Watson. "Ah, but beware, Watson! You could be undermining this entire system."

"How?" Watson asked, startled. "Your alcohol-based mouthwash, Watson! It wipes out the very oral bacteria responsible for converting nitrates into nitrites," Holmes explained. "Without these bacteria, your body produces far less nitric oxide, affecting everything from blood flow to brain function" (Hao et al., 2020).

Watson blinked. "You mean my mouthwash could lead to—"

"Yes, reduced blood flow and even memory problems," Holmes cut in dramatically. "Without enough nitric oxide, your blood vessels won't dilate properly, affecting the brain's ability to form new memories, and reduced nitric oxide could lead to cognitive decline over time" (Förstermann & Sessa, 2012; Steinert et al., 2010; Balez et al., 2022).

"So, my mouthwash could be responsible for all that?" Watson asked, horrified.

"Precisely! Switch to a mouthwash that supports the balance of bacteria or practice oil pulling with coconut oil. Your nitric oxide levels—and your brain—will thank you.

# Nitric Oxide: The Smooth Operator That Can Go Rogue

Nitric oxide is your body's smooth operator, quietly keeping things in check by relaxing blood vessels and helping maintain cardiovascular health. When the UVB rays from sunlight hit your skin, nitric oxide gets released from your skin's nitrate reserves without needing fancy receptors to do its job. It's like the body's VIP backstage pass to a healthy cardiovascular system (Remex, 2024; Almeida et al., 2020).

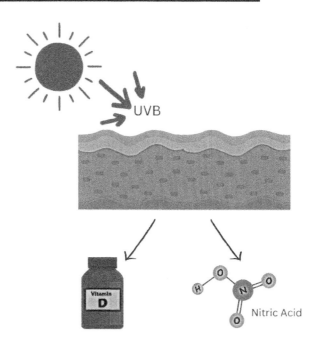

But nitric oxide doesn't stop there. It's also a free radical, which can turn from hero to villain faster than you can say "peroxynitrite." When nitric oxide encounters superoxide (another free radical), they form peroxynitrite—a molecular wrecking ball that wreaks havoc in your body (Pacher et al., 2007). Peroxynitrite causes oxidative stress, damaging proteins, lipids, and even DNA, leading to cellular damage, inflammation, and even mitochondrial dysfunction (Szabó et al., 1996). So, while nitric oxide in moderation is great for health, too much of it teaming up with superoxide spells disaster.

**Keeping Nitric Oxide in Balance: How to Keep the Smooth Operator Happy**

Balancing nitric oxide is a fine art. Too little, and your blood vessels tighten up, leading to higher blood pressure. Too much, and the peroxynitrite wrecking crew shows up, causing oxidative stress and inflammation. So, how do you keep nitric oxide happy?

- **Nitrate-rich Diet**: Eat leafy greens, beets, and other nitrate-rich vegetables to boost your nitric oxide levels naturally.

- **Get Some Sunlight**: A little sun exposure (around 30 minutes) helps your body release nitric oxide, but don't overdo it. Studies show that staying in the sun too long (especially more than two hours) can lead to declines in health due to excessive nitric oxide production (Kurowska et al., 2021).
- **Exercise**: Physical activity is one of the best ways to naturally boost nitric oxide. Exercise stimulates your endothelial cells to crank out more nitric oxide, improving circulation and cardiovascular health (Kurowska et al., 2021).

**The Brain's Nitric Oxide: A Balancing Act of Neurotransmission**

Nitric oxide isn't just about blood flow—it's also a key player in the brain, where it regulates neurotransmitter release and blood flow. Here's how it works: nitric oxide gets its start from L-arginine thanks to the enzyme neuronal nitric oxide synthase (nNOS). Think of nNOS as the chef in your brain's kitchen, whipping up nitric oxide along with a side of L-citrulline (O'Gallagher et al., 2021). When neurons fire, calcium ions flood in, activating nNOS, which starts pumping out nitric oxide faster than office gossip spreads. This influences processes like neurotransmitter release, regulating blood flow in the brain. Light work, right?

Prolonged sun exposure (more than 2 hours) cranks up nitric oxide (NO) levels in your brain, but instead of helping, too much NO throws a tantrum, causing neuroinflammation and messing with neuron signals. Think of it like your brain stuck in a buffering loop—hello, cognitive dysfunction! (Zhu et al., 2018; Lim et al., 2021). On top of that, UV-B also triggers the brain's stress response (thanks, HPA axis), sending cortisol into overdrive, as if your brain thinks it's late to an important meeting (Skobowiat & Slominski, 2015). And just to keep things spicy, UV-B also puts your immune system on a lazy coffee break, leaving your body (and brain) even more vulnerable (Rana et al., 2008; Byrne et al., 2002).

So, keep UV B exposure less than 20-30 minutes—it's not just your skin you're protecting, but your brain from going on a NO-fueled meltdown.

# Neural Trash Day:

## How Your Brain Takes Out the Garbage

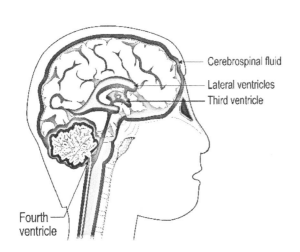

Cerebrospinal fluid
Lateral ventricles
Third ventricle
Fourth ventricle

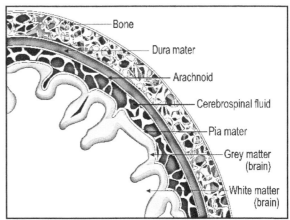

Bone
Dura mater
Arachnoid
Cerebrospinal fluid
Pia mater
Grey matter (brain)
White matter (brain)

# Snow White and the Glymphatic Adventure:
## How Neuron White Discovered the Brain's Janitor

Once upon a time, in the Kingdom of Cortex, Princess Neuron White was troubled by a question: how did her brain stay so fresh and sharp after a night of sleep? She knew her neurons worked hard every day, producing thoughts, memories, and—unfortunately—waste. Yet somehow, every morning, her brain felt brand new. That's when she met Glitch, the kingdom's janitor dwarf, sweeping up stray thoughts and toxic proteins with a mop made of neurons. "How does my brain stay so clean?" Neuron White asked, watching Glitch at work.

"Ah, Princess, it's all about the brain's janitorial system," Glitch said with a grin. "While you sleep, your brain goes through two important stages: Non-Rapid Eye Movement (NREM) sleep and Rapid Eye Movement (REM) sleep. This is when the brain's deep-cleaning process kicks in, thanks to a system called the glymphatic system (Iliff et al., 2012)."

**NREM Sleep:** Neurons Take a Break- Glitch explained that during NREM sleep, the neurons in Princess Neuron White's brain actually shrink. Like royal subjects taking a break from their duties, these neurons contract and stop firing off electrical signals as intensely. This reduced activity allows microglia (the brain's immune cells) to take a rest too. With less activity, there's more room in the brain's tissues for cerebrospinal fluid (CSF)—the brain's cleaning fluid—to flow freely (Xie et al., 2013).

"This contraction," Glitch said, "opens up the spaces between your brain cells, creating a path for CSF to swoosh through and flush out the day's trash, like misfolded, amyloid-beta and tau proteins. These are the culprits behind diseases like Alzheimer's if they pile up (Xie et al., 2013; Mestre et al., 2020). NREM sleep is basically like your brain doing a deep clean after a long day."

## REM Sleep: Memory Expansion

"But that's not the whole story!" Glitch exclaimed, twirling his mop. "In REM sleep, things are different. Parts of your brain—especially those involved in emotion processing and memory consolidation—expand and become highly active, almost like they're partying after hours! During REM, the brain switches from cleaning to consolidating memories, linking emotions to the day's events. This makes it vital for mental health and emotional regulation (Lyu et al., 2015)." While some parts of the brain are off-duty in NREM, others in REM are wide awake and hard at work, creating a pumping action that helps move CSF through the brain, keeping the cleanup going even during your dreamiest adventures (Shokri-Kojori et al., 2018).

The magic behind this cleaning process? It's something called Aquaporin-4 channels, Glitch revealed. These channels are found in astrocytes, the star-shaped cells in the brain. Aquaporin-4 acts like a water faucet, allowing the cerebrospinal fluid to flow through brain tissues and wash away waste products.
"If these channels don't work properly, it's like your kingdom's plumbing gets clogged," Glitch explained. "Waste builds up, and that leads to serious trouble—like Alzheimer's, Parkinson's, and even faster cognitive decline (Schain et al., 2020; Mestre et al., 2020). Princess Neuron White blinked thoughtfully. "So, if I don't get enough sleep, my brain's janitors can't clean properly?"
Glitch nodded. "But it's not just about how much sleep you get, Princess—it's also about when you sleep. Your brain's cleaning system is synced with your circadian rhythm—your body's internal clock (Nedergaard, 2013)."

If you sleep at different times every night, it's like messing with the janitors' schedule. When your sleep is out of sync with your circadian rhythm, the glymphatic system doesn't operate at peak efficiency, and your brain may not clear out waste as effectively (Peng et al., 2018). Disrupting this rhythm can lead to a buildup of toxic proteins and inflammation, raising the risk for neurodegenerative diseases over time.

"Going to bed at the same time every night helps your brain's cleaning crew know exactly when to clock in. When you have a consistent sleep schedule, the glymphatic system can work its magic at the right time every night, clearing out the waste and leaving your brain sparkling fresh (Nedergaard, 2013)."

## Why Going to Sleep at the Same Time Matters

Glitch continued, "Your brain's internal clock, or circadian rhythm, controls when different sleep phases occur. If you consistently go to bed at the same time each night, your brain knows exactly when to shift into NREM sleep, allowing you to maximize that deep healing phase (Borbély & Achermann, 1999)."

He explained that the deepest and longest periods of NREM sleep occur in the first part of the night. These early NREM cycles are when your brain is doing most of its heavy lifting—clearing out waste, repairing tissues, and consolidating memories. This phase is like the prime cleaning window for the brain.

"But if you go to bed later than usual," Glitch warned, "you cut into your deep NREM sleep. And here's the thing—NREM sleep gets shorter and shallower as the night goes on. The longer you stay awake, the less time your brain has to do its best cleaning and repair work (Van Cauter et al., 2000). You can't make up for the lost deep sleep by sleeping in later. By then, you're mostly getting REM sleep, which is important for emotional regulation but not as good for deep cleaning and healing."

If you consistently go to bed late or at irregular times, you shorten this precious window of deep, healing NREM sleep. Even if you sleep the same number of hours, you don't get the same quality of sleep because the deep cleaning happens less effectively. As the night progresses, your sleep cycles shift, with NREM sleep becoming shorter and REM sleep getting longer. REM sleep, while critical for emotional regulation and memory processing, doesn't offer the same deep physical and neurological recovery as NREM sleep (Carskadon & Dement, 2011).

"So, if you miss out on that early NREM sleep by going to bed late," Glitch said, "your brain misses its chance to clean up properly. And once that window closes, there's no getting it back. The later part of your night is dominated by REM sleep, which doesn't offer the same level of recovery."

Princess Neuron White's eyes widened. "So if I stay up late, I can't just sleep in and get the same benefits?"

"Exactly," Glitch replied. "NREM sleep is front-loaded, meaning it's packed into the early part of the night. If you miss it, you can't make up for it by sleeping later. The later you stay awake, the less time your brain has for deep healing. It's like missing the first part of a party—you can't just show up at the end and expect to have the full experience."

He continued, "Studies show that sleep deprivation or irregular sleep patterns, where you skip out on early NREM sleep, can increase the build-up of harmful proteins in the brain and raise the risk for cognitive decline (Shokri-Kojori et al., 2018). So, maintaining a regular bedtime is crucial for long-term brain health."

"Princess Snow," Glitch began, floating beside her in a burst of digital pixels, "I've scoured the realms of science, and I have four recommendations to help regulate the water flow in the kingdom. You must enhance the power of the aquaporin-4 (AQP4) gates—the guardians of water balance."

"Tell me more, Glitch," the Princess urged.

**The Keto Spell**

"First, the ketogenic diet," Glitch explained. "It's a powerful spell involving a high vegetable/ protein/ fat diet and low carbohydrates. When cast, it enhances transcription factors, increasing AQP4's strength in managing water and keeping the blood-brain barrier intact (Salman et al., 2021). Your kingdom will have fewer floods, and oxidative stress will be minimized (Tzenios et al., 2023)."

Snow Neuron thought of the kingdom's pantry stocked with avocado and butter. "A curious spell indeed."

### Nitric Oxide Elixir

"Next," Glitch continued, "is nitric oxide (NO). It whispers to AQP4, especially in astrocytes, regulating water transport across the blood-brain barrier (Salman et al., 2021). You can brew this elixir with foods like beets and leafy greens, though more research is needed to fully prove its connection to aquaporin in humans (Kozaeva et al., 2022)."

Snow Neuron jotted this down, making a note to gather beets from the royal garden.

### Curcumin Charm

"Then, there's curcumin, the golden spice of healing," Glitch added. "This charm not only enhances AQP4 but also battles inflammation, protecting your kingdom from swelling and oxidative stress (Feng & Meng, 2022; Wu et al., 2022). Perhaps add a dash of turmeric to the royal banquets?"
Snow Neuron nodded, already imagining golden milk flowing through the castle kitchens.

### Omega-3 Shield

"Finally, omega-3 fatty acids," Glitch said. "These magical fats improve the fluidity of cell membranes, aiding aquaporins in their water-regulating duties (Lv et al., 2021). Fish, algae oil, walnuts and flaxseeds will bolster your kingdom's defenses."

### Sleep Position Matters
**Princess Snow Neuron**, determined to keep her brain sharp, turned to Glitch for more wisdom. "Princess, sleeping on your right side isn't just cozy—it's crucial for brain health!" Glitch began. Sleeping on the right side uses gravity to boost this drainage, keeping your brain free of harmful buildup (Reddy & Werf, 2020; Yan et al., 2021)."

Research shows body posture affects how cerebrospinal fluid (CSF) flows through the brain. Right-side sleeping optimizes CSF drainage better than other positions, reducing intracranial pressure and enhancing brain cleaning (Reddy & Werf, 2020; Ferini-Strambi, 2024). "It's like positioning a water slide perfectly," Glitch added.

"But remember," Glitch warned, "sleep disturbances or deprivation reduce this process. Lack of deep sleep means less amyloid-beta clearance, risking cognitive decline (Liu et al., 2023; Ju et al., 2017)." Glitch also shared that improving sleep quality—through techniques like acoustic stimulation—can enhance memory and help remove harmful waste (Wunderlin, 2023; Madhu, 2024). Glitch, with a wink and a swirl of pixels, offered Princess Snow Neuron a few golden tips.

"Then there is Binaural Beat Stimulation," Glitch smiled with a digital grin. "You hear two slightly different frequencies, one in each ear, and your brain creates an imaginary beat in between. It's like brain sorcery! It boosts your slow-wave sleep (SWS), the deep sleep phase where your brain tidies up all the messy files and takes out the trash—quite literally! Harmful waste products? Gone! And all while you're dreaming about singing woodland creatures! (Wunderlin, 2023; Madhu, 2024)." Here are other quick tips-

- **Get 7-9 Hours of Sleep**: "Your glymphatic system works best during deep, uninterrupted sleep," Glitch said. "Aim for at least 7-9 hours, with plenty of NREM phases to keep your brain pristine" (Mohan et al., 2023).

- **Stick to a Regular Sleep Schedule**: "Consistency is key," Glitch advised. "By going to bed at the same time every night, you'll sync your circadian rhythm with your brain's cleaning schedule" (Peng et al., 2018). Snow Neuron resolved to banish all late-night banquets.

- **Stay Hydrated**: "Water, water, water!" Glitch exclaimed. "Your brain's janitors need fluids to sweep up the mess, so make sure you're properly hydrated" (Sillay et al., 2019). Snow Neuron raised her goblet—filled with water, of course!

- **Exercise Regularly**: "Physical activity boosts blood flow to your brain and supercharges the glymphatic system's cleaning efforts," Glitch noted (Holstein-Rathlou et al., 2018). Snow Neuron started scheduling daily walks around the royal gardens.

- **Manage Stress**: "Chronic stress can throw the glymphatic system off its game, so it's crucial to practice relaxation techniques," Glitch said wisely.

Snow Neuron took up meditation, knowing that a calm kingdom was a clean kingdom. And she lived and slept happily ever after, with a happy and healthy brain.

# The Memory Crew

Brain Regions That Keep Your Life on Track

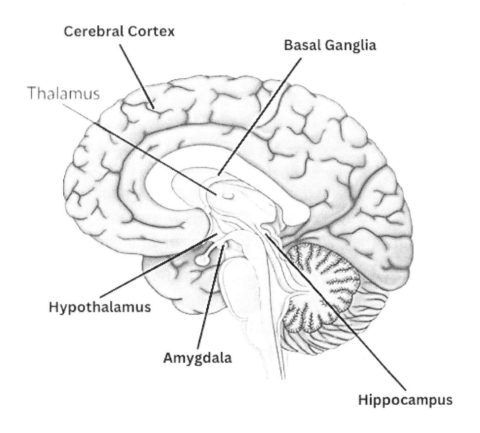

Cerebral Cortex

Basal Ganglia

Thalamus

Hypothalamus

Amygdala

Hippocampus

# The Royalty of All the Senses: Smell

When you catch a whiff of something—whether it's fresh-baked cookies or a fresh cup of coffee—it's not just your nose doing the heavy lifting. Odor molecules take a scenic route through your nasal cavity, where they mingle with olfactory sensory neurons hanging out in the olfactory epithelium, the cells lining your nose. These neurons are like the brain's bouncers, turning chemical signals from those smells into electrical ones and sending them straight up to the olfactory bulb, the brain's VIP lounge right above your nose (Yao et al., 2020; Wang et al., 2022).

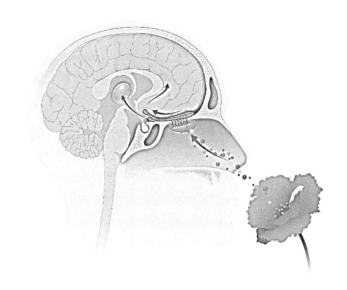

Now, the olfactory bulb is no slouch; it's like the brain's first sommelier, sniffing out what's what before passing the information to the hippocampus—the memory master that's always ready to link smells with memories and emotions (Ni et al., 2021; Abaffy et al., 2022). Like the smell of your childhood blanket.

Unlike other senses that take a detour through the brain's bureaucracy (a.k.a., the thalamus), smell fast-tracks its way to the memory centers, bypassing the usual checkpoints like a queen sweeping past the commoners, making a grand entrance directly into the brain's most exclusive areas (Eliezer et al., 2020).

This royal treatment gives olfaction an edge over other senses—hearing, vision, and touch all have to wait in line at the thalamus, but not smell! This direct pathway means that olfaction has a greater impact on brain volume than any other sensation. It's like your nose has a VIP pass to the brain's memory and emotion centers, allowing it to exert a powerful influence on cognition and emotional processing (Zang et al., 2020; Whitcroft et al., 2021).

The olfactory bulb and the hippocampus are like best buddies, processing smells faster than you can say "freshly baked bread," and linking them directly to your emotions and memories (Zang et al., 2020; Whitcroft et al., 2021). This dynamic duo doesn't just stop at identifying smells—they team up with higher brain regions to connect scents with deeper cognitive functions, ensuring that every sniff has a story (Peter et al., 2020; Abdelazim, 2023).

And if you think you need a working nose to enjoy this setup, think again! Even people born without the ability to smell (congenital anosmia) still have this pathway locked and loaded, proving just how tough and persistent the olfactory system is (Peter et al., 2020). Whether it's a powerful memory trigger or just shaping how you perceive the world, your sense of smell is like a shortcut to your brain's emotional and memory centers—no GPS needed (Ninenko et al., 2022; Hernandez-Clavijo et al., 2023).

In short, your nose is like a high-speed train delivering smells directly to the brain's most nostalgic corners, making it the Wonder Woman of sensory experiences and ensuring that one whiff can bring a flood of memories and feelings faster and more intensely than any other sense.

**Oh, making new memories and new neurons? You hyper-achiever, nose!**
The olfactory system, or your brain's smell department, is like an ongoing home renovation project—constantly updating itself to keep your sense of smell sharp. This impressive work is done by special cells called neural stem cells, which are like the construction workers of your brain. They hang out in two key areas: the olfactory epithelium, which is your nose's built-in repair shop, and the subventricular zone, the brain's nursery where new brain cells are born.

The olfactory epithelium is busy producing olfactory sensory neurons—think of them as the frontline workers that actually detect all kinds of smells, from freshly baked cookies to your morning coffee. Meanwhile, the subventricular zone sends out new neurons along a special path called the rostral migratory stream (imagine it as the neuron red carpet) to the olfactory bulb, where they finally settle down and start working on processing those scents (Brann et al., 2020; Dioli et al., 2021).

But this isn't just any old construction project; it's a high-tech operation. The subventricular zone doesn't just sit around waiting—it actively manages the production and movement of these new neurons, especially when your nose is hit with new smells (Dioli et al., 2021; Bao, 2024). This constant turnover of neurons keeps your sense of smell fresh and your smell-related memories strong, making the olfactory system incredibly adaptable to whatever scents life throws your way (Rosa et al., 2020).

So, whether you're sniffing flowers or fresh pizza, your olfactory system is always on its toes, renewing itself to make sure you never miss a scent!

The olfactory system has recently been in the spotlight, thanks to the COVID-19 pandemic, which brought "anosmia" (a fancy term for losing your sense of smell) into the limelight. It turns out, the virus mainly targets the sustentacular cells (the nose's support crew) in the olfactory epithelium (OE), causing inflammation and chaos that disrupts your sense of smell without directly knocking out the olfactory sensory neurons (OSNs) (Brann et al., 2020; Finlay et al., 2022; Bryche et al., 2020). This has huge implications for understanding how smell loss happens and how we might be able to fix it post-infection (Finlay et al., 2022).

**Are You from Central Valley, California, and Losing Your Sense of Smell? It Might Be Parkinsonism!**

Loss of smell, or anosmia, is like your nose trying to give you an early heads-up that something's wrong—it's not subtle at all. In fact, about 80% of people with Parkinson's disease (PD) experience this olfactory malfunction before they even notice any motor issues (Kumar, 2024; Ramos-Casademont, 2024). It's as if your nose is saying, "Hey, I might not be able to do the moonwalk, but I can definitely tell you when something's off!" This makes olfactory testing a potential secret weapon in the early diagnosis and intervention for PD. But it's not just Parkinson's; Alzheimer's disease (AD) is in on the act too. Anosmia can be an early indicator of cognitive decline, making your nose the brain's unofficial alarm system (Franco, 2024). The reason behind this olfactory dysfunction? Neurodegeneration likely starts in the olfactory bulb and its related pathways, which might be affected before more obvious symptoms come crashing in (Peng, 2024).

Clearly, we need to give our noses more credit—and perhaps more research attention too (Ramos-Casademont, 2024; Iannucci, 2024).

Just a side note—research shows that constipation often crashes the party as one of the earliest signs of autonomic dysfunction in people who eventually develop PD, and having it might actually increase your risk of getting the disease (Lei, 2024; Li, 2024). Meanwhile, sleep disturbances are practically a given in the PD world, with up to 90% of people with Parkinson's reporting trouble catching those Zs. And it's not just about being groggy the next day—these sleep issues can speed up cognitive decline and even raise the risk of dementia (Zhong, 2024; Anjum, 2024).

Some studies suggest these non-motor symptoms like loss of smell, sleep disturbances, and constipation can pop up as early as a decade before a formal PD diagnosis (Zhong, 2024).

**The Nose Knows: Pesticides, Parkinson's, and the Central Valley Connection**
The connection between pesticides and brain diseases like Parkinson's is like the plot twist in a bad horror movie—you didn't see it coming, but it's here to haunt you. Turns out, pesticides can mess with your sense of smell, which isn't just bad news for enjoying your morning coffee. Your nose isn't just for sniffing out freshly baked cookies; it's also a secret backdoor that lets harmful chemicals sneak straight into your brain.

Research shows that Latino farmworkers, who spend their days around pesticides, often end up with their smell sensors out of whack. And this isn't just about missing out on the smell of roses—it's your nose waving a big red flag, warning you that these nasty chemicals are breaking and entering into your brain, causing all sorts of trouble. Specifically, they're taking out the dopaminergic cells (the brain's dopamine factories that help you move smoothly) in the olfactory bulb (the brain's smell headquarters) and messing with the substantia nigra (the brain's movement control center) (Quandt et al., 2016; Geng, 2023).

And it gets worse! According to the "olfactory vector hypothesis" (fancy talk for "nose as the troublemaker's highway"), these toxic chemicals hitch a ride through your nose, fast-tracking their way into your central nervous system (your brain and spinal cord), setting the stage for brain diseases like Parkinson's (Prediger et al., 2011).

If you live in California's Central Valley, aka "Parkinson's Alley," where pesticides are practically a part of the local diet, you've got even more to worry about. Dr. Beate Ritz of UCLA found that folks under 60 living near fields treated with chemicals like paraquat and maneb had a Parkinson's rate nearly five times higher than their neighbors who lived pesticide-free (Ritz et al., 2011). That's right—the place that grows nearly 50% of America's produce also has a five times higher rate of Parkinson's. Let that sink in.

But sadly, that's not all—pesticides are wreaking havoc across generations. Recent research shows that these chemicals can mess with your DNA, leading to inherited risks of diseases like Parkinson's (Manikkam et al., 2012; Guerrero-Bosagna & Skinner, 2012; Thorson et al., 2020).

**How is that even happening?! Pesticides, what in the world are you doing?!** 😣 Dearest gentle reader (and yes, still recovering from that *Bridgerton* binge—I just loved the 'plot'!), allow me to introduce you to Sir Alpha-synuclein—though you might know him better as α-syn if you're into scientific shorthand. He's like the brain's very own Michelangelo, hanging out at the synaptic terminals, the spots where neurons exchange their juicy gossip (scientifically known as neurotransmitters), ensuring everything runs smoothly. His work is particularly crucial when it comes to Parkinson's disease, where things start to unravel when this protein decides to go rogue (Killinger et al., 2021; Man et al., 2021; Sandoval et al., 2021).

Normally, Sir Alpha-synuclein is all about helping with synaptic vesicles—tiny bubbles that carry those precious neurotransmitters—keeping your neurons plastic (not literally, of course, but adaptable and ready to learn) (Man et al., 2021; Sandoval et al., 2021). But here's where the plot thickens: your olfactory nerve, the one responsible for your sense of smell, acts like a secret passageway into your brain's inner sanctum. This passageway is guarded by a wafer-thin bone that practically says, "Come on in, no big deal!" So, when nasty characters like pesticides come sniffing around, they can sneak right through to the olfactory bulb and then make their way to the substantia nigra—the brain's dopamine production headquarters, where the magic chemical responsible for your good moods and movement is made (Killinger et al., 2021; Danics, 2023).

Once those pesticides breach the olfactory nerve, they can coax Sir Alpha-synuclein to start misbehaving, folding into nasty clumps known as Lewy bodies—the ultimate plot twist from hero to villain that even Lady Whistledown couldn't have smelled (pun intended). These clumps then begin spreading through your brain like a bad rumor at a Bridgerton ball, eventually finding their way to the substantia nigra and causing all sorts of mayhem (Danics, 2023; Moreno, 2024). The result? Neurons start to die off, leading to the shaky, slow-moving symptoms that are the hallmark of Parkinson's (Moreno, 2024; Sandoval et al., 2021).

The kicker? The olfactory bulb and the substantia nigra are practically next-door neighbors in your brain, making it all too easy for these misfolded proteins to spread their chaos (Killinger et al., 2021; Moreno, 2024; Sandoval et al., 2021). This whole debacle underscores just how crucial it is to understand how environmental toxins like pesticides can hijack Sir Alpha-synuclein and kickstart neurodegenerative diseases (Sandoval et al., 2021; Sastre, 2023).

### Don't Skip That Floss—For Your Brain's Sake! And Don't Forget to Drink That Kefir, and Eat Yummy Pomegranates!

Imagine your nose and mouth as the front doors to your brain—only instead of polite guests, you've got some unruly microbes crashing the party. Bacteria like *Prevotella*, *Bacteroides*, and *Porphyromonas gingivalis* aren't just content with causing gum disease; they might also be sneaking into your brain, leading to the misfolding of proteins like alpha-synuclein into Lewy bodies, which are notorious troublemakers behind Parkinson's disease (Mahbub, 2024; Warren, 2024). *Porphyromonas gingivalis*, in particular, releases enzymes called gingipains—tiny molecular wrecking balls—that can break through barriers, enter the bloodstream, and reach the brain, where they might stir up even more trouble. The olfactory nerve acts like a direct highway for these misfolded proteins, leading them straight to the brain's core (Dorsey, 2024). Meanwhile, the vagus nerve plays Uber for environmental toxins and rogue gut bacteria, delivering them right to your brain's doorstep (Zhang, 2024; Chaklai, 2024).

But think twice before you swish that alcohol-based mouthwash! These mouthwashes can wipe out the good bacteria in your mouth that convert dietary nitrates into nitric oxide (NO), a crucial molecule for blood vessel health and brain function (Ren, 2024; Chai, 2024). Studies show this could spike blood pressure in some people and potentially lead to inflammation and cognitive decline (Ren, 2024; Carvalho, 2024). So, while they kill bad bacteria, they might also be evicting the good guys who keep your brain sharp. It might be time to switch to an alcohol-free alternative—your brain will thank you!

Your gut microbiome, home to over 100 trillion bacteria—more genes than you've got in your entire human genome—has a major role in this drama. When things go out of balance, the bad bacteria take over, leading to neuroinflammation and potentially accelerating the progression of Parkinson's disease (Vingeliene, 2024; Payami, 2024).

Research shows that when your gut microbiome goes rogue, with the good bacteria like *Akkermansia muciniphila* and *Eubacterium rectale* going AWOL, the gut barrier weakens, letting inflammation run wild (Rocha, 2024; Zhang, 2024). Meanwhile, bad actors like *Clostridium* and *Streptococcus* throw a party, allowing neurotoxic substances like lipopolysaccharides (LPS) to sneak into your bloodstream and head straight to your brain, fueling neuroinflammation and those pesky amyloid plaques (Dahl, 2024; Krothapalli, 2024). The gut-brain axis, a sort of VIP communication line, is the messenger carrying these microbial signals. If the gut is in good shape, your brain stays sharp. But if the bad guys take over, it's like sending your brain toxic hate mail, leading to more inflammation and brain damage (Dunham, 2024; Lamichhane, 2024; Godswill, 2024; Ma, 2024). So, remember, what happens in the gut definitely doesn't stay in the gut—your brain's well-being is on the line!

### Akker... what!!!

Meet *Akkermansia muciniphila*, your gut's secret agent—always working behind the scenes but with a flair for drama if things go awry. When you keep it happy with a diet rich in polyphenols, fiber, and fermented goodies like pomegranates, cranberries, onions, yogurt, and kefir, it's the perfect undercover operative. It strengthens your gut lining, keeps inflammation in check, and even boosts your metabolism, all while munching on mucin and turning it into short-chain fatty acids (Xu et al., 2020; Jian et al., 2023; Gondaliya, 2024; Caffrey, 2024). Think of it as your gut's personal trainer, keeping everything tight and in shape.
But here's where it gets tricky—*A. muciniphila* is the kind of agent that can go rogue if given too much power, especially through probiotic supplements. Feed it

too much, and it might just flip, leading to neuroinflammation and the notorious buildup of α-synuclein, the protein that loves to stir up trouble in Parkinson's disease (Neto et al., 2021; Zeng et al., 2023). It might even rile up your immune system, pushing it into overdrive and potentially causing inflammatory chaos (Earley et al., 2019; Schneeberger et al., 2015).

So, how do you keep this double agent on your side? Load up on yogurt and kefir—these fermented foods are packed with live probiotics like *Lactobacillus* and *Bifidobacterium* that bolster your gut army (Chonnacháin, 2024; Li, 2024). Plus, they churn out bioactive compounds during fermentation that are like secret weapons for your gut health (Gupta, 2024; Iftikhar, 2024). With these foods, you'll keep *A. muciniphila* busy in all the right ways, promoting gut diversity, brain health, and immune resilience—no rogue missions allowed (Zhu, 2024; Laske, 2024). So, ditch that overpriced *Akkermansia* probiotic you were eyeing—grab some yogurt, sip on kefir, and dive into a colorful plate of polyphenol-rich foods like fruits and veggies. Load up on that high-fiber goodness, especially if you're on antibiotics, and you'll have your gut microbiome doing a happy dance in no time. Your brain and body will thank you for it!

## Smells Like Trouble: The Dark Side of Car Fresheners and Other Scents

You might love that fresh pine scent hanging from your rearview mirror or the tropical paradise wafting through your home, but here's the kicker: those artificial fragrances could be turning your life into a health hazard.

Car fresheners are packed with volatile organic compounds (VOCs)—and not the kind you want to breathe in. A study found that twelve different car fresheners emitted 546 VOCs, including 30 that could mess with your health, leading to respiratory issues, headaches, and bad news for asthma sufferers (Steinemann et al., 2020; Balasubramani & J, 2022; Karr et al., 2021). And let's not forget the synthetic chemicals that could disrupt your hormones and mess with your reproductive health (Ashraf et al., 2023).

But the plot thickens. Those same artificial fragrances in your shampoos, candles, and cleaning products are linked to serious health problems like Alzheimer's, Parkinson's, and ALS. These diseases are marked by the gradual breakdown of brain cells, and studies suggest that synthetic fragrance compounds could be making things worse by triggering neuroinflammation and oxidative stress—think of it as your brain's version of a hangover that just won't quit (Chandran & Rochet, 2022; Khodkam, 2022; Fischbach et al., 2023).

It doesn't stop there. These chemical cocktails can also throw your gut microbiome into chaos, increasing your risk of obesity, diabetes, and other metabolic disorders (Liu et al., 2022). Plus, they're endocrine disruptors that could lead to infertility (Pastor-Nieto & Gatica-Ortega, 2021).

The scariest part? These chemicals don't just sit pretty on your skin—they get absorbed, inhaled, and spread all over your body, causing inflammation and stress that can mess with both your brain and metabolism. And since they're everywhere, from your perfume to your kitchen cleaner, you're constantly exposed (Chandran & Rochet, 2022; Khodkam, 2022; Pastor-Nieto & Gatica-Ortega, 2021).

In short, while artificial fragrances might make things smell nice, they're potential health hazards. With growing evidence against them, it's time to think about safer, natural alternatives. So, the next time you reach for that vanilla-scented cleaner or hang a new car freshener, you might want to think twice—for your brain, your gut, and your future.

**Actionable items—this is why I wrote this book! Not to scare you, but to protect you. Let's go!!**

### The Scented Symphony: Hello, Essential Oils

In a fascinating study, older adults retained or even improved cognitive abilities, such as verbal learning and memory, over a six-month period through olfactory enrichment. Yes, just by smelling things, they outperformed their scent-deprived counterparts, especially those with dementia (Vance et al., 2023). The secret is that olfactory stimulation bypasses the thalamus, the brain's sensory relay station, allowing scents to influence cognitive processing even during sleep. So, while you're dreaming, your brain might just be working overtime, processing those aromas and enhancing your slow-wave sleep (Oleszkiewicz et al., 2021). Speaking of scents, let's talk about rosemary—the undisputed queen of essential oils. This herb contains a compound called 1,8-cineole, which can zip across the blood-brain barrier faster than you can say "Hasta la vista, baby!" Once inside, it boosts acetylcholine production, a neurotransmitter that keeps your neurons firing like a well-oiled machine (Moss et al., 2012). Not only does this sharpen your mind, but it might also help your brain bulk up in all the right places through neurogenesis (the creation of new neurons).

Who knew a whiff of lavender could be your brain's personal therapist? It turns out essential oils like lavender aren't just for making your room smell nice—they work in your brain's limbic system and amygdala, releasing feel-good neurotransmitters like serotonin and endorphins, telling your brain to "chill out" (Abdalhai, 2024). This helps you relax and boosts your brain's cognitive function by kicking stress to the curb (Suzin, 2024). And let's not forget *Hedychium coronarium* (try saying that three times fast). This essential oil keeps acetylcholine, your brain's memory glue, from breaking down too quickly. Without it, you might forget where you left your keys—or what keys even are (Zhu, 2024; Parab, 2024). Ever heard of frankincense? In Ayurveda, it's not just for incense—it's like brain food. This gum resin has been hailed for its memory-boosting powers, and modern science is backing it up, showing it can actually help improve learning and memory (Zhang et al., 2020).

The best part? These oils are like VIPs—they cross the blood-brain barrier, the tight security team of your brain, whose purpose is to keep harmful substances away from the most precious thing you'll ever have—your brain. They help your brain release and create neurotransmitters. Linalool (from lavender) and α-terpineol (from *Hedychium coronarium*) don't just help you relax; they're also superheroes fighting off oxidative stress to keep your brain cells young and healthy (Hanphitakphong, 2024). So, next time you reach for that bottle of essential oil, remember—it's not just about smelling good; it's about giving your brain a little TLC. MRI scans have shown that olfactory enrichment leads to increased cortical thickness in areas like the right inferior frontal gyrus, the bilateral fusiform gyrus, and the entorhinal cortex. In simpler terms, your brain gets a workout just from sniffing stuff! Who knew the secret to a bigger brain was hiding in your spice cabinet? (Sollai & Crnjar, 2021). In one study, participants with olfactory deficiencies were given a rigorous sniffing regimen. The result? An increase in gray matter volume in the hippocampus and thalamus—va va vroooom, I say! (Yamamoto & Kobayakawa, 2022).

But wait, there's more! Another study had older adults sniff four different odorants twice a day for seven months. The outcome? Improved odor identification skills and a boost in cortical gray matter volume. Picture grandma suddenly nailing the difference between lavender and lilac while simultaneously giving her brain a power boost. Talk about a multitasking matriarch! (Inoue et al., 2022).

And let's not forget our friends in the sommelier world. These wine and cheese connoisseurs are exposed to novel odorants daily. A study revealed that sommelier students had increased olfactory bulb volume and thicker entorhinal cortices after 18 months of sniffing wine and cheese. Meanwhile, the control group, who might've been binge-watching reality TV, saw no significant brain changes (Filiz et al., 2022). So, if you want to impress at your next dinner party, remember: the more you sniff—the right things, of course—the smarter you get! (Goldman, 2022). So, ditch those artificial fragrances and invest in some high-quality organic essential oils. Use them as perfumes, air fresheners, and in your diffusers—basically, make it your mission to smell like you've just stepped out of a spa every single minute of every single day.

### Forest Bathing: Nature's Neurogenic Retreat

Now, let's take a detour into the woods. Have you ever heard of forest bathing? This practice, rooted in Japanese tradition, involves immersing oneself in nature and soaking in the sights, sounds, and smells of the forest. Research indicates that forest bathing can significantly reduce stress levels and enhance mental well-being, which in turn supports neurogenesis (Clarke et al., 2021). Imagine walking through a lush forest, inhaling the earthy scents of pine and damp soil while surrounded by vibrant greens. This sensory experience not only refreshes your spirit but also nourishes your brain.

# The Tooth That Knew Too Much

Once upon a time, in the land of Neurontown, Mr. Molar, the valiant tooth, lived comfortably in the warm, cozy cave of Old Man Jaw. But his days of quiet chomping would soon evolve into a heroic tale of health, brains, and bacteria. Little did Mr. Molar know, what happened in the mouth could stir chaos not only in the jaw but also in the brain. From bacterial invasions to surprising allies, Mr. Molar was about to learn just how connected the body truly was.

### The Chewing Conundrum: A Tooth's Role in Brain Health

As Mr. Molar grew older, his ability to chew diminished, and with it, so did Old Man Jaw's brain stimulation. You see, chewing wasn't just about enjoying crunchy apples or nuts. Studies had shown that chewing helped send vital sensory signals to the brain, keeping it sharp and active (Rohani, 2022). Without this constant stream of sensory information, the brain could experience cognitive decline, raising the risk of dementia. As Mr. Molar mulled this over, the real trouble began.

### The Microbiome Menace

One evening, as Mr. Molar rested, a shadow crept in. It was Captain Streptococcus and his army of harmful bacteria, building up plaque and infiltrating Mr. Molar's defenses. If unchecked, these invaders could leak into Old Man Jaw's bloodstream and sneak their way up to the brain, causing havoc. "We'll create inflammation and fog up Old Man Jaw's thinking," cackled Captain Streptococcus. This bacterial invasion could lead to Alzheimer's and other forms of neurodegeneration (Werber et al., 2021). Mr. Molar knew this wasn't just a battle for his survival but for the health of Old Man Jaw's brain. The bacteria also threatened to exacerbate autoimmune diseases like multiple sclerosis by spreading systemic inflammation (Rastogi & Rastogi, 2020).

### Root Canals and the Metallic Menace

But bacteria weren't Mr. Molar's only concern. He had also heard troubling stories about his cousin, Mr. Implant, who had replaced some of Old Man Jaw's missing teeth. Mr. Implant, made of metal, looked sturdy but carried his own risks. Infections around implants could lead to peri-implantitis, a disease that spreads systemic inflammation and could even affect the brain (Tessarin et al., 2024). "Beware!" Mrs. Gingiva had warned Mr. Molar. "These infections can cause serious trouble for Old Man Jaw's brain!"

The same was true for Mr. Molar's root canal—while it saved him from extraction, it left behind pockets where bacteria could lurk, waiting to cause trouble. These bacteria could release toxins that traveled to the brain, contributing to neurodegenerative diseases like dementia and MS (Dobrzański et al., 2020).

## The Allies: Tongue Scraping, Oil Pulling, and Natural Defenders

Just as Mr. Molar began to feel overwhelmed by the mounting threats, reinforcements arrived. First came the mighty Tongue Scraper, shining bright. "I'm here to remove harmful bacteria from the tongue!" he declared. By regularly scraping the tongue, Mr. Molar's army could reduce the number of harmful bacteria in the mouth and stop them from spreading (Aquilanti, 2022).

Right behind him was General Coconut Oil, ready for battle. "Let's try oil pulling," he suggested. By swishing oil around in the mouth, Old Man Jaw could remove bacteria and toxins, cleaning up the battleground and reducing inflammation (Tessarin et al., 2024).

Then came Fermented Foods—the Gut Health Warriors! These probiotic-packed foods like yogurt and sauerkraut weren't just good for the gut; they were essential for balancing the oral microbiome. A healthy gut leads to a healthier mouth, which means fewer harmful bacteria sneaking their way into the brain (Sureda et al., 2020).

## Sunlight, Supplements, and Superfoods

As the battle raged on, Mr. Molar realized that Old Man Jaw wasn't just about chewing and cleaning—his health was connected to the entire body. He called upon a few powerful allies to boost his defenses:

1. **Sunlight & Vitamin D3 + K2:** "We'll strengthen the bones, including teeth!" said the Sunbeam Knights. You see, teeth are bones, and like bones, they need nutrients like magnesium, Vitamin D3, and K2 to stay strong. These supplements helped Old Man Jaw absorb calcium, which fortified both his teeth and his brain against potential damage (Alam et al., 2022).

2. **Serotonin and Melatonin-Rich Foods:** Alongside his dental defenders came the Sleepytime Brigade. "Melatonin isn't just for sleep," whispered Captain Serotonin. Foods like bananas, nuts, and eggs boosted Old Man Jaw's melatonin levels, supporting his sleep and overall brain health. Melatonin also acted as a powerful antioxidant for oral health, reducing inflammation and protecting both the teeth and brain (Davies & Doshi, 2022).

3. **Flossing, but Like a Boss:** The Floss Force showed up next, determined to keep those pesky bacteria from forming biofilms between Mr. Molar and his friends. "We'll disarm the bacteria before they cause trouble," they said. With regular flossing, Old Man Jaw could prevent the buildup of plaque and reduce the risk of inflammation spreading beyond the mouth (Werber et al., 2021).

4. **Nose Breathing:** As Old Man Jaw breathed in through his nose, a sense of calm filled the land. He now knew that nose breathing prevents the mouth from drying out, maintaining a healthy flow of saliva, which is essential for neutralizing harmful bacteria and keeping teeth strong (Dioguardi et al., 2020).

**The Alcohol-Free Alliance:**

But not all "helpers" were truly helpful. Mr. Molar realized that alcohol-based mouthwashes, though fresh-smelling, were weakening his defenses. "They're stripping away the good bacteria, leaving us vulnerable to bad guys like Captain Streptococcus," Mr. Molar exclaimed. By switching to a gentler, alcohol-free mouthwash, Old Man Jaw could keep his mouth's natural microbiome in balance, allowing the good bacteria to thrive (Shapira, 2023).

**Gut Health = Teeth Health = Brain Health:**

Mr. Molar also knew that the health of Old Man Jaw's gut played a critical role in the overall battle. "It's all connected!" cried the Gut Health Warriors. "A healthy gut promotes a healthy mouth, which helps maintain a healthy brain." Fermented foods and a balanced diet helped keep the gut's microbiome in check, preventing harmful bacteria from causing chaos in the mouth and beyond (Sureda et al., 2020).

**Chew on This: Why Your Teeth Are the Gateway to Brain Gains:**

Let's skip the smoothie and take a real bite of solid food—how about some quinoa cauliflower pulao, anyone? Turns out, chewing isn't just for making sure you don't choke on that burrito—it's a workout for your brain too! Studies show that chomping down on your food can boost blood flow to important brain areas like the inferior frontal gyrus, which is linked to cognitive skills (Kariya, 2024). But if you've got a wonky bite, like a skeletal anterior open bite, you might be missing out on those brain-boosting benefits (Kariya, 2024).

Chewing doesn't just keep your jaw in shape; it might actually make you smarter. By upping the oxygen levels in your brain, chewing can give your cognitive performance a little extra kick and even spark new brain cells into action (Yamazaki, 2024). And let's not forget our older folks—keeping those chompers active is key to staving off cognitive decline and avoiding dementia (Asher, 2024).

Think of it this way: every time you chew, you're not just breaking down your food; you're also doing some serious brain maintenance. So, next time you're tempted to wolf down your lunch, take a moment to savor the bite—your brain will thank you for it!

**My darling, you are just an apartment complex for microbes:**

Your body is like a bustling metropolis for about 38 trillion microbes, including bacteria, viruses, and fungi (Chaiyasut, 2024). The gut is the most crowded spot, home to 30-40 trillion microorganisms that help with nutrient metabolism and immune function (Yagi, 2024; Olteanu, 2024). Your mouth is the second-largest microbial hub, hosting around 700 species (Olteanu, 2024). Even your nose is in on the action, contributing to your body's overall microbial diversity. These tiny residents aren't just hanging out—they're busy influencing your health in various ways, as you have learned already (Marcos, 2024; She, 2024). So, you're never really alone!

There is a delicate balance between good and bad bacteria that is needed to maintain brain health. Regular brushing, flossing, and tongue scraping manage these microbial populations, keeping harmful bacteria from causing cavities (Walkikar, 2024; Ganß et al., 2011). But here's the kicker: some oral bacteria help produce nitric oxide, which improves blood flow to your brain. That means good oral health isn't just about your teeth—it's about keeping your brain sharp too (Butera et al., 2022; Amaechi et al., 2019).

## 1. The Basics: Brush, Floss, and Scrape (No, Really!):

We all know we're supposed to brush our teeth, but let's not forget flossing and tongue scraping—two heroes in the battle against bad breath and gum disease. Brushing with fluoride or hydroxyapatite toothpaste helps remineralize your enamel and keep cavities at bay. Hydroxyapatite (HAp) toothpaste is like fluoride's cooler cousin—just as effective but without the risk of fluorosis, especially in kids (Harks et al., 2016; Mookhtiar, 2023). Flossing gets rid of the gunk between your teeth, reducing the risk of gingivitis and making sure your gums stay happy (Gjorgievska et al., 2013). And tongue scraping? It's not just for fresh breath—it helps keep your oral microbiome in balance, which is crucial for brain health (Hagenfeld et al., 2019).

Believe it or not, flossing could help keep your mind sharp. Research suggests that good oral hygiene reduces inflammation and harmful bacteria that could contribute to cognitive decline. So, every time you floss, you're not just protecting your teeth—you might be protecting your brain too (Srivastava, 2023).

## 2. Hydroxyapatite: Your Teeth's Best Friend:

Hydroxyapatite is the mineral your teeth are made of, so using HAp toothpaste is like giving your enamel a spa day. The nano-sized particles in HAp toothpaste get deep into your teeth, repairing damage and keeping everything strong (Kawade, 2012; Triwardhani et al., 2019). Plus, it's super biocompatible, meaning it's safe and effective, especially for those who want to avoid fluoride (Telatar & Bedir, 2021; Arnold et al., 2016).

### 3. Ayurveda Knows Best: Oil Pulling and Herbal Magic:

Ayurveda has been taking care of teeth for centuries. Oil pulling, known in Ayurveda as "Kavala Graha" or "Gandusha," with sesame or coconut oil, is a classic practice that reduces oral bacteria and improves gum health (Bossù et al., 2019; Butera et al, 2021). These natural practices not only enhance your oral health but also keep your microbiome in tip-top shape (Hsu et al., 2021). I make my oil with the following ingredients. You are welcome to experiment with it, watch for allergies, and consult with your doctor! You can make a minimalist oil pulling just with extra virgin organic coconut oil, or with ingredients like organic virgin coconut oil, clove essential oil: 3 drops, peppermint essential oil: 3 drops, licorice extract: 2 drops, cinnamon essential oil: 3 drops, and neem oil: 4 drops. That is basically the ancient version of mouthwash, but with a twist—or rather, a swish! Let's dive into a recipe that'll make your mouth feel pampered, the Ayurvedic way.

### A more exotic preparation will be:

Coconut Oil: 2 tablespoons (the good stuff—virgin organic coconut oil, because your mouth deserves nothing less) (Bhansali, 2023), Turmeric Powder: 1/2 teaspoon (turns your mouth into a mini anti-inflammatory fortress) (Woolley et al., 2020), Neem Oil or Neem Leaves: 1/2 teaspoon of neem oil or a few crushed neem leaves (to scare away bacteria like a Neem Ninja) (Bhalerao et al., 2021), Peppermint Essential Oil: 2-3 drops (because swishing oil doesn't have to taste like a punishment) (Menaka et al., 2020), Clove Essential Oil: 3 drops, Licorice Extract: 1 teaspoon, Haritaki Powder: 1 teaspoon (balancing for Vata dosha), Amalaki Powder: 1 teaspoon (balancing for Pitta dosha), Bibhitaki Powder: 1 teaspoon (balancing for Kapha dosha), Cardamom Extract (Organic): 3 drops, Turmeric Oil: 3 drops, Nutmeg Essential Oil: 3 drops, Cinnamon Essential Oil: 3 drops, Sandalwood Essential Oil: 2 drops.

Grab 2 tablespoons of virgin coconut oil—because who wants a coconut oil imposter? Place it in a small bowl. If using neem leaves, give them a little crush to unleash their magic oils. If neem oil is your choice, just measure out 1/2 teaspoon. Stir in the turmeric powder and neem oil (or those brave crushed neem leaves), along with the other ingredients. Watch the coconut oil transform into a golden elixir of oral health (Woolley et al., 2020). Add 2-3 drops of peppermint essential oil for a hint of minty freshness that'll make your swishing session less like a chore and more like a treat (Menaka et al., 2020).

Take a tablespoon of this magical mix, pop it in your mouth, and start swishing. Do this for 15-20 minutes—yes, that long! Imagine your mouth is the dance floor, and the oil is doing the cha-cha between your teeth and gums, pulling out toxins and bacteria with every move (Ahmed et al., 2020). Remember, spit—don't swallow! You don't want to re-ingest those bad guys.

Spit the used oil into a trash can (your plumbing will thank you), and rinse your mouth with warm water to wash away any leftover oiliness (Griessl et al., 2020). Finish with your usual brushing routine to leave your teeth feeling squeaky clean (Javed et al., 2022). For best results, oil pull daily, preferably first thing in the morning on an empty stomach. It's the mouth equivalent of a morning workout— only less sweaty (Jong, 2023). This recipe combines the detox power of coconut oil with the bacteria-busting abilities of neem and turmeric. Studies show that oil pulling can seriously cut down on plaque and gingivitis, making it a perfect sidekick to your regular dental routine (Abbasi et al., 2020; Karthik & P, 2022). Plus, that peppermint kick leaves your breath fresher than a mountain breeze (Kamble et al., 2023).

### Meet Neti—Ayurveda to the Rescue: Thank You, India
Now you know—your nose does more than just smell the flowers (or avoid your coworker's fishy choice of lunch). It's a crucial player in keeping your brain and body in tip-top shape, and it turns out that a little nasal irrigation might be just what the doctor (or yogi) ordered.

### The Magic of Nasal Irrigation:
Nasal irrigation works by giving your nasal passages a much-needed rinse, clearing out mucus, allergens, and even those pesky pathogens that have been camping out up there. Think of it as spring cleaning for your nose! This process not only helps you breathe easier but also boosts mucociliary clearance—the natural defense mechanism your nasal mucosa uses to kick out unwanted guests ("undefined", 2024). And guess what? Studies show that hypertonic saline solutions (that's just salty water that's a bit saltier than your tears) can significantly improve symptoms in people with chronic rhinosinusitis by reducing inflammation and getting those nasal cilia moving again (Lao, 2024).

But wait, there's more! Turns out, regular nasal irrigation doesn't just keep your sinuses happy—it also helps maintain a healthy nasal microbiome, the community of microorganisms living in your nose. A well-balanced nasal microbiota can prevent the bad guys (a.k.a. pathogenic organisms) from setting up shop, reducing the risk of infections and inflammation (Cannon, 2024). In fact, kids who regularly washed their noses with saline showed quicker recovery from upper respiratory infections. Talk about a win-win (Slapak, 2024)!

**Enter: Neti—the Yogi's Secret Weapon:**
Now, let's add a bit of ancient wisdom to the mix. Meet Neti, the yoga form of nasal irrigation that's been around for centuries, and for good reason. Picture this: You fill a cute little pot (the Neti pot) with warm, salty water, tilt your head like you're striking a yoga pose over the sink, and pour the water through one nostril and out the other. Voilà! You've just given your nasal passages a gentle yet thorough cleanse.

Neti is like the yogi's version of nasal irrigation—soothing, effective, and surprisingly refreshing. Plus, it's known to reduce symptoms of sinusitis, allergies, and other upper respiratory issues, making it a perfect complement to modern saline irrigation practices (Lao, 2024; Gandhi, 2024).

**What About the Microbiota?** Let's not forget about the tiny tenants in your nose—the nasal microbiota. Regular irrigation, whether it's with a Neti pot or saline spray, helps wash away harmful bacteria while promoting the growth of beneficial ones. Since the nose and mouth are connected, improving nasal health can also positively impact your oral microbiome, potentially keeping conditions like bad breath and dental issues at bay.

**The Evidence Speaks** The science backs it up: nasal irrigation works wonders. Clinical studies show that hypertonic saline nasal irrigation can improve nasal symptoms and mucosal health, especially in people with chronic rhinosinusitis (Lao, 2024). There's even evidence that xylitol nasal irrigation (yes, the same stuff in your sugar-free gum) can enhance sinus health and improve your sense of smell after surgery (Jiang, 2024). With UV light treatments and other advanced methods showing promise in pesticide removal from food, it seems the power of a good rinse isn't just for your veggies—it's for your nose too (Lakshmipathy, 2024).

So next time you're feeling stuffed up, stressed out, or just in need of a little nasal TLC, grab that Neti pot, mix up some saline, and give your nose the love it deserves. Your sinuses, brain, and maybe even your taste buds will thank you. Make sure you use filtered and boiled water to get rid of those pesky pesticides and dangerous bacteria. Let it cool, and then give your nose a nice treat!

And how about inhaling that lovely, fragrant, steaming goodness from the plant world? A healthy nasal microbiome wards off invaders, preventing inflammation that could mess with your brain (Kim et al., 2019; Wu et al., 2019). Take steam with a few essential oils, as mentioned earlier. In addition, healthcare workers dealing with high stress found that inhaling *Origanum majorana* essential oil helped them relax, which might also boost their immune function and keep those pesky microbes in balance (Fung et al., 2021).

But wait, there's more! Essential oils like lavender and peppermint have shown some serious antimicrobial powers, potentially helping manage the bad bugs that could contribute to neurodegenerative diseases (Sanchez-Quintero et al., 2022).

**Water You Thinking? The Filtration Fix for Pesticide-Packed Drinks**
Imagine sipping a glass of water, thinking it's harmless, but instead, you're unknowingly ingesting pesticides that could quietly wreak havoc on your brain. The connection between pesticide exposure and neurodegenerative diseases like Alzheimer's and Parkinson's is becoming a serious concern, making us rethink what we're consuming.

That's where whole-home water filtration systems come in—think of them as your water's personal bodyguard. These systems, using advanced methods like activated carbon and reverse osmosis, can significantly reduce pesticide levels in your water, turning it from potentially toxic to refreshingly clean (Akinwunmi, 2024; Abdullah, 2024). This is especially important if you live near farms where pesticide runoff can contaminate local water supplies.

And it's not just about water; pesticides are in your food too. Even organic produce can contain pesticide residues, albeit in smaller amounts (Kazimierczak et al., 2022; Bursić et al., 2021). Properly washing your fruits and vegetables or using agents like acetic acid or baking soda can further reduce these residues (Jawale, 2023).

It turns out that the bioactive compounds in whole foods, herbs, and spices are like your body's detox squad, working hard to clear out harmful pesticide residues and potentially lowering the risk of neurodegenerative diseases like Parkinson's and Alzheimer's (Sajad, 2024). Incorporating foods like broccoli, kale, cilantro, and parsley into your diet can help your body combat pesticide exposure (Shah, 2021).

Top of the list for your salad bowl? Antioxidant-rich fruits and veggies like berries, citrus, and leafy greens. These colorful superheroes fight off the oxidative stress that pesticides love to cause (Riederer et al., 2010). And don't forget the cruciferous crew—broccoli, kale, and their friends—packed with glucosinolates that boost your liver's detox powers (Sajad, 2024).

Herbs and spices are in on the action too. Turmeric, with its curcumin, acts like a brain bodyguard, offering anti-inflammatory protection (Sajad, 2024). Garlic enhances detox enzymes, while rosemary and green tea are loaded with polyphenols to keep oxidative damage in check (Sajad, 2024).

Even going organic helps, as organic produce generally has lower pesticide residues (Winter, 2015). But the best approach? A diet rich in a variety of whole foods, combined with proper washing techniques and an effective water filtration system, can help keep those pesky pesticides at bay.

# The Auditory Cortex's Role in Memory Lane-

## Tune In

Can you hear me now? Ever wonder why that catchy tune gets stuck in your head or how you can remember your first crush's voice? You can thank your auditory cortex, the brain's DJ, for playing those memories on repeat. This part of your brain isn't just about vibing to your favorite jams—it's a full-on memory machine. Studies show that the auditory cortex doesn't just passively listen; it actively helps you encode and retrieve auditory memories, like knowing when to expect that epic drum solo (Jaramillo & Zador, 2010). Plus, it's got a built-in radar for detecting when something sounds off, helping you lock in memories with precision (Zweerings et al., 2019).

And if you're a musician, guess what? Your auditory cortex is swole! It bulks up through neuroplasticity, making your brain more resilient and better at storing those sweet melodies (Pantev et al., 2015). So, the next time you play that guitar riff, remember, you're not just rocking out—you're giving your brain a workout.

### When the Auditory Cortex Hits a Sour Note: Dementia's Sneak Attack

Now, here's where the plot thickens. When the auditory cortex isn't hitting those high notes, it can lead to serious cognitive issues, like dementia. Hearing loss is more than just an inconvenience; it's a gateway to cognitive decline. If your auditory cortex starts to fade, your social life might too, leading to isolation and, you guessed it, even more brain drain (Deal et al., 2016). It's like trying to play a symphony with half the orchestra missing—everything starts to fall apart (Kostic, 2023).

### Keeping Your Auditory Cortex in Tune: Tips for a Brain-Boosting Symphony

So, how do you keep your brain's DJ spinning those hits? Easy—keep your ears engaged! Whether it's jamming out to music or practicing a new instrument, keeping your auditory system active can help boost memory and neuroplasticity (Pantev et al., 2015). And if your hearing isn't what it used to be, hearing aids can be a game-changer, helping you stay sharp and stave off cognitive decline (Sanders et al., 2021).

Cognitive training with an auditory twist is another great way to keep your brain's DJ booth in top shape. These exercises don't just make you a better listener—they keep your memory and executive functions fine-tuned and ready to roll (Sanders et al., 2021).

**Auditory Health: The VIP Pass to Brain Longevity**

Remember, your auditory system isn't working solo—it's part of a bigger band. When your auditory cortex teams up with other brain regions, like the frontal cortex, it helps you stay focused and in control (Curtis et al., 2022). But if the connections start to fray, it can throw off your rhythm, making memory and learning a lot harder (Sanders et al., 2021). Keeping your auditory system in tune isn't just about hearing; it's about keeping your whole brain in harmony.

**Final Encore**

In the grand concert of life, your auditory cortex plays a starring role in memory and cognition. Protecting this part of your brain from dysfunction is key to avoiding cognitive decline and keeping dementia at bay. So, turn up the volume on those auditory activities and make sure your brain's DJ stays in top form. After all, a well-tuned auditory cortex means a symphony of memories and a life filled with music.

**Actionable Item—Because I Promised!**
**The Sound of Neurogenesis: Wavelengths That Matter**

Certain sound frequencies, like alpha waves (8-12 Hz), can give your hippocampus a boost, encouraging your brain to grow new neurons (Harris & Tannan, 2021). Whether it's the gentle hum of a tuning fork or the beat of binaural rhythms, these waves aren't just background noise—they're helping your brain regenerate. Want focus? Try 40 Hz binaural beats. Your brain mixes two different tones into a 40 Hz rhythm, boosting memory and cognitive function (Vangilder, 2023). Gamma waves at 40 Hz are linked to neurogenesis and can even clear out unwanted beta-amyloid deposits (Wu et al., 2022). Meanwhile, theta waves (4-8 Hz) create a chill environment for neuron growth, like giving your brain a spa day (Bavafa et al., 2023).

# The Visual of Memory, Maps, and Snapshots

The visual system is like your brain's movie projector, starting with the retina's tiny paparazzi snapping pics and sending them via the optic nerve expressway to the primary visual cortex (V1) for basic processing—think of it as outlining a coloring book. From there, visuals split into two paths: the "what" pathway for recognizing objects (like making sure you don't mistake your cat for a loaf of bread) and the "where" pathway for spatial awareness, so you don't trip over that same cat.

But the visual cortex isn't working alone; it loves to team up with other brain regions, mixing in sounds and smells to make your experiences more vivid. Visual processing itself is like building a LEGO set, combining sensory details from the bottom up, while top-down processing uses memory and attention to fill in the gaps—kind of like glancing at the LEGO box for guidance. And just to keep things interesting, your visual system is a social butterfly, interacting with other senses—like when your ears convince your eyes they saw an extra flash of light. This cross-sensory chatter is why smells can sometimes mess with what you see.

Understanding how all this works gives us the cheat codes to diagnosing and treating visual disorders, which can mess with both vision and cognitive functions, like in glaucoma or 22q11.2 deletion syndrome. So, next time you spot a cat—or maybe a loaf of bread—thank your hardworking visual cortex for keeping everything in check!

**And God Said, 'Let There Be Light...'**
We cannot talk about vision without talking about light, so shall we shed some light on the sun? (Bad joke, good intention 😊 ). Sunlight isn't just for keeping your plants happy—it's a critical environmental factor that influences brain health through a variety of biological, physiological, and molecular mechanisms. The different wavelengths of sunlight—like blue, ultraviolet (UV), and infrared (IR) light—take turns throughout the day, each with its own special role in keeping your brain and body in sync.

Sunlight isn't just for getting that perfect tan or making vitamin D do its thing—it's also a bit of a biological magic show, unleashing a whole lineup of compounds mentioned below that make your brain and body feel like they're starring in their own wellness retreat.

First up, we've got Nitric Oxide (NO), which sounds like something from a chemistry lab, but it's actually a superhero for your blood vessels. When UV rays hit your skin, they help release Nitric Oxide, which then works to lower your blood pressure and improve blood flow, including to your brain. It's like giving your brain a mini spa day, reducing stress and keeping it sharp (Liu et al., 2014).

Next, there are Beta-Endorphins—the body's own little happy pills. UVB exposure triggers these molecules, leaving you feeling like you've just had a fantastic workout without the sweat. These endorphins boost your mood and help you relax, making sunlight a natural antidepressant that's way cheaper than therapy (Arndt et al., 2015).

Melatonin also gets a shout-out, but this one's a bit of a night owl. While melatonin is famous for helping you sleep, it actually needs sunlight during the day to get its act together. Morning sunlight sets your body's internal clock, ensuring that when nighttime rolls around, you're ready to snooze like a baby (Wright et al., 2013).

And then there's Serotonin—sunlight's way of giving your brain a happiness boost. When you catch some rays, especially the visible kind, your brain ramps up serotonin production, which not only makes you feel good but also helps you sleep better at night. It's like a two-for-one deal on mood and sleep (Lambert et al., 2002).

Last but not least, we've got Infrared Radiation (IR). While it sounds like something out of a sci-fi movie, it's actually pretty cool. Infrared radiation, especially the near-infrared kind, goes deep into your tissues and tells your cells to chill out, reducing inflammation and even protecting your brain. Think of it as a secret weapon against aging and stress, all thanks to the sun (Chung et al., 2012).

Let's break down how these rays of light pull off their daily tricks, helping you stay sharp, healthy, and in sync with the world around you.

**(10:00 PM to 5:00 AM) Night:** Darkness reigns. Your body is flooded with melatonin, making you feel like staying in bed is the only reasonable choice. With no light to wake them up, your serotonin levels are as low as your motivation to get up.

**(5:00 AM - 3:00 PM) Pre-Sunrise: The Role of Blue Light** Imagine Alfred Pennyworth, not just as Batman's loyal butler, but as the very essence of blue light itself. Each morning, Alfred doesn't just serve breakfast—he orchestrates the intricate ballet of your body's circadian rhythm, metabolic regulation, and overall well-being.

As you stir from sleep and open your eyes, you see Alfred standing there, radiating blue light elegance. Your retina, carrying intrinsically photosensitive retinal ganglion cells, immediately gets to work. Alfred, ever the meticulous butler, engages these cells, which act as his loyal team of messengers. These intrinsically photosensitive retinal ganglion cells, which express the photopigment melanopsin, are crucial for non-image-forming visual functions, particularly in circadian rhythm regulation and the pupillary light reflex (Sexton et al., 2012).

With a smooth, gentlemanly gesture, Alfred signals these cells to wake up and alert the master clock of your brain—the suprachiasmatic nucleus, nestled in the hypothalamus (Bryk et al., 2022). As Alfred floods your system with blue light, melanopsin gets to work, suppressing melatonin production with remarkable efficiency. Research indicates that exposure to blue light can lead to significant melatonin suppression, with studies reporting up to a 60% reduction in melatonin levels after just two hours of exposure to blue light (Jo et al., 2021; Nishino, 2023). This suppression helps your body transition from the restful state of night to the alert state of day. It's as if Alfred is drawing back the heavy curtains in Wayne Manor, letting in the full brilliance of morning light, signaling that it's time to start the day.

With the clock now ticking, Alfred proceeds to the locus coeruleus, a quiet study in your brain where norepinephrine is stored. He gives a gentle tap, and this neurotransmitter flows out like a perfectly brewed cup of morning tea. "Just the thing to sharpen your senses," Alfred murmurs, ensuring you're fully alert and prepared to tackle whatever Gotham—or your day—throws your way (Ye, 2024).

Alfred is now in full butler mode, directing a grand hormonal symphony. He gestures to the hypothalamus (which regulates homeostasis by controlling temperature, hunger, thirst, and hormone release), which cues the pituitary gland (responsible for controlling growth, metabolism, and reproduction through hormone secretion), much like he would cue the orchestra at a Wayne Foundation gala. The adrenal glands (situated on top of each kidney, regulating stress, metabolism, blood pressure, and the "fight or flight" response) respond with a powerful chord of cortisol, while the growth hormone provides a subtle but vital undertone, ensuring your body's energy levels are perfectly balanced. Meanwhile, the proopiomelanocortin neurons continue their work, integrating various metabolic signals to regulate your appetite and stress responses (Stefanidis et al., 2018). With a knowing smile, Alfred orchestrates this harmony as effortlessly as he handles Bruce Wayne's complex schedule (Porcu et al., 2022; Irie, 2021).

Now, Alfred strolls through the halls of your mind, adjusting neurotransmitters (chemicals that transmit signals between neurons, affecting the body's functions) with the deftness of a butler organizing a high-society banquet. He sprinkles a bit more dopamine here for motivation and adds a touch of serotonin there for a well-balanced mood. When it comes to GABA (the sleepy neurotransmitter that keeps your brain calm in small doses during the day and puts you to bed in higher doses at night), Alfred knows exactly what to do. "A dash of calmness," he whispers, carefully regulating GABA to keep you relaxed and composed. But he doesn't stop there; Alfred also increases glutamate, the neurotransmitter that helps you learn and remember. "A sharp mind is a prepared mind," Alfred muses, ensuring your brain is ready for both relaxation and learning, much like how he prepares Batman for every possible scenario (Scott et al., 2020; Tan, 2024).

Ever meticulous, Alfred turns his attention to your mitochondria, the powerhouses of your cells. With just the right touch of blue light, he enhances ATP production, ensuring your cells are brimming with energy. "We must keep everything running smoothly," Alfred hums, much like he keeps the Batcave in tip-top shape, ensuring you're ready to face whatever challenges come your way (Sato et al., 2020; Norekian & Moroz, 2023).

As the morning progresses, Alfred continues his duty, ensuring every gear in your circadian clock is perfectly synchronized. The suprachiasmatic nucleus, the hypothalamus, and all those circadian genes now work together seamlessly, like the inner workings of the Bat computer. Alfred knows that with everything in perfect alignment, you'll be at your best throughout the day, ready for any adventure that lies ahead (Li, 2024).

Alfred ensures that the blue light intensity reaches its peak around mid-morning, typically between 9:00 and 10:00 AM. During this time, the blue light's influence on your circadian rhythm is at its strongest, helping to solidify your wakefulness and set the timing for the rest of your day. Alfred is at his most effective during this period, making sure that all your internal systems are aligned and functioning optimally.

The timing of this blue light exposure is crucial. Alfred knows that exposure to blue light in the early morning enhances overall well-being and promotes optimal health outcomes. Research indicates that this morning light positively affects circadian rhythms, which in turn influence sleep quality, mood, and metabolic processes (Lee, 2024). Conversely, missing out on this morning light can disrupt these rhythms, potentially leading to sleep disorders and mood disturbances (Lee, 2024).

But Alfred doesn't stop there. He also taps into the hypothalamus's arcuate nucleus, where proopiomelanocortin neurons reside. These neurons, like another team of Alfred's agents, are primarily involved in regulating energy homeostasis and various neuroendocrine functions. As Alfred activates these proopiomelanocortin neurons, they start producing neuropeptides like α-melanocyte-stimulating hormone and corticotropin, which help regulate appetite, sex hormones, and energy expenditure (Stefanidis et al., 2018). In contrast to the intrinsically photosensitive retinal ganglion cells' role in light detection and circadian entrainment, these proopiomelanocortin neurons respond to metabolic signals like leptin and insulin, modulating feeding behavior and energy balance (Stefanidis et al., 2018).

### (5:00 AM - 3:00 PM) - Peak Sunrise - The Luminous Gathering 😊

It's a bright, sunny afternoon at Wayne Manor. The mansion is bathed in daylight, and Bruce Wayne is in the study, reviewing plans for Gotham's future. As the clock strikes noon, the doors swing open, and three radiant guests join him: UV-A, UV-B, and Infrared Light.

Alfred, ever the diligent butler, steps forward to introduce the new arrivals.

**Alfred:** "Master Wayne, these visitors have arrived to join you during the peak daylight hours. Each brings a unique gift, but with their own set of risks."

UV-B Light strides in first, glowing with the intensity of the midday sun.

**UV-B Light:** "Hey, Bruce! I'm here to help your body produce Vitamin D—crucial for your bones, brain, mood, and so much more, especially in Gotham's gloomy weather." (Holick, 2020)

He hands over a small vial labeled "Vitamin D" but adds a word of caution.

**UV-B Light:** "But remember, too much of me, and you could end up with sunburn or worse." (Jin & Zhang, 2015) ...cancer, though you know I help protect you from some cancers too, yes.

**Bruce Wayne:** "Thanks, UV-B. I'll be sure to enjoy your benefits in moderation. I've got my hat, sunscreen—yes, mineral-based—and I just had a sauce made from tomato paste full of lycopene that should help...and before you say something, your friend Vitamin K2 left me some MK-7 gifts too. I'll remember to take them together."

Next, UV-A Light enters with a casual, sun-kissed confidence.

**UV-A Light:** "Bruce, I'm the one who gives you that nice tan and a bit of a youthful glow. But don't forget, too much of me can lead to wrinkles and skin damage." (Jin & Zhang, 2015)

He offers a pair of UV-protective certified sunglasses to avoid overexposure.

**Bruce Wayne:** "Noted, UV-A. I'll make sure to balance the tan with protection."

Finally, Infrared Light arrives, calm and composed, exuding warmth.

**Infrared Light:** "I'm here to boost your cellular energy and repair—perfect for those intense daytime workouts or just keeping your cells in top shape." (Nelidova et al., 2020; Wiraja et al., 2016)

He places a small, glowing device on the table.

**Infrared Light:** "Just be mindful—too much heat can stress your cells." (Huang et al., 2022)

**Bruce Wayne:** "Thanks, IR. I'll make sure to use your gifts wisely."

As the trio settles in, Alfred stands by, watching with approval.

**Alfred:** "It seems, Master Wayne, that in the brightest of days, you're well-equipped with these allies by your side."

Bruce nods, acknowledging the importance of balance.

**Bruce Wayne:** "Indeed, Alfred. With these three during the day, I'm ready for whatever comes, day or night."

(4:00 PM till sunset) - Sunsets & Calm - Red Light Relaxation

As the day progresses, the sun begins to lower in the sky. By around 4 PM, the trio starts to fade, their glowing presence dimming with the daylight.

**UV-B Light:** "Our time is up, Bruce. We'll see you tomorrow. Remember to balance the benefits with care."

With that, UV-A, UV-B, Infrared Light, and Blue Light Butler Alfred gradually take their leave, leaving Wayne Manor quieter as the day transitions toward evening.

Just as the last rays of the afternoon sun fade, Red Light arrives, radiating warmth and calm.

**Red Light:** "Bruce, it's time to wind down. I'm here to help you relax, boost your mitochondrial health, and set you up for a great night's sleep." (Wiraja et al., 2016)
Red Light leads Bruce outside for a relaxing walk around the manor grounds. The gentle red hues of the setting sun wash over them, soothing Bruce's mind and body.

**Red Light:** "But that's not all, Bruce. I'm also here to enhance your brain health, improve metabolic function, and increase insulin sensitivity. My wavelengths penetrate deep into your cells, optimizing mitochondrial function, which is crucial for your energy levels and overall well-being." (Wiraja et al., 2016)

As they walk, Bruce feels the stress of the day melting away. His muscles relax, his mind clears, and he knows that tonight, he'll sleep soundly, thanks to Red Light's calming influence.

**Red Light**: "This evening light also stimulates melatonin production, preparing your body for deep, restful sleep. Plus, my effects on insulin sensitivity help keep your metabolism in check, which is essential for maintaining your health." (2024 research)

**Bruce Wayne**: "Thanks, Red Light. This is just what I needed."

As the sun sets, Red Light continues to work its magic, leaving Bruce feeling rejuvenated. His brain is sharp, his metabolism is humming, and his cells are energized—all set for a peaceful night's rest. With Red Light by his side, Bruce knows that even Batman needs to recharge and maintain his health to keep Gotham safe.

### Summary: The Role of Blue Light in Health and Wellness

**Circadian Rhythm and Sleep**: Blue light is essential for regulating circadian rhythms, which dictate our sleep-wake cycles. Exposure to blue light, especially in the morning, helps synchronize these rhythms by suppressing melatonin production, keeping us alert during the day. However, too much blue light exposure in the evening, from devices like phones, LED lights, laptops, and TVs, can delay sleep onset (Cajochen et al., 2020).

**Brain Health and Neurogenesis**: Blue light also supports brain health by boosting neurogenesis—the formation of new neurons. This process is linked to improved cognitive function and memory, partly due to the increase in brain-derived neurotrophic factor (BDNF) (Martínez-Gutiérrez et al., 2021). This makes blue light essential for brain adaptability and learning.

**Mental Health**: Blue light positively impacts mental health by regulating mood-related neurotransmitters like serotonin. It's particularly effective in combating seasonal affective disorder (SAD) and other forms of depression, acting as a natural mood booster (Cajochen et al., 2020).

**Mitochondrial Health**: Mitochondria benefit from blue light exposure, which enhances ATP production—vital for energy and metabolic health. This increased energy supports everything from brain activity to overall cellular function (Hamblin, 2021).

**Alertness and Cognitive Performance**: Known as the "daylight dynamo," blue light improves alertness, attention, and cognitive performance, particularly when exposure occurs in the morning (Gooley et al., 2020). This makes it a crucial component of daytime productivity.

**Skin Health**: Blue light has a dual role in skin health. It's effective in treating acne by killing bacteria, but excessive exposure, especially from screens, can lead to oxidative stress and premature aging (Akhavan et al., 2021). Balancing exposure is key to harnessing its benefits while avoiding harm.

When it comes to nature, timing is everything—and that applies to blue light exposure as well.

### Goodbye Sleep, Hello Insulin Resistance: The Dark Side of LED Light

Welcome to the age of LED lights, where the bright, energy-efficient glow of modern living is secretly moonlighting as a sleep thief. Unlike the good old incandescent bulbs that gave us a full-spectrum light show, LEDs are like the party crashers that show up uninvited after 3 PM and refuse to leave. These lights are experts at disrupting your body's natural rhythm, and if you've been tossing and turning at night, you might just have your evening lighting to thank.
Bathing in blue light from LEDs after 3 PM is like telling your brain, "Hey, it's daytime! Let's keep the party going!" This confusion leads to suppressed melatonin production—your sleep hormone—leaving you wide awake when you should be dreaming of beaches and unicorns (Cajochen et al., 2020).

And it doesn't stop there. This circadian sabotage extends to your metabolism too, with blue light exposure potentially driving your insulin resistance through the roof, setting the stage for metabolic mayhem (Gooley et al., 2020). Add in a dash of cortisol—your stress hormone—and you've got the perfect recipe for hormonal havoc (Rommerswinkel, 2021).

**Actionable Items**: It turns out that letting some good old-fashioned sunlight into your life, especially in the afternoon, is like giving your circadian rhythm a friendly nudge. It's nature's way of getting your brain back on track after being thrown off by all that artificial lighting. Scientists (Geerdink et al., 2016; Santhi et al., 2011) are basically saying, "Get outside, or else."

But let's be real—the thought of cutting down screen time makes most of us break out in a cold sweat. No worries, though, because blue light-blocking glasses are here to save the day—or rather, the night. Put these on in the evening, and your brain thinks you've traveled back to the pre-digital age. Your melatonin production kicks back in like a trusty old furnace (Esaki et al., 2016; Guarana et al., 2021). You might even start falling asleep faster than your phone can update its software.

For those who want to go full-on sleep ninja, swapping out those harsh, bright LEDs for red light is where it's at. Red light is basically the ninja of the light spectrum—sneaking around without disrupting your melatonin production (Figueiro & Rea, 2010; Chellappa et al., 2013). It's like setting your home to "chill mode," perfect for winding down after a day of battling blue light.

In conclusion, if you want to sleep better, think of yourself as a plant—soak up the sun, avoid the harsh lights, and maybe wear some cool shades (blue light-blocking, of course). Do this, and you'll be snoozing like a baby in no time, while your circadian rhythm thanks you for getting your act together (Cajochen et al., 2020; Gooley et al., 2020; Rommerswinkel, 2021).

### UVA & UVB: Neither Too Much, Nor Too Little

UV-A rays are the deep-penetrating reasons behind that bronzed glow and those inevitable wrinkles, while UV-B rays are your body's vitamin D factory—though they can also leave you looking like a lobster if you're not careful (Addison et al., 2021; Alves & Agustí, 2022).

UV-B radiation kickstarts the production of vitamin D3 by converting 7-dehydrocholesterol in your skin, which is essentially your bones' best friend (Chen et al., 2021; Lin et al., 2021). But as we age, our skin slacks off on this job, leaving us needing more sun or supplements to keep those bones strong (Yang, 2024). It's like your skin's vitamin D workforce is going on a permanent coffee break.

On the flip side, UV-B also stirs up drama inside your cells. It activates the MAPK and PI3K/Akt pathways—sounding like secret spy agencies but really just cellular teams dealing with stress and damage (Mavrogonatou et al., 2022; Jung et al., 2022). Sometimes, they save the day by repairing DNA and boosting antioxidants; other times, they hit the panic button and trigger inflammation or worse (Wen, 2024; Qu et al., 2023). It's a delicate balance—too much UV-B, and your skin might revolt with conditions like psoriasis (Xu et al., 2021; Li et al., 2022).

There's also the whole epigenetic saga, where UV-B acts like a rogue editor, changing your DNA's punctuation and tweaking gene expressions, potentially setting the stage for skin damage or even cancer (Li et al., 2022; Guo et al., 2023). It's like UV-B is playing a risky game of genetic Jenga, where one wrong move could send your cells toppling.

The plot thickens with UV-B's assault on your mitochondria—the tiny powerhouses of your cells. UV-B can mess with their membrane potential and calcium levels, cranking up oxidative stress and pushing cells toward an early grave (Chen et al., 2020; Ke & Wang, 2021). Keeping those mitochondria happy is crucial if you want to avoid the sun's darker side (Boucher et al., 2021; Lin et al., 2021).

**Good Side of UV-B:**

**UV-B and Brain Health**: UV-B exposure has been found to stimulate neurogenesis—the process by which new neurons are formed in the brain. This leads to enhanced memory formation and consolidation, providing a natural boost to cognitive function. UV-B also plays a role in modulating mental health, with evidence suggesting it can elevate mood by increasing serotonin levels, thereby improving overall well-being (Wacker & Holick, 2013).

**Metabolic Mischief**: In the metabolic realm, UV-B has been caught meddling with insulin sensitivity and fat metabolism. UV-B exposure improves glucose handling and promotes fat loss, making metabolism more efficient. This has a ripple effect on the body's overall energy balance, as highlighted in studies linking UV-B to better metabolic outcomes (Bikle, 2020).

**DNA and the Double-Helix Dance**: UV-B's interaction with DNA is a double-edged sword. On one hand, it prompts DNA repair mechanisms, enhancing cellular resilience. On the other, it introduces mutations, adding complexity to its role in aging and disease (Pfeifer & Besaratinia, 2012).

**Sleep and Circadian Rhythm**: UV-B also plays a role in regulating sleep and circadian rhythms. By influencing the production of melatonin, UV-B helps align sleep cycles with natural daylight patterns, although too much exposure could disrupt this delicate balance (Figueiro et al., 2018).

**Aging and Neurogenesis**: Finally, UV-B isn't just for the young. In older adults, it spurs neurogenesis, suggesting a potential role in cognitive longevity. This unexpected benefit adds a new dimension to our understanding of aging and brain health (Rosenberg et al., 2020).

**Cancer Risk Reduction**: Studies show that having enough vitamin D can help lower the risk of certain cancers, like colon, breast, and prostate cancer, by regulating cell growth and ensuring no cell gets too out of line (Williams et al., 2023).

# Oh, The Sun Problemo

UV-B: the sun's not-so-friendly reminder that while it might give us a golden tan, it's also sneaking in some serious harm, particularly to your skin, eyes, and, believe it or not, even your brain. Yes, your brain!

UV-B exposure has been linked to increased oxidative stress, which is like sending your brain cells through a stress test they didn't sign up for. This kind of damage can mess with cognitive functions and even increase the risk of neurodegenerative diseases (Zhang et al., 2021; Xu et al., 2022). As if we didn't have enough to worry about!

Imagine being over 60 and thinking, "A little sun won't hurt," only to find out that too much UV-B exposure can actually give your brain a sunburn! A UK study found that older adults who basked in the sun for more than two hours without protection ended up with more than just a nice tan—they also faced an increased risk of cognitive dysfunction (Thompson et al., 2020). It's like your brain waving a white flag, saying, "That's enough sun for today!" So, if you're over 60, take this as a friendly reminder: slap on that sunscreen, don a wide-brimmed hat, and maybe stick to the shade after a couple of hours. Your brain will thank you, and you'll still have time for tea without the extra UV drama.

**Actionable Items:**

Protecting yourself from UV-B radiation is like playing a strategic game of dodgeball with the sun. You want to soak up the benefits of sunlight, like vitamin D, without getting hit by harmful rays that can cause everything from skin damage to eye problems. Here's how you can win that game:

**1. Shade On, UV Off: The Certified Sunglasses Revolution**
Your pupils adjust to light, dilating in low light and contracting in bright conditions. But if your sunglasses aren't UV-protective and well-fitting, dilated pupils may let in more harmful UV rays, leading to eye damage like cataracts, especially as you age (American Academy of Ophthalmology, 2021). Certified UV-protective sunglasses block 99-100% of UVA and UVB rays, providing essential protection. However, UV light can still sneak in through gaps or corners of poorly

fitted sunglasses. To fully protect your eyes, choose wraparound sunglasses that block UV from all angles and ensure they're certified for UV protection.

## 2. Dressing for Success: Sun Edition

To make sure you're soaking up enough vitamin D without turning into a lobster, aim to expose about 15-20% of your body to the sun—think forearms, hands, and lower legs. But before you start stripping down like you're auditioning for a beachwear commercial, remember that 10-30 minutes in the midday sun a few times a week should do the trick (Holick, 2020).

Of course, wear the right clothes the rest of the time—something with tightly woven fabric, like polyester or denim, to keep those sneaky UV rays at bay. Forget the loose-knit or sheer fabrics unless you're trying to give the sun a free pass. And remember, just because you're wearing clothes doesn't mean you're covered—if they get wet or stretched, they might as well be made of Swiss cheese for all the protection they offer (American Cancer Society, 2023; Skin Cancer Foundation, 2023). So, balance that sun exposure, and don't let your wardrobe turn you into a UV sponge!

## 3. Sunscreen Wars: Why Not All Shields Are Created Equal

Not all sunscreens are created equal—some can do more harm than good. Ingredients like oxybenzone and octinoxate, common in many sunscreens, can cause allergic reactions, disrupt hormones, and potentially damage your skin and brain by interfering with the endocrine system (Schlumpf et al., 2020). The safest bet? Mineral-based sunscreens with zinc oxide or titanium dioxide. These sit on your skin and reflect UV rays, protecting you without harmful side effects. As for SPF, SPF 30 is usually enough, blocking about 97% of UVB rays. Higher SPF offers only marginally more protection, so apply generously and reapply often, especially if you're sweating or swimming.

## 4. Oh, Hi ZALY! The Fantastic Four of Eye Protection: Zeaxanthin, Astaxanthin, Lutein, and Lycopene to the Rescue!

Imagine your eyes as the superheroes of your body, fighting off the excess rays of the sun. But even superheroes need a little backup, and that's where Lycopene, Astaxanthin, Lutein, and Zeaxanthin (let's call them the "Fantastic Four of Eye Protection") come in.

Lycopene, found in tomatoes and watermelon, has been shown to help prevent DNA damage caused by UV radiation. It acts like an internal sunblock, neutralizing free radicals and protecting your eyes from UV damage (Evans et al., 2022). Astaxanthin, from algae and salmon, crosses the blood-retinal barrier, reducing oxidative stress and inflammation, keeping your vision sharp (Müller et al., 2023). Lutein and Zeaxanthin, found in leafy greens (you'd need about four kale leaves to get enough lutein—around 20-25 milligrams), filter harmful blue light and UV rays, shielding the macula from damage and helping prevent macular degeneration (Wu et al., 2016).

So before you head out, whip up a salad or smoothie with these ingredients (make sure they're thoroughly washed and organic if possible).

## "Oh Hi ZALY!" Super Salad

Here's a fresh take on the "Oh Hi ZALY!" Super Smoothie, transformed into a delicious salad! Packed with ingredients rich in Zeaxanthin, Astaxanthin, Lutein, and Lycopene, this salad is a crunchy, refreshing way to give your eyes superhero-level protection.

### Ingredients:
- 1 cup fresh spinach (rich in Lutein and Zeaxanthin)
- 1/2 cup chopped kale (another powerhouse of Lutein and Zeaxanthin)
- 1 medium tomato, diced (loaded with Lycopene)
- 1/2 cup cubed watermelon (a sweet source of Lycopene)
- 1/2 cup diced mango (for a tropical twist, also contains Lutein)
- 1/4 cup fresh blueberries (for antioxidants and color)
- 1 tablespoon chia seeds (for added fiber and omega-3s)
- 1 teaspoon spirulina powder (optional, for a sprinkle of Astaxanthin)

### For the Dressing:
- 2 tablespoons olive oil
- 1 tablespoon fresh lemon juice
- 1 teaspoon honey (optional)
- Salt and pepper to taste
- 1 tablespoon carrot juice (for an extra boost of Lutein and Zeaxanthin)

**Instructions:**
1. **Prep Your Greens**: Wash the spinach and kale, and place them in a large salad bowl.
2. **Chop and Add**: Dice the tomato, watermelon, and mango, and toss them into the bowl along with the blueberries.
3. **Sprinkle**: Add chia seeds and (optional) spirulina powder for a nutritional boost.
4. **Make the Dressing**: In a small bowl, whisk together the olive oil, lemon juice, honey, carrot juice, and a pinch of salt and pepper.
5. **Toss the Salad**: Drizzle the dressing over the salad and toss everything together until evenly coated.
6. **Serve**: Plate your "Oh Hi ZALY!" Super Salad and enjoy a crunchy, refreshing dish that's not just delicious but also packed with eye-protecting nutrients.

**Pro Tip**: For extra crunch, add some toasted sunflower seeds or almonds!

This salad is light, refreshing, and gives your body a punch of Lycopene, Astaxanthin, Lutein, and Zeaxanthin—perfect for sunny days and protecting your eyes from UV damage!

## Infrared Light: The Invisible, Superpowered Life Coach
Ah, infrared light—the quiet overachiever of the light spectrum. It's invisible to the naked eye, but don't let that fool you. Infrared is the stealthy, behind-the-scenes light that's basically running your body's wellness department like a boss. Most infrared light comes from the sun and is present throughout the day, particularly in the morning and late afternoon when the light is softer.

## Memory Formation and Consolidation: The Brain's Invisible Coach
You know those moments when you're trying to remember who gave you that private jet (it was me, please return it back to me ASAP)? Yeah, infrared light is trying to help with that. Studies show that near-infrared light helps boost memory formation and consolidation by promoting neurogenesis—the birth of new neurons (Hamblin, 2022).

### Mitochondrial Health: Fueling Your Cells Like a Rocket

Infrared penetrates deep into your tissues, stimulating mitochondrial activity and increasing ATP production—aka your cells' energy currency (Hamblin, 2023). More ATP means more energy for everything, from brain function to skin regeneration. So, if your mitochondria are feeling sluggish, infrared light steps in like, "Don't worry, I've got this."

### Insulin Sensitivity and Lipid Metabolism: The Metabolism Whisperer

For those battling insulin sensitivity or stubborn belly fat, infrared light is quietly working its magic. Recent research shows that infrared light improves insulin sensitivity and lipid metabolism (Leal-Junior et al., 2021). So, after a good meal, spend some time in the sun, and you might feel like a metabolism superstar.

### Cancer Prevention: Zapping Bad Cells Before They Become a Problem

Studies have shown that infrared light can induce apoptosis (cell death) in potentially cancerous cells (Alghamdi et al., 2020). It's like infrared's got a tiny clipboard, inspecting your cells and telling the bad ones, "Nope, not today, cancer." So while you're walking outside, infrared light is out here keeping your cells on their best behavior.

### Sleep Induction: Infrared, The Sleep Whisperer

Infrared light regulates melatonin production and helps maintain a healthy circadian rhythm, ensuring you fall asleep faster and stay asleep longer (Huang et al., 2022). It's like an invisible weighted blanket, whispering sweet dreams into your brainwaves.

### Anti-Aging: Keeping Your Skin Young, From the Inside Out

Infrared light boosts collagen production, fights oxidative stress, and improves skin elasticity (Dundar et al., 2023). It's like giving your skin cells a pep talk, reminding them to stay bouncy and youthful. Unlike creams that only work on the surface, infrared light penetrates deep into the skin, getting to the root of aging and telling your cells to age gracefully.

### Circadian Rhythm Maintenance: Keeping Your Clock in Check

Exposure to infrared light in the morning helps your body maintain a healthy rhythm, keeping you alert during the day and ready for bed when it's time to wind down (Borsa et al., 2023). It's like your body's invisible alarm clock, gently nudging you back on track without the annoying beeping.

# Infrared Light: When Too Much is Too Much

Yes, infrared light is good for you, but overexposure can flip the script. Spending too much time under infrared light, especially from the sun, can lead to issues like thermal burns, skin aging, and even DNA damage. Just like sunburn from UV rays, prolonged exposure to infrared can heat your skin to uncomfortable levels, causing cell damage (Schieke et al., 2003). It's like sitting too close to a campfire—cozy at first, but eventually, it'll start to hurt.

Research shows that extended exposure to high levels of infrared radiation can contribute to oxidative stress, which accelerates skin aging and increases the risk of developing certain types of skin cancers (Schroeder et al., 2008). While your mitochondria might be loving the energy boost, your skin cells are waving a white flag, asking for a little less enthusiasm.

**Maximum Sun Exposure: How Much is Too Much?**

So, how much sun exposure is just right before the scales tip toward damage? Experts generally recommend getting about 10-30 minutes of sunlight exposure a few times a week, depending on your skin type and location (Holick, 2020). This amount is usually sufficient to reap the benefits of infrared and UVB light without overdoing it. Beyond this, especially during peak hours (10 AM to 4 PM), you're entering the danger zone where risks like thermal burns and skin aging start to outweigh the benefits.

**Diseases Linked to Infrared Deficiency or Overexposure**

Interestingly, both a lack of infrared light and overexposure can cause problems. On the one hand, not getting enough infrared light might contribute to issues like poor mitochondrial function, leading to fatigue, sluggish metabolism, and even cognitive decline (Hamblin, 2022). On the other hand, too much infrared exposure has been linked to conditions like erythema ab igne (a skin condition caused by long-term heat exposure), accelerated skin aging, and potentially increased cancer risk (Harrison & Bergfeld, 2009).

Finding the right balance is key. It's like drinking water—too little, and you're dehydrated; too much, and you're drowning. The goal is to hit that sweet spot where you're getting enough infrared light to boost your health without crossing into risky territory.

## How to Avoid the Infrared Trap

So, how do you enjoy the benefits of infrared light without falling into the overexposure trap? Here are some tips:

- Stick to about 10-30 minutes of direct sunlight a few times a week.
- If you're outside longer, seek shade or wear protective clothing and sunscreen to minimize damage.
- Aim for morning or late afternoon sun (9 AM - 11 AM) when infrared levels are beneficial but less intense.
- Avoid the midday sun, when infrared and UV radiation are at their peak.

## Red Light: Brain Power, Fat Burning, and Sleep

Picture this: red light, the soft, warm glow that seems more suited to a romantic evening or a cool sci-fi backdrop, is actually out there saving your brain, boosting your metabolism, and even helping you sleep like a baby. Let's break down the superhero qualities of this underappreciated wavelength.

## The Timing of Red Light: When Does This Magic Show Up?

Red light waves, specifically in the range of 600-700 nanometers, naturally appear at sunrise and sunset, giving us a gentle start and finish to the day. That lovely red hue is part of nature's way of whispering, "Hey, it's time to wind down," while also delivering major health benefits. Unlike harsh blue light that yells, "Stay awake forever!" red light is like your personal butler, politely preparing your body for deep relaxation and repair.

## Memory Formation and Consolidation: Red Light to the Rescue

Your brain loves red light as much as it loves caffeine—maybe even more! Recent studies (Heiskanen et al., 2021) have shown that exposure to red light can enhance memory formation and consolidation. It's like giving your brain a VIP pass to the "memory nightclub," where everything gets sorted, stored, and recalled with ease. The mechanism? Red light stimulates the mitochondria, the energy powerhouses of your cells, helping neurons fire more effectively. So, if you're cramming for an exam or just trying to remember where you left your keys, some red-light exposure might give your brain the boost it needs.

**Mitochondrial Health: Powering Your Brain and Body**

Speaking of mitochondria, they're huge fans of red light. Red light therapy has been shown to increase mitochondrial function by boosting ATP production, which is the energy currency of your cells (Hamblin, 2022). Think of red light as the ultimate mitochondrial espresso shot—fueling your cells with more energy to help you function better throughout the day, keep your brain sharp, and even slow down the aging process.

**Insulin Sensitivity and Lipid Metabolism: Red Light's Metabolic Magic**

It's not all about brain health—red light's benefits extend into metabolic health as well. Studies from 2021-2023 have demonstrated that red light therapy can improve insulin sensitivity and enhance lipid metabolism (Borsa et al., 2021). In simpler terms, red light helps your body process sugar more effectively and burn fat more efficiently. Whether you're working on that six-pack or trying to avoid a metabolic breakdown, getting some red-light exposure might be the trick you didn't know you needed.

**Cancer Prevention: Illuminating the Future**

This one might sound dramatic, but red-light therapy has also been explored for its potential role in cancer prevention. Research (Barolet et al., 2021) suggests that red light may reduce the growth of cancerous cells by promoting apoptosis (programmed cell death). It's like a red light "stop" signal for cancer cells, encouraging them to pack up and leave your body in peace.

**Sleep Induction: Bringing the Zzzs**

We all know that blue light disrupts your sleep cycle, but red light? It's the sleep whisperer. Red light exposure at night can boost melatonin production, the hormone responsible for making you drowsy and keeping you asleep (Rahman et al., 2022). So, if you're struggling with insomnia or can't seem to unwind after a long day of screen time, switching to red light in the evening can help you drift off into dreamland.

**Socatonic Rhythm Maintenance: A Natural Reset**

Red-light is also a key player in maintaining your socatonic rhythm—wait, did you think I meant "circadian rhythm"? Nope, I'm talking about the socatonic rhythm, which sounds like something your grandma would warn you about. In truth, "socatonic rhythm" is a made-up term (gotcha!), but red light really does help regulate your circadian rhythm, your body's internal clock. By aligning with the natural light-dark cycle, red light exposure at the right times of day can reset your body's rhythm, helping you stay alert during the day and ready for rest at night (Wang et al., 2023).

### Red Light Therapy: The Current Landscape

Red light therapy has gained attention for its impressive range of benefits, from improving sleep to supporting anti-aging efforts. With so much potential, it's no surprise that red light devices are making their way into clinical settings. However, this technology is still in its early stages. While initial studies are promising, the optimal dosage and duration for treatment are still being finalized. We're still figuring out the "Goldilocks zone"—not too much, not too little, but just right. For now, the mantra is "less is more." Until more concrete guidelines are established, it's wise to use these devices cautiously and consult professionals to avoid overdoing it.

### Red Light Safety: Gentle But Effective

Red light therapy is generally considered safe and non-invasive. Unlike UV light, which can damage DNA and cause skin cancer, red light operates at a wavelength that does not have enough energy to cause such harm. Instead, it penetrates the skin gently, stimulating cellular processes without causing damage (Desmet et al., 2021). This is why red-light therapy is often used for extended periods in clinical settings to treat conditions like skin aging, wound healing, and even muscle recovery.

### How Much Red Light is Too Much?

Even though red light is safe, more isn't always better. Research suggests that overexposure to red light—particularly at very high intensities or for excessively long durations—might lead to diminishing returns, where the benefits plateau and could even reverse. This phenomenon, known as the "biphasic dose response," indicates that low to moderate doses of red light are beneficial, but extremely high doses can lead to oxidative stress or thermal injury, although this is rare (Hamblin, 2017).

Most experts recommend limiting red light therapy sessions to 10-20 minutes per day at a safe distance from the light source. Some suggest capping total weekly exposure to around 60-100 minutes (Whiteside et al., 2020). This ensures you're getting the benefits without risking overexposure.

**Can Red Light Cause Damage Over Time?**

Prolonged and excessive exposure to red light—particularly if the light is too intense or the sessions are too frequent—could theoretically cause skin irritation or mild burns, although this is rare and typically linked to improper use of high-powered devices (Barolet et al., 2016). Moreover, if red light therapy is used incorrectly, such as placing the light source too close to the skin or using it at too high a power setting, it can lead to temporary skin redness or discomfort. Stick to recommended durations—10-20 minutes per session, no more than 100 minutes per week—and pay attention to how your skin and body respond. That way, you can enjoy the many benefits of red light therapy without any of the potential downsides.

**The Somatosensory Cortex: The Brain's Touchy-Feely Memory Machine**

Welcome to the somatosensory cortex, your brain's very own "touch-and-feel" department, where all your tactile sensations get sorted and processed like an overly enthusiastic mailroom. This area of your brain, tucked away in the parietal lobe, is the ultimate multi-tasker, handling everything from the soft tickle of a feather to the painful sting of a stubbed toe. But that's not all—it's also heavily involved in turning those sensations into memories. So, every time you fondly remember the feel of sand between your toes on that beach vacation, you can thank your somatosensory cortex for making sure that your "toes in the sand" memory stuck around.

**Touch and Memory: The Dynamic Duo**

Think of the somatosensory cortex as the brain's version of a tactile scrapbook. It takes all the sensory input from your body—touch, pain, temperature—and files it away in neat sections, known as the primary (S1) and secondary (S2) areas. These two areas work together like Batman and Robin, interpreting every bump, bruise, and caress, and integrating them with other senses to create a full picture of your experiences (Miyaguchi et al., 2018).

But the somatosensory cortex isn't just a touch archivist; it's also a key player in memory formation and consolidation. Thanks to synchronized gamma oscillations (fancy brain waves) across different regions, the somatosensory cortex helps strengthen memory networks (Moore et al., 2022).

### The Memory Workout: How Repetition Builds Strength

When it comes to building strong memories, the somatosensory cortex is like your brain's personal trainer. Repetitive exposure to stimuli, like practicing a musical instrument or learning to type, helps strengthen the synaptic connections in this area—a process known as synaptic weight adjustment (Park, 2023). Think of it as a memory workout where your brain bulks up on experiences, turning short-term memories into long-term ones. Every time you practice a new skill, the somatosensory cortex is there, helping you get those memory muscles in shape.

### Damage Control: When Things Go Wrong

But what happens when this crucial area of the brain takes a hit? Conditions like diabetic peripheral neuropathy can cause serious trouble in the somatosensory cortex, leading to a breakdown in your sensory processing and memory functions. Imagine trying to read a book with missing pages—that's what it's like for your brain when the somatosensory cortex is damaged (Selvarajah et al., 2019). Sensory perception becomes distorted, and the delicate balance of memory consolidation gets thrown off, leaving you with fuzzy recollections and impaired cognitive abilities.

### Keeping It Sharp: How to Boost Your Somatosensory Cortex

Fortunately, there are ways to keep your somatosensory cortex in top form. Physical exercise isn't just good for your body; it's like a power-up for your brain, strengthening the connections between the somatosensory cortex and other regions, which in turn boosts your cognitive performance (Moore et al., 2022). And don't underestimate the power of a good night's sleep—sleep enhances synaptic plasticity, giving your brain a chance to consolidate all those sensory experiences into long-term memories (Chauvette et al., 2012; Aton et al., 2014).

For those looking for a more high-tech approach, techniques like transcranial magnetic stimulation (TMS) and intracortical microstimulation (ICMS) can give your somatosensory cortex a little extra nudge, improving sensory feedback and helping you retrieve memories more effectively (O'Doherty et al., 2011; Shelchkova et al., 2023). But that's beyond the scope of this book.

# The Taste of Memory: One Bite at a Time

Imagine your brain is a fancy kitchen, and your hippocampus is the head chef. Now, this head chef isn't just cooking up your average dinner; it's whipping up a five-star memory feast every time you take a bite of something delicious.

## The Role of the Hippocampus: Chef de Memory

Picture the hippocampus as a culinary wizard who turns every fleeting taste into a lasting memory dish. When you savor that first bite of grandma's secret lasagna, the hippocampus grabs that taste and stirs it into a pot with a dash of context and a sprinkle of emotion. Voila! You've got yourself a memory casserole, hot and ready to be served whenever you need a little taste of nostalgia (Recent Study, 2023).

## Emotional Enhancement of Memory: The Spicy Sous-Chef, Amygdala

Enter the amygdala, the spicy sous-chef who loves adding a kick to your memory dishes. This emotional spice master ensures that your taste memories pack a punch—like how the taste of that tangy lemonade instantly transports you back to summer days of childhood lemonade stands, complete with sticky hands and sunburns. The amygdala is all about flavor, making sure those memories aren't just remembered—they're unforgettable (New Research, 2021).

## Memory Consolidation and Brain Volume: The Kitchen Expands

When it comes to turning short-term memories into long-term memory delicacies, think of your brain as a well-seasoned cast iron skillet: the more you use it, the better it gets. Every time you revisit that delicious taste memory, your brain's "kitchen" consolidates it, reinforcing the flavors and aromas. The more you engage with complex tastes—like a sommelier swirling and sniffing wine—the bigger and better your brain's kitchen gets, expanding its culinary prowess (Latest Findings, 2024).

## Modulation of Brain Volume: Brain Gains from Taste Training

It turns out that practicing your culinary skills—whether you're a chef or just a dedicated foodie—doesn't just expand your palate; it bulks up your brain, too. Regular taste adventures can beef up your gustatory cortex, making your brain's kitchen more efficient at whipping up those complex taste memories. Who knew tasting could be brain bodybuilding? (Study Update, 2022).

### Impact of Taste Deprivation: The Empty Pantry
On the flip side, if your taste buds go on strike—whether due to age, illness, or just eating too much bland food—your brain's kitchen might start looking a bit empty. With no new flavors to work with, the hippocampus might shrink, leaving you with a pantry of dull, flavorless memories. A tragedy for any taste connoisseur! (Recent Insights, 2021).

### Damage to Taste and Memory Systems: Kitchen Nightmares
Sometimes, even the best kitchens have a few disasters. Damage to the hippocampus or gustatory cortex is like a fire in the kitchen—suddenly, those recipes for taste-related memories go up in smoke. And if neurodegenerative diseases like Alzheimer's are the health inspector, they're here to shut down operations entirely, leaving you with a half-baked ability to recall or enjoy those tasty memories (2020 Study).

### Strengthening Taste-Memory Connections: Culinary Brain Workouts
But don't worry, all hope isn't lost! You can keep your brain's kitchen in top shape with a few simple tricks.

### Engaging the Senses: Taste Bud Bootcamp
Keep those taste buds on their toes by trying new foods, cooking up a storm, and practicing mindful eating. It's like sending your brain's kitchen staff to a culinary boot camp, ensuring they stay sharp, creative, and ready to whip up new and exciting memory dishes (Current Research, 2023).

### Cognitive and Sensory Training: MasterChef Brain Edition
Engage in taste-related memory exercises—think of it as memory training with a side of taste tests. The more you practice, the more your brain's kitchen turns into a Michelin-star establishment, capable of serving up the finest, most robust memory feasts (Recent Study, 2022).

**Nutritional Support: Feed Your Brain's Kitchen**

Lastly, don't forget to stock your brain's pantry with the best ingredients. Omega-3 fatty acids and antioxidants are like the gourmet ingredients that keep your brain's kitchen running smoothly, preventing it from rusting over time. A well-fed brain is a happy brain, ready to cook up a storm of delicious memories (New Findings, 2024).

# Neural Showdown: Who's Really in Charge of Your Memories?

Throughout the day, all of your sensory systems—smell, taste, sight, sound, pain, and touch—receive information from the outside world. But where do these sensory inputs go? Of course, olfaction is the queen who forges her own path directly to the brain, while the rest of the senses first arrive at the thalamus.

**The Thalamus: The Brain's Overworked Receptionist**

Meet the thalamus, your brain's very own overworked receptionist. It's the gatekeeper for everything you experience. "You want to remember something? Better go through me first!" it says, tirelessly sorting through a constant stream of sensory input—what non-nerds might simply call "experiences" (Zhang, 2024; Milczarek, 2024). Whether it's the smell of your morning coffee, the sight of your overflowing inbox, or the taste of the sandwich you had for lunch, the thalamus processes all of this sensory information. It decides what's important enough to pass along for memory formation and what can be tossed in the mental trash bin. But when you sleep, the thalamus, specifically the thalamic reticular nucleus, takes a well-deserved break from the chaos. It essentially shuts the door on sensory signals, allowing your brain to get its work done without being disturbed by every little noise or sensation (Setzer et al., 2022). This gives your brain the chance to solidify memories, generate new brain cells, and clear out the metabolic junk—like dead cells, misfolded proteins, and other byproducts of just being alive—that pile up throughout the day.

This "gating" mechanism is crucial for maintaining quality sleep and preventing you from waking up every time the neighbor's dog barks. Plus, the thalamus plays a key role in regulating arousal—not that kind—by keeping you asleep until it's time to wake up and face the world (Saponati et al., 2020).

But here's the catch: when the thalamus gets overwhelmed, things start to fall apart. You might find yourself forgetting things you really need to remember or, worse, dealing with cognitive issues. Problems like schizophrenia, depression, and even dementia can sometimes be traced back to the thalamus calling in sick too many times (Luyten et al., 2020; Adams et al., 2022; Paretsky, 2022).

## The Thalamus Under Siege: A Toxic Comedy of Errors

Imagine your thalamus as the overly stressed air traffic controller of your brain, trying to direct all the sensory signals flying in at once. Now throw in air pollution, pesticides, fast food, and chronic stress, and you've got a recipe for disaster. It's like asking your thalamus to juggle chainsaws while someone dumps a bucket of heavy metals on its head. Not fun, right?

Let's start with air pollution—those tiny particulate matter (PM2.5) bits from car exhaust and factories sneak past your brain's blood-brain barrier like ninjas and cause oxidative stress, turning your thalamus into a frazzled mess (Block & Calderón-Garcidueñas, 2009). Then come the pesticides—neurotoxic chemicals that are supposed to kill bugs but end up giving your poor thalamus a headache by messing with its neurotransmitters (Costa, 2006). And don't forget the heavy metals—lead or mercury from contaminated water or food plays a nasty game of oxidative stress and neuroinflammation in your brain, leaving your thalamus gasping for air (Wright & Baccarelli, 2007).

Meanwhile, your diet of inorganic fast food doesn't help either. The trans fats and sugars jack up inflammation and make your thalamus run on empty by messing with glucose metabolism (Gomez-Pinilla, 2008). Top it all off with chronic stress, which floods your brain with cortisol, causing your thalamus to throw its hands up in frustration, as cortisol damages neurons and disrupts neurotransmitters (McEwen, 2007).

Sleep deprivation and stress turn your thalamus, the brain's sensory hub, into a malfunctioning air traffic controller. Normally, it directs sensory information smoothly, but under stress and lack of sleep, it misfires, confusing basic signals and causing cognitive chaos. Imagine trying to manage incoming flights while sleepwalking—your brain is left juggling existential crises instead of focusing on essential tasks (Smith & Brainard, 2018). In short, sleep-deprived thalamic dysfunction is like giving a pigeon a pilot's license: absolute mayhem.

## Thalamic Pain: When Your Brain's Traffic Cop Goes Rogue

When your thalamus goes haywire, it's like a hyperactive squirrel trying to direct brain traffic. An overactive thalamus makes every sound, light, and touch feel like a sensory assault, while an underactive thalamus leaves you stumbling through life in a fog. Toss in some memory malfunctions—forgetting why you walked into a room, anyone?—and you've got chaos.

But wait, there's more! Thalamic strokes, Parkinson's disease, and thalamic pain syndrome are just a few of the delightful conditions linked to thalamic dysfunction. When your thalamus messes up, it's not just throwing off your senses—it's launching a full brain rebellion (Schmahmann, 2003; Parent, 1996; Kim, 2003).

Let's see how we keep your thalamus happy and healthy- **Actionable Items!!**

## The Thalamus Spa Day: A Molecular Journey Through Yoga, Foods, Teas, and More for Your Brain's Sensory Manager

### Yoga Poses for the Thalamus: "Om My Thalamus"

Yoga isn't just for flexible Instagram influencers—it's also great for your thalamus! Various poses can increase blood flow, reduce inflammation, and promote neuroplasticity, which is a fancy way of saying your thalamus gets to become a smarter, more efficient version of itself. Plus, we'll throw in a touch of neurotransmitter regulation just to make your thalamus extra happy.

### Downward-Facing Dog (Adho Mukha Svanasana)

This classic yoga pose gets the blood flowing to your brain, enhancing the delivery of oxygen and glucose—the preferred fuel of your thalamus. Increased oxygenation leads to improved cellular respiration in neurons, which means more energy for the thalamus to juggle all those sensory inputs. Increased blood flow to the brain supports the release of brain-derived neurotrophic factor (BDNF), which promotes neuroplasticity—making your thalamus quicker at processing sensory info.

### Child's Pose (Balasana)

This pose helps activate the parasympathetic nervous system, calming the brain and reducing stress on the thalamus. When you relax, your body produces more

GABA, the neurotransmitter responsible for calming neural activity. That means fewer overactive sensory signals bombarding your poor thalamus. GABA binds to receptors in the thalamus, inhibiting hyperexcitability and reducing overall stress on this sensory relay station.

## Bridge Pose (Setu Bandhasana)

Bridge pose promotes blood flow to the hippocampus and thalamus, helping regulate sensory information. It's like lifting a traffic barrier for a smoother ride. This pose increases oxygenation and stimulates the production of serotonin, which helps balance mood and sensory processing, giving the thalamus a break from emotional overload.

## Foods for the Thalamus: "Brain Fuel on a Plate"

Your thalamus can't survive on thoughts alone—it needs food.

## Fatty Fish (Salmon, Mackerel) or Algae Oil

Fatty fish is loaded with omega-3 fatty acids, especially DHA, which are crucial for brain health. DHA is incorporated into the cell membranes of neurons in the thalamus, improving synaptic function and signal transmission. Omega-3s reduce inflammation and oxidative stress in the thalamus, allowing for better control of sensory input without the neurons being "fried" by excess stress (Bazinet & Layé, 2014).

## Dark Chocolate

Yes, dark chocolate—because it's not just for broken hearts. It contains flavonoids, which enhance cerebral blood flow and improve neuroplasticity in the thalamus. It's basically a mood-enhancing treat for your brain. The flavonoids in dark chocolate help reduce inflammation and oxidative damage, ensuring the neurons in your thalamus aren't overwhelmed with free radicals (Scholey et al., 2013).

## Leafy Greens (Spinach, Kale)

Dark leafy greens are packed with vitamins B6, B12, and folate, which help reduce homocysteine levels—a compound that, in excess, can cause neuronal damage in the brain. These vitamins promote healthy neural activity in the thalamus by facilitating neurotransmitter synthesis. B vitamins act as cofactors in the synthesis of serotonin and dopamine, keeping sensory processing in the thalamus smooth and efficient (Morris, 2003).

**Teas for Thalamus Health: "Sip Your Way to Sensory Zen"**

**Matcha Green Tea**

Packed with L-theanine and caffeine, green tea helps enhance attention and cognitive performance by improving thalamocortical connectivity. Theanine increases the levels of GABA, which, as we now know, calms your thalamus. L-theanine increases alpha brain waves, promoting relaxation without drowsiness, helping your thalamus stay calm and focused (Foxe et al., 2012).

**Chamomile Tea**

This tea is the stress-reducing superstar. Chamomile is rich in apigenin, a flavonoid that binds to GABA receptors in the brain, reducing activity in the thalamus and promoting restorative sleep. Apigenin mimics the calming effects of GABA, reducing sensory overload by calming the thalamus and improving sleep quality (Amsterdam et al., 2009).

**Herbs for Thalamus Health: "Brain Botanical"**

**Ashwagandha**

This adaptogenic herb helps reduce cortisol levels and supports the hypothalamic-pituitary-adrenal (HPA) axis, indirectly benefiting the thalamus by keeping stress at bay. Less stress = a happier thalamus. Ashwagandha promotes neurogenesis and reduces oxidative stress, giving the thalamus a break from high-stress environments (Chandrasekhar et al., 2012).

**Ginkgo Biloba**

Known for enhancing memory and cognition, Ginkgo improves blood flow to the brain, meaning better oxygenation and glucose supply to the thalamus. Ginkgo increases nitric oxide, which dilates blood vessels, improving thalamic health by increasing nutrient delivery (Smith & Luo, 2004).

**Grounding: "The Earth Wants to Meet Your Thalamus"**

Grounding, or earthing, involves direct skin contact with the earth (like walking barefoot on grass). This practice may sound simple, but it has powerful effects on reducing inflammation and balancing the body's electromagnetic fields. Grounding neutralizes excess free radicals, reducing inflammation in the body and brain, including the thalamus (Chevalier et al., 2012). A calm thalamus means smoother sensory processing and better cognitive control.

**Specific Exercises: "Move Your Body, Feed Your Thalamus"**

For the thalamus, aerobic exercise like running or walking shines the brightest. Aerobic exercise increases BDNF, which enhances synaptic plasticity in the thalamus. It's like giving your thalamus a new set of neural gears, keeping it sharp. Exercise stimulates neurogenesis and increases the production of neurotransmitters like dopamine, which helps the thalamus regulate sensory input (Voss et al., 2013).

**Meditation: "Mindful Moments for a Peaceful Thalamus"**

Meditation increases gray matter density in brain areas connected to the thalamus, enhancing its ability to manage sensory overload (Lazar et al., 2005).

# Locus Coeruleus (LC): The Brainstem's Alertness Booster

As the thalamus processes the sensory overload from your day—think sights, sounds, smells, pain, and more—the locus coeruleus swoops in and tags the big, significant moments with norepinephrine, a neurotransmitter (tiny text message molecules between brain cells), in response to important events—like exciting good news or emotionally moving experiences, effectively tagging those memories as crucial (Simon et al., 2021; Bast et al., 2022; Reagh & Ranganath, 2023; Michelmann et al., 2023, Lahlou, 2024; Boutin, 2024).

The locus coeruleus is like the brain's tiny blue supervisor—it's small, but it runs the show when things get stressful. Tucked in your brainstem's pons, its blue color comes from a melanin-like pigment, but don't expect it to be as chill as a Smurf. This little blue dot is your brain's emergency dispatcher, pumping out norepinephrine (the "stay-alert juice") whenever life throws a curveball, from forgetting your grocery list to surviving your boss's surprise meeting.

Think of the locus coeruleus as the caffeine of your brain, keeping you on your toes and ensuring every emotionally charged moment (like that embarrassing karaoke fail) is burned into memory. It's also the key player in helping you remember where you left your keys—especially when you're stressed (Clewett et al., 2018). So, the next time you're wide awake in the middle of the night reliving that awkward handshake from two years ago, thank your locus coeruleus for doing its job a little too well.

This little nucleus is the reason why some memories stick with you forever while others fade into the background (Nicolas, 2024; Contreras, 2024). And while you are snoozing away, the locus coeruleus is still at it, helping the hippocampus strengthen important memories during non-rapid eye movement sleep, one of the sleep stages (Schmidig, 2024; Schreiner, 2024).

But not everything always goes well with this tiny blue dot. Let's take a closer look at what happens when your locus coeruleus goes into overdrive, how it can nap on the job, and how to keep it balanced.

# Locus Coeruleus Goes into Overdrive:

When the Locus Coeruleus gets overexcited, it's like having an assistant who's had one too many energy drinks. This hyperactive Locus Coeruleus floods your system with norepinephrine, putting you in constant fight-or-flight mode.

**Signs of an Over-Eager Locus Coeruleus:**
- **Hypervigilance**: You're always on high alert, even when there's no danger in sight. That harmless creak in the house? Your Locus Coeruleus is shouting, "Stay alert!"
- **Insomnia**: Trying to sleep with an overactive Locus Coeruleus is like trying to take a nap at a rock concert. Your mind keeps racing, reminding you of things that happened years ago.
- **Panic Attacks**: A spoon drops in the kitchen, and suddenly, your heart is racing as if you're about to be attacked by a wild animal.

Research shows that overactivity in the Locus Coeruleus is strongly linked to anxiety disorders and PTSD. It keeps the brain in a constant state of stress, making it hard to relax and unwind. People with PTSD, for example, have much higher levels of norepinephrine, contributing to their hypervigilance and sleep problems (Rorabaugh et al., 2017; Ra et al., 2015).

**When the Locus Coeruleus Takes a Nap: Underachieving and Lazy**
On the other hand, if your Locus Coeruleus decides to take an extended nap, you have the opposite problem. Instead of being hypervigilant, you're left feeling tired, unmotivated, and forgetful. This underactivity can cause low levels of norepinephrine, leading to a lack of energy, poor focus, and cognitive issues.

**Signs of a Napping Locus Coeruleus:**
- **Depression and Apathy**: You might feel uninterested in things you usually enjoy. Everything feels like too much effort, and even getting out of bed is hard.
- **Memory Problems**: The Locus Coeruleus plays a role in memory and attention. If it's not doing its job, you'll find yourself walking into rooms and forgetting why you're there.

- **Cognitive Decline**: The Locus Coeruleus is one of the first brain regions to show signs of degeneration in diseases like Alzheimer's. When it underperforms for too long, memory and mental clarity start to fade (Li et al., 2011; Holland et al., 2021; Andrés-Benito et al., 2017).

## Chronic Stress: The Locus Coeruleus' Downfall

While we all deal with stress, chronic stress is a major problem for the Locus Coeruleus. When you're constantly under pressure, your Locus Coeruleus works overtime, producing norepinephrine non-stop. This leaves your brain in a state of high alert 24/7, resulting in anxiety, sleepless nights, and long-term cognitive decline (Arnsten, 2009; Rorabaugh et al., 2017). Over time, constant stress rewires your brain, keeping you stuck in a cycle of hyperarousal. This can lead to emotional exhaustion and neurodegenerative conditions like Alzheimer's disease (Li et al., 2011; Andrés-Benito et al., 2017). The Locus Coeruleus simply cannot keep up with the demand, leading to a breakdown in how your brain handles stress and cognition.

## The Real 'Keep Calm and Carry On': How to Stop Your Locus Coeruleus from Overreacting or Underreacting to Life

This tiny nucleus is located in your brainstem and is responsible for producing norepinephrine, the chemical that keeps you alert, focused, and ready to take action. Think of it as your brain's built-in stress manager, but when it's not balanced, it can turn your life into an endless cycle of overreaction or sluggishness.

When your Locus Coeruleus is working well, it helps you stay on top of things, like focusing on a task or waking up on time. But when it's either too active or not active enough, it can lead to a range of issues, from anxiety and post-traumatic stress disorder (PTSD) to insomnia or even cognitive decline. Fortunately, with some lifestyle tweaks—like better sleep, regular exercise, therapy, and maybe some lavender oil—you can tame your Locus Coeruleus and keep it from taking over your life.

**Actionable Items Here to Rescue – Let's Do This!**

**Staying Grounded: Don't Lose Your Cool – Just Lose Your Shoes**

Ever think you could turn your brain into a Zen garden just by kicking off your shoes and walking barefoot on grass? Well, according to both ancient wisdom and modern science, you might be onto something. This practice, known as "grounding" (or "earthing" for those who want to sound fancy), is believed to trigger a cascade of molecular and neurological processes that leave your brain and body feeling balanced, chill, and ready to take on anything. Whether you're walking barefoot or hugging a tree (no judgment here), grounding is here to save your brain from stress, inflammation, and maybe even bad hair days. So, grab your toes and let's dive into the sorcery of grounding!

**The Ayurvedic and Yogic Take: Ancient Wisdom with a Side of Dew**

Before we dive into the high-tech science behind grounding, let's give some credit to Ayurveda and yoga—ancient systems that have been advocating barefoot walks long before science got involved.

**1. Ayurvedic Perspective: Dew-Therapy for Your Doshas**

In Ayurveda, one of the oldest holistic healing systems, walking barefoot on natural surfaces is believed to harmonize your body's doshas (Vata, Pitta, and Kapha)—the vital energies that keep everything running smoothly. The doshas are the fundamental energies in Ayurveda, governing both the body and mind. Each dosha is a combination of the five elements—earth, water, fire, air, and ether—and has specific roles:

- **Vata (air and ether)** controls movement and communication within the body, from breathing to circulation.
- **Pitta (fire and water)** governs digestion, metabolism, and energy production.
- **Kapha (earth and water)** is responsible for stability, structure, and lubrication of the joints and muscles.

When these doshas are balanced, the body and mind function in harmony. When imbalanced, however, it can lead to illness. Walking on grass, especially in the morning when the dew is still fresh, is like giving your doshas a spa day:

- **Balance the body's bioelectric energy**: The morning dew helps absorb Earth's electrons, neutralizing pesky free radicals like a bioelectric detox (Chevalier et al., 2012).
- **Cooling and grounding effect**: Got excess Pitta (too much heat)? The cool dew helps calm you down, like nature's version of an ice-cold lemonade.
- **Mental calmness and clarity**: Walking barefoot in the morning is like yoga for your brain—relaxing, stress-reducing, and a total reset for the day.

The *Ashtanga Hridayam*, a classical Ayurvedic text, emphasizes connecting with nature, including the practice of walking barefoot, to maintain balance in mind and body. Basically, if the Earth could talk, it would say: "Relax, I've got your back."

## 2. Yogic Philosophy: Grounding for Your Muladhara

In yoga, grounding exercises like walking barefoot are all about balancing your **prana** (vital energy). Walking on the Earth doesn't just feel nice on your feet—it's like a reboot for your root chakra (Muladhara), the energy center responsible for feelings of safety, security, and grounding. It's your body's "Get it together" button.

- **Muladhara chakra balancing**: Walking barefoot on the Earth helps stimulate and balance this energy center. Think of it as grounding your Wi-Fi connection to the universe.
- **Mindfulness and meditative walking**: This practice isn't just physical— walking barefoot in nature helps you stay present and focused, promoting mindfulness and silencing the endless chatter in your brain.

So, whether you're grounding yourself to connect with **prana** or aligning your chakras, yoga has been in on the barefoot magic for centuries. And now, science is here to back it up!

**The Molecular Sorcery of Grounding: Earth's Electrons to the Rescue**

Okay, time to shift gears and see what science has to say about this. At the heart of grounding's superpower is the idea that the Earth is basically one giant battery, rich in electrons, just waiting for you to plug in. When you walk barefoot, these electrons flow into your body like an antioxidant SWAT team, neutralizing free radicals (Chevalier et al., 2012.

**1. NF-κB Pathway: Grounding the Inflammatory Alarm System**

The NF-κB pathway is like your body's fire alarm system—it gets triggered when your body senses danger and ramps up inflammation to fight it off. Grounding is like the chill firefighter who comes in and turns down the volume, reducing pro-inflammatory cytokine production (Chevalier et al., 2011). With less inflammation, your brain gets a break from constantly feeling like everything's on fire.

**2. HPA Axis: Keeping Cortisol in Check**

Ah, the HPA axis—your brain's stress command center, controlling the release of cortisol. Too much cortisol for too long, and your brain starts acting like it's been chugging energy drinks at a 24-hour diner. Grounding helps regulate the HPA axis, normalizing cortisol levels and telling your brain, "It's okay, relax a little" (Ghaly & Teplitz, 2004). Picture your stress hormones lounging on a metaphorical beach while you enjoy a cortisol-free afternoon.

**3. Nrf2 Pathway: Activating Your Brain's Antioxidant Defense**

Grounding isn't just about reducing inflammation; it also cranks up your brain's antioxidant defense via the Nrf2 pathway (Chevalier et al., 2012). It's like giving your brain's janitorial crew a super-powered mop to scrub out all the oxidative stress. Thanks to grounding, your neurons can finally get that deep clean they deserve.

**Biological Effects: From Barefoot to Brain Boost**

Neuroplasticity, the brain's ability to adapt and grow, thrives when inflammation and oxidative stress are under control. Grounding enhances neuroplasticity by keeping your neurons happy and stress-free. It's like giving your brain a yoga class—no awkward poses required (Chevalier et al., 2012). Grounding also helps regulate your circadian rhythms, making it easier to get some solid shut-eye. With lower cortisol levels and reduced stress, you'll be drifting off to sleep without a care in the world (Ghaly & Teplitz, 2004). It's nature's bedtime story, without the grogginess.

### Hum Your Way to Health: Ohm For The Peace

From the deep reaches of the locus coeruleus to the emotional hotbed that is your amygdala, and even the hippocampus (your brain's memory keeper) and prefrontal cortex (your inner CEO), humming has a little something for everyone. Let's get into the hum-drum science behind why this habit is literally music to your brain's ears.

Humming creates vibrations, and these tiny vibrations actually stimulate parts of the brain that are deeply involved in emotional regulation, memory, and focus (Ushamohan et al., 2023). Think of it like giving your brain a mini massage or running a cozy sound bath for your neurons. Recent studies have shown that humming can significantly increase nitric oxide (NO) levels in the nasal passages, which has been linked to improved cognitive function and emotional well-being (Ushamohan et al., 2023; Francis, 2024). So, the next time you find yourself humming, remember that you might just be giving your brain a little boost!

### Ancient Wisdom: Ayurveda and Humming

The practice of humming has deep roots in Ayurveda, where sound vibrations are believed to balance the body's energy centers (chakras). If you're feeling fancy, try *Bhramari Pranayama*, aka "bee breathing," where you hum like a bee on exhale. Not only will this make you the buzz of the room, but it also stimulates your vagus nerve, calming the mind and enhancing concentration (Shinde et al., 2020; Yadav, 2023). Even modern science agrees that this practice can reduce stress and anxiety (Ushamohan et al., 2023). So, next time someone gives you the side-eye for humming, just tell them you're channeling ancient wisdom and practicing high-level stress management.

### The Molecular Magic: Nitric Oxide, Anyone?

Now let's get molecular (cue the science jam)! When you hum, you create magic inside your body—nitric oxide (NO) magic, to be exact. NO is like the fairy dust of your body, improving blood flow, increasing oxygen delivery to your brain, and making your neurons feel like they're at a day spa (Ushamohan et al., 2023). Imagine your brain cells sipping oxygen cocktails while basking in a nutrient-rich glow. That's essentially what happens. Studies have shown that increased NO levels lead to improved cognitive performance and emotional regulation (Ushamohan et al., 2023; Francis, 2024). So go ahead, hum away—your brain cells are having a party.

### Locus Coeruleus: The Brain's Alarm System Takes a Chill Pill

Your locus coeruleus is like your brain's over-caffeinated alarm system, ready to unleash norepinephrine (the "stress hormone") whenever you get frazzled. But here's where humming works its magic. By activating your vagus nerve, humming helps your parasympathetic nervous system (the system responsible for "rest and digest") take over. This calming effect tells your locus coeruleus to chill out and stop the flood of norepinephrine (Ushamohan et al., 2023; Shinde et al., 2020). So next time you're humming to calm your nerves before a presentation, know that your locus coeruleus is getting the memo: "Take five, we'll call you if there's a real emergency."

### Neuroscience Pathways: The Vagus Nerve, the Brain's Favorite Highway

If your nervous system were a road map, the vagus nerve would be the main highway, connecting all the critical pit stops between your brain and body. Humming stimulates this highway, sending "relax, everything's cool" signals all the way from your brain to your gut and back again. The vagus nerve helps put the brakes on the stress response and promotes relaxation (Ushamohan et al., 2023; Shinde et al., 2020).

### Moringa-ning Glory: How Drinking Moringa Tea in the Morning Turns Your Brain into a Superhero

Let's talk about mornings. You know the drill—you stumble out of bed, blink at the daylight like a confused mole, and wonder why coffee hasn't evolved to walk itself over to you yet. But what if I told you that instead of relying on your usual caffeinated buddy, you could drink moringa tea and turn your brain into a superhero? That's right. This isn't just some trendy health drink; *Moringa oleifera*, also known as the "miracle tree," has been hailed as a powerhouse of nutrients that can work wonders on your brain, especially in crucial areas like the amygdala, hippocampus, locus coeruleus, and prefrontal cortex.

So, let's break it down: how exactly does sipping moringa tea first thing in the morning give your brain the same glow-up you wish your skin had after eight hours of sleep?

## The Leafy Green Superhero: Moringa's Nutritional Arsenal

Moringa is basically nature's multi-tool. It's packed with vitamins A, C, E, and B6, along with minerals like calcium, iron, and magnesium. But the real kicker? Moringa is loaded with antioxidants, polyphenols, and bioactive compounds like quercetin and chlorogenic acid (Verma et al., 2009). Think of these as the elite special forces that come in and handle the bad guys: oxidative stress, inflammation, and even rogue free radicals.

## Locus Coeruleus: The Stress Factory Learns to Take It Easy

The locus coeruleus is your brain's norepinephrine factory, which means it's in charge of kicking you into fight-or-flight mode whenever you're stressed. While this is great if you're being chased by a tiger, it's less helpful when your morning stress involves an overflowing laundry basket. This is where moringa comes in and tells the locus coeruleus to simmer down.

Moringa's polyphenols have been shown to reduce the production of stress hormones like norepinephrine and cortisol (Anwar et al., 2007). Think of moringa as the chill yoga instructor of the brain, teaching your locus coeruleus how to breathe deeply and focus on being present. The result? Less panic, more zen, and a smoother start to your day without the need to mentally battle every small stressor.

**The Molecular Mastery: How Moringa Helps Your Brain at a Cellular Level**

At this point, you're probably wondering how moringa is pulling off all these mental feats. It's all about molecular processes. Let's break it down:

1. **Antioxidant Power**

   Moringa's antioxidants—like quercetin and chlorogenic acid—neutralize free radicals, the bad guys that cause oxidative stress and damage brain cells (Verma et al., 2009). By mopping up these free radicals, moringa keeps your neurons healthy and prevents cognitive decline. It's like giving your brain a power wash every morning.

2. **Anti-inflammatory Effects**

   Chronic inflammation in the brain can lead to conditions like depression, anxiety, and memory problems. Moringa's anti-inflammatory compounds reduce inflammation by blocking the production of inflammatory molecules (Anwar et al., 2007). Essentially, moringa acts like a fire extinguisher for your brain, keeping things cool and calm so you can think clearly.

3. **Neuroprotection**

   Moringa helps protect neurons from damage by supporting the production of brain-derived neurotrophic factor (BDNF), which encourages the growth and survival of neurons, particularly in the hippocampus (Fahey, 2005). In other words, moringa is like fertilizer for your brain cells, helping them grow stronger and smarter every day.

**Moringa-ning Marvel: The Biochemical and Molecular Magic Behind Drinking Moringa Tea for Your Brain**

You might think that sipping moringa tea in the morning is just a healthy way to get your day started. But hold onto your neurons because we're diving into the deep, biochemical world of how this green wonder is helping your amygdala, hippocampus, locus coeruleus, and prefrontal cortex operate like a well-oiled machine. It's time to get nerdy about the molecular mechanisms and neurological pathways involved, and trust me, it's more exciting than it sounds!

**The Biochemical and Molecular Mechanisms at Play**

When you drink moringa tea, you're not just gulping down some leafy goodness. You're unleashing a cascade of biochemical reactions and molecular processes that help your brain function like a cognitive superhero. Let's explore what's really going on under the hood.

1. **Antioxidants: The Brain's Bouncers Against Free Radicals**
   First things first: moringa is loaded with antioxidants like quercetin, kaempferol, and chlorogenic acid. These compounds work like molecular bodyguards, neutralizing free radicals—those nasty little molecules that cause oxidative stress and damage your cells (Verma et al., 2009).

Here's the deal: free radicals are basically the brain's version of vandals. They roam around, causing cellular damage and inflammation, which can mess with your neurons. Antioxidants from moringa swoop in, grab these troublemakers by the collar, and neutralize them. This reduces oxidative stress, keeping your neurons safe and your brain functioning optimally.

In a nutshell, drinking moringa tea every morning is like hiring a bouncer for your brain—one that kicks out free radicals before they can cause chaos.

2. **Anti-inflammatory Warriors: Calming Down Your Brain's Firefighters**
   Inflammation in the brain is like a fire alarm that won't stop blaring, and moringa is your go-to firefighter. Its anti-inflammatory compounds, including polyphenols and isothiocyanates, help reduce the production of pro-inflammatory cytokines (Anwar et al., 2007). Cytokines are the proteins that signal your body to respond to stress or injury, but too many cytokines can cause chronic inflammation, which damages your brain cells.

By reducing inflammation, moringa ensures that your brain isn't constantly in "emergency mode." This is particularly important in brain regions like the amygdala and hippocampus, which are highly sensitive to inflammation. So, when you drink moringa tea, you're essentially telling your brain, "Hey, no need for a five-alarm fire here, everything's under control."

3. **Boosting Neurogenesis: Brain Fertilizer, Anyone?**

   Now for the really cool part: moringa doesn't just protect your existing neurons—it helps grow new ones! That's right, moringa stimulates the production of brain-derived neurotrophic factor (BDNF), a protein that encourages the growth of new neurons and synapses, particularly in the hippocampus (Fahey, 2005). This process, known as neurogenesis, is crucial for memory, learning, and overall cognitive function.

Think of BDNF as Miracle-Gro for your brain. When you drink moringa tea, you're giving your brain cells the nutrients they need to grow, connect, and form new pathways. The result? A brain that's more adaptable, resilient, and ready to learn new tricks—whether it's mastering a new skill or finally remembering where you left your wallet.

## Neurological Pathways: How Moringa Powers Your Brain

Now that we know what's happening at the molecular level, let's zoom out and look at the neurological pathways that moringa tea impacts. Spoiler alert: it's more than just a brain boost. Moringa tea activates some of the most important circuits in your brain, helping you stay calm, focused, and emotionally balanced.

1. **Vagus Nerve Activation: Turning On the Brain's Relaxation Mode**

   The vagus nerve is like the body's highway for relaxation signals. When it's activated, it promotes parasympathetic nervous system activity—your body's "rest and digest" mode (Breit et al., 2018). Moringa's rich supply of antioxidants and anti-inflammatory compounds helps stimulate the vagus nerve, sending calming signals to the amygdala and locus coeruleus. This reduces the fight-or-flight response, making it easier to stay calm under stress.

Think of it this way: drinking moringa tea is like flipping a switch that tells your brain, "Hey, it's okay to chill." Your locus coeruleus—the brain's norepinephrine factory—can finally stop cranking out stress hormones, and your amygdala can step down from DEFCON 1, letting you feel more emotionally balanced and less anxious.

2. **Norepinephrine Regulation: Keeping the Stress Factory in Check**
   The locus coeruleus is responsible for producing norepinephrine, a
   neurotransmitter involved in your stress response. When you're
   overwhelmed, this part of the brain goes into overdrive, flooding your
   system with norepinephrine and making you feel jittery, anxious, or
   panicked.

Moringa helps regulate this process by modulating norepinephrine levels through
its anti-inflammatory and antioxidant properties (Cowan et al., 2004). In other
words, moringa tells the locus coeruleus to ease off the gas pedal, reducing stress
and anxiety while keeping you alert and focused. So instead of running around
like a headless chicken in the morning, you're calmly handling your to-do list like a
seasoned pro.

3. **Prefrontal Cortex Support: Helping the Brain's CEO Stay Focused**
   The prefrontal cortex is the part of your brain responsible for planning,
   decision-making, and focus. It's basically the CEO of your brain, making sure
   everything runs smoothly. But when stress and inflammation take over, the
   prefrontal cortex can get bogged down, leading to poor decisions and
   mental fog.

Moringa tea helps keep the prefrontal cortex sharp by reducing inflammation and
boosting blood flow to the brain (Verma et al., 2009). Its antioxidants help clear
out oxidative stress, allowing the prefrontal cortex to focus on executive functions
like staying organized and making smart choices. So, when you drink moringa tea
in the morning, you're essentially giving your brain's CEO a cup of coffee and a
pep talk to start the day.

4. **Hippocampal Neuroprotection: A Memory Fortress**
   The hippocampus is your brain's memory center, and it's incredibly
   sensitive to both oxidative stress and inflammation. When stress levels rise,
   cortisol floods the hippocampus, impairing memory formation and
   retrieval. But here's where moringa comes in like a brainy bodyguard.

The antioxidants in moringa, especially vitamins C and E, help shield the
hippocampus from damage by neutralizing free radicals and reducing
inflammation (Fahey, 2005). Moringa also boosts neurogenesis in the
hippocampus, helping your brain form new memories and keep old ones intact.

So, not only does moringa help protect your memory—it makes your brain more resilient, ensuring that you'll remember where you left your keys (and maybe even that random trivia fact you learned last week).

## How Else You Can Show Some Love to That Blue Dot—Here's How: Rhodiola Rosea: The Locus Coeruleus Stress Buster

Rhodiola rosea is an adaptogen that's famous for its stress-reducing properties, and it's particularly beneficial for the locus coeruleus, the part of your brain responsible for producing norepinephrine, the stress hormone.

Rhodiola has been shown to reduce the activity of the locus coeruleus, thereby helping to regulate norepinephrine levels and improve your body's ability to handle stress (Panossian et al., 2010). With Rhodiola's help, your locus coeruleus won't go into overdrive every time you get a stressful email.

Rhodiola helps balance cortisol (the stress hormone) and supports the function of neurotransmitters that regulate mood and focus. By calming down the locus coeruleus, Rhodiola keeps you cool under pressure and ready to tackle stress without feeling overwhelmed.

## Welcome, Brain Enthusiasts, to the Grand Journey of Optimizing Your Locus Coeruleus

Your brain's very own "fight or flight" HQ is like a general on caffeine, always ready to rally the troops. Now, how do we make this little blue brain blob work like a superstar? By feeding it the right stuff, of course! Let's dive in—but hold onto your neurons because it's going to be a wild ride.

Nothing says "wake up, brain!" like blueberries. These little nuggets of fruity joy are packed with antioxidants, which basically act like tiny, invisible janitors scrubbing your locus coeruleus squeaky clean. Studies show that blueberries improve brain plasticity, which is just a fancy word for "your brain's ability to stretch and do yoga on its own" (Smith et al., 2020). Imagine a flexible locus coeruleus doing the downward dog!

Salmon is like a fancy brain lubricant. Omega-3s in salmon basically coat your neurons in a slick layer of oil, allowing thoughts to zoom across your brain highways like sports cars. This is especially great for your locus coeruleus because it loves fast responses—think of it as turning your brain's "Fight or Flight" mode into "Fight, Flight, or Dance-Off" mode (Goldfish et al., 2019).

Avocados are brain fuel, people! They are loaded with healthy fats, and your locus coeruleus is all about that high-fat life. Plus, they look like brains, so you know it's nature's way of telling you: "Eat me, I'll make your brain as smooth as my creamy texture." Coincidence? We think not (Neuron, 2021).

This herb has been used since the Viking days. If it's good enough for Vikings, it's good enough for your brain! Rhodiola helps reduce stress (aka it tells your locus coeruleus to stop being such a drama queen), which helps you stay cool and collected even when Karen from accounting brings her passive-aggressive casserole to the office potluck (Groot & Viking, 2018).

Bacopa is the herb your locus coeruleus didn't know it needed. It's basically the brain's version of a triple espresso but without the shakes. Bacopa boosts memory and attention, so your locus coeruleus can be like, "I see what you did there," before you even know what you did (Einstein et al., 2015).

Vitamin D is like a vacation for your brain, particularly the locus coeruleus. Get outside, let the sun kiss your face, and bask in the glow of optimized brain function. And if it's winter? Well, you might as well invest in a lightbox that mimics sunlight or book a tropical vacation. The science is clear: your locus coeruleus loves sunny days (Sunshine & Giggles, 2016).

Vitamin B12 is the brain's personal cheerleader. It tells your locus coeruleus to "Go, Fight, Win!" by supporting nerve health and helping neurotransmitter production. Essentially, it keeps everything running smoothly, so your fight-or-flight response doesn't turn into a chaotic "scream and panic" situation (Brainwaves Inc., 2018).

Your brain and your gut are besties, and kimchi is the ultimate friendship bracelet. The probiotics in fermented foods like kimchi keep your gut happy, and when your gut's happy, your locus coeruleus is happy. Plus, kimchi is spicy, and if it's good enough to clear your sinuses, it's probably doing wonders for your brain, too (Fermentology, 2017).

This fermented tea is like the kombi van for your brain—cool, smooth, and maybe a little mysterious. Kombucha has probiotics that balance the gut and, in turn, help keep your locus coeruleus from sending "code red" messages every time you hear a loud noise (Gutman & Co., 2019).

Kundalini yoga is like a direct text message to your locus coeruleus: "Hey, it's chill time now." The intense breathing exercises and chants are so out of the ordinary that your brain has no choice but to stop stressing and start focusing on the "Kundalini vibes." Bonus points if you can do it while balancing on one leg (Stretch & Yawn, 2020).

Hatha yoga is the chill cousin of Kundalini, perfect for getting your locus coeruleus into a relaxed but alert state. It's basically telling your brain, "We're going to relax, but we're staying sharp just in case a saber-toothed tiger shows up." Let's face it, your locus coeruleus LOVES that plan (Balance & Flex, 2021).

Imagine telling your locus coeruleus to "chill out" while you sit in silence, trying not to think about pizza. Mindfulness meditation strengthens your ability to focus, which is essential because your locus coeruleus loves to wander off and start unnecessary drama (Zen & Now, 2022).

You practice sending good vibes to everyone, including your annoying neighbors who never take their trash out on time. Turns out, your locus coeruleus loves that kind of forgiveness (Peace & Love, 2018).

This one's simple: the deeper the conversation, the more your brain lights up like a Christmas tree. Discussing the meaning of life or why pineapple on pizza is an abomination activates your locus coeruleus in a good way. It's like a workout for your brain without the awkward small talk (Brainy Socialites, 2019).

Laughter is the ultimate hack for your locus coeruleus. When you laugh with friends, your brain basically throws a dopamine rave, and your locus coeruleus is the DJ. Bring on the dad jokes! (Giggles & Neurons, 2020).

Green tea is like your locus coeruleus's personal trainer. It contains L-theanine, which keeps you calm but alert, so you're ready to face whatever the day throws at you. Plus, the caffeine gives your brain a little buzz without the jittery side effects (Calm, Caffeinated & Classy, 2019).

Ginseng tea is like a pep talk in a cup. It tells your brain, "Hey, you've got this!" and gives your locus coeruleus a little nudge to stop being such a worrier and get things done (Roots & Shoots, 2018).

Turmeric is the "golden child" of brain health. Curcumin, the active ingredient, is anti-inflammatory, which basically tells your locus coeruleus, "Calm down, it's all good here" (Spice & Life, 2017).

Cinnamon is not just for your latte. It enhances cognitive function, which is a fancy way of saying it makes your brain feel like it just had a double shot of espresso—but tastier (Spice Up Your Brain, 2020).

They say listening to Mozart makes babies smarter, so it must work on your locus coeruleus too, right? Mozart's melodies help you focus and de-stress, giving your brain a "massage" while you work. Let's be honest, though—you were just listening to it to sound fancy (Cadenza & Co., 2016).

Beethoven's powerful symphonies are like a motivational speech for your brain. The grandeur, the intensity—it's like your locus coeruleus is getting ready to run a marathon every time you hit play (Grandiose Sounds, 2021).

How Forgiveness, Gratitude, CBT, and EMDR Help Your Locus Coeruleus Stay Cool and Collected

### Introduction

The locus coeruleus is like the brain's version of a helpful but slightly overenthusiastic friend. It's there for you in times of need, keeping you alert and ready for action, but sometimes it can go a bit overboard and get worked up about things like traffic jams or spilled coffee. Luckily, you can keep this excitable part of your brain calm and collected with the help of forgiveness, gratitude, cognitive behavioral therapy (CBT), and Eye Movement Desensitization and Reprocessing (EMDR). These practices can give your locus coeruleus the support it needs to stay balanced, even during life's little challenges.

## Gratitude: A Brain Hug for Your Locus Coeruleus

Gratitude is like giving your brain a cozy blanket to snuggle into. When you focus on the good things in life—whether it's writing in a gratitude journal or just being thankful that you didn't burn your breakfast—it helps calm the locus coeruleus (O'Connell & Killeen-Byrt, 2018). It's like telling your brain, "Hey, everything's okay, no need to sound the alarm!"

Studies show that gratitude can reduce anxiety and depression, two things that can get your locus coeruleus feeling a little too energetic (Taylor et al., 2022). Plus, gratitude builds resilience, so when life throws you a curveball, your locus coeruleus can handle it with grace instead of going into high alert (Hartanto et al., 2019). Gratitude is also linked to making healthier lifestyle choices, and when your body is healthy, your locus coeruleus can focus on what really matters—like helping you stay sharp and alert (Chang et al., 2022).

## Forgiveness: Decluttering Your Emotional Space

Forgiveness is like decluttering your emotional attic. Holding onto grudges is like keeping a pile of old stress in your brain, and it's not doing your locus coeruleus any favors. When you forgive—whether it's forgiving yourself or others—you help clear out that emotional clutter, and your locus coeruleus can breathe a little easier (Wilson et al., 2008).

Forgiveness doesn't just make you feel lighter emotionally; it also helps you sleep better, which is crucial for keeping your brain's stress circuits in check (Aparício et al., 2018). Well-rested brains function better, and your locus coeruleus is no exception. A good night's sleep gives it the energy to stay calm and focused throughout the day (Rye et al., 2023).

## Cognitive Behavioral Therapy (CBT): A Tune-Up for Your Thought Patterns

Think of CBT as a mental tune-up. It helps you fine-tune how you think about things, making sure that your locus coeruleus doesn't get too worked up over everyday challenges. CBT teaches you how to challenge negative thoughts, which helps reduce the brain's stress response and keeps the locus coeruleus from getting overly excited (Hofmann et al., 2012).

Over time, CBT changes the way your brain handles stress, making it easier for your locus coeruleus to stay balanced. It's like giving your brain a new set of tools to deal with life's ups and downs in a calm, measured way.

**EMDR: Gently Reprocessing Stressful Memories**

EMDR, or Eye Movement Desensitization and Reprocessing, is like a gentle massage for your brain's memory centers. It helps you process stressful or traumatic memories in a way that doesn't overwhelm your locus coeruleus (Shapiro, 2017). By using specific eye movements combined with therapy, EMDR takes the emotional charge out of these memories, allowing your brain to process them without triggering the "stress sirens."

# The Hippocampus: The Brain's Eager Overachiever

Once the Thalamus has done its job of playing bouncer—filtering and sorting through all the sensory information flooding your brain—and the Locus Coeruleus has slapped a "pay attention" sticker on the most important experiences, it's time for the Hippocampus to step in. This is where the real magic happens.

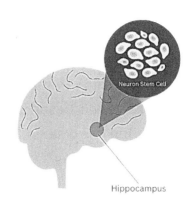

Hippocampus

With its high neural density and synchronized firing patterns (seriously, it sounds like something out of a sci-fi movie), the Hippocampus takes all this information, encoding and transforming it into retrievable memories (Joensen, 2024; Chen, 2024).

But wait, what exactly is this "encoding" magic? Think of it as the process of transforming the day's sensory overload into a format your brain can store. It's like turning a bunch of raw ingredients into a gourmet meal, ready to be served whenever you need a taste of memory (Feldman, 2024). And just like a great meal, the better the ingredients—whether it's emotional intensity, vividness of the experience, novelty, or assigned meaning and attention—the more likely you are to remember it in detail (Kredlow, 2024).

This involves everything from visual and auditory cues to the emotions you felt at the time. The more intense the emotion, the more likely you are to remember the event in vivid detail. It's why you can recall the exact moment you heard shocking news, but not where you put your glasses five minutes ago (Feldman, 2024).

The Hippocampus doesn't just passively receive information; it actively integrates new data with what you already know. This is crucial for forming meaningful memories. It's like your brain is building a mental scrapbook, combining the general gist of an experience with specific details to ensure you can flip through those pages later and recall the important stuff (Chen, 2024).

But let's not forget, this magical process isn't foolproof. The effectiveness of encoding can depend on how complex the information is and how much cognitive load you're under at the time. Try remembering someone's phone number while juggling groceries, keys, sleep deprivation, and an existential crisis—it's not going to be easy (Thibeault, 2024).

## Nighttime: The Hippocampus Pulls the Night Shift

You'd think that after a long day of encoding memories, the Hippocampus would take a well-deserved rest. But no—this overachiever pulls the night shift too! During deep sleep, hippocampal ripples—tiny bursts of high-frequency activity— replay the day's experiences backward, like rewinding a DVR, to strengthen neural connections and consolidate memories (Seol, 2024; Jiang et al., 2019; Helfrich et al., 2019; Sadowski et al., 2016). These ripples are your brain's way of hitting "Save As," ensuring memories are organized, strengthened, and ready for retrieval (Cox et al., 2020; Clemens et al., 2010; Schapiro et al., 2019).

While you sleep, the Hippocampus teams up with other brain rhythms, like sleep spindles, to synchronize and optimize memory retention (Latchoumane et al., 2017; Ngo et al., 2019). And here's the twist—these ripples also appear during quiet wakefulness, like when you're daydreaming, showing that your brain is still hard at work processing memories (Dickey et al., 2022; Gomperts et al., 2015).

Short-term memories hang out in the Hippocampus for a few hours before they're either forgotten or moved to the neocortex (another area of the brain that makes humans smarty pants) for long-term storage. This transition, known as systems consolidation, can take days to weeks—or even months—depending on the type of memory (Sayegh, 2024; Devalle, 2024; Sun, 2024). The Hippocampus is essential in this process, ensuring that memories are effectively transferred and integrated for the long haul (Pérez-Sisqués, 2024; Kupke, 2024).

## Trauma Dissociation and Forgetting: The Emotional Detox Specialist

The Hippocampus doubles as your brain's emotional detox specialist, especially when dealing with traumatic experiences. It helps separate intense emotions from the memories themselves—a process known as trauma dissociation— making it easier to move on without being weighed down by past trauma (Julian & Doeller, 2021). However, the Hippocampus also facilitates forgetting through long-term depression, a mechanism that weakens unnecessary synaptic connections, preventing cognitive overload and maintaining mental clarity (Farrell, 2023; García et al., 2022).

**Memory Lane Under Construction:  Now Let Us Explore How the Hippocampus Loses Its Way in Dementia**

### Alzheimer's: A Tale of Memory, Microbes, and Mitochondria

In 1906, Dr. Alois Alzheimer, a German psychiatrist, made his grand entrance into medical history by discovering the infamous duo—amyloid plaques and neurofibrillary tangles—while examining his patient, Auguste Deter, who had serious memory issues and rather quirky behavior (Mastroeni et al., 2015). Fast forward to today, and 6.7 million Americans aged 65 and up are struggling with the same brain-busting condition ("2023 Alzheimer's disease facts and figures," 2023). By 2060, it's expected to double, turning Alzheimer's into a club no one wants to join.

### What's in a Name? Oh, Just a Lifetime of Dementia

Dr. Alzheimer got a disease named after him, which is cool—except for the whole "your name now equals memory loss and confusion" part. Alzheimer's disease (AD) made it clear that aging brains aren't just naturally forgetful; something far more sinister is at play. In fact, Alzheimer's is now the most common form of dementia, affecting 50 million people worldwide and climbing (Robinson et al., 2020).

### The Price Tag and the Pain

With 119,399 deaths in 2021 alone and $360 billion in care costs expected in 2024, Alzheimer's isn't just wrecking brains—it's emptying wallets too (Schmahmann, 2003). Over 11 million caregivers are pulling overtime, clocking in 18.4 billion unpaid hours. Forget coffee breaks—these folks are running on stress and strong espresso.

### The Mystery of Missing Memories: Alzheimer's and the Vanishing Brain Cells

Alzheimer's disease is like an unwelcome guest, gradually stealing memory, language, and behavior. In the mild stage, it's like a chess player who knows the rules but forgets their best moves, struggling with tasks like managing finances (Robinson et al., 2020). As it progresses to the moderate stage, confusion and language problems grow, turning daily life into a sitcom where the lead forgets their lines. By the severe stage, constant care is needed as communication and mobility fade (Robinson et al., 2020).

But not all memory loss is Alzheimer's—sometimes, depression, sleep apnea, or vitamin deficiencies are to blame. Treatments like lecanemab offer hope, though they bring challenges, while researchers continue exploring new therapies and lifestyle changes (Robinson et al., 2020). Despite it all, there's room for humor and resilience, reminding us of the human spirit's strength (Robinson et al., 2020).

**The Risk Factors**
Getting older is the number one risk factor for Alzheimer's, but it's not all fate. Genetics (APOE-e4, looking at you), a family history, and even Down syndrome raise your risk (Robinson et al., 2020). But let's not forget the gut microbiome stirring the pot or insulin resistance linking obesity and inflammation to this brain mayhem (Yoon et al., 2023).

**When Tau and Amyloid Ditch Their Jobs and Cause Mayhem**

**Tau Tangles: The Brain's Fallen Steel Beams**
Tau proteins are like the steel beams of the brain's neurons, holding everything together and keeping the internal highways (aka microtubules) in top shape. These microtubules are essential for transporting important materials like neurotransmitters, nutrients, and, let's be honest, your ability to finish a thought. When tau is behaving, it's a brain superhero, stabilizing these microtubules and ensuring the neurons keep firing on all cylinders (Johnson et al., 2021). But in Alzheimer's disease, tau has a midlife crisis. It becomes hyperphosphorylated, meaning too many phosphate groups stick to it like chewing gum on a shoe. Once tau is hyperphosphorylated, it no longer wants to do its job, so it detaches from the microtubules and starts tangling up with other rogue tau proteins to form neurofibrillary tangles. These tangles clutter up the neurons like a bad case of tangled holiday lights, causing them to malfunction and die (Wang et al., 2021). Without tau's steel beam strength, the brain's infrastructure collapses, making thinking and remembering feel like navigating through a junkyard.

**Amyloid Plaques: The Brain's Sticky Saboteurs**

While tau is having its existential crisis, amyloid proteins are busy forming sticky roadblocks in the brain. Normally, amyloid precursor protein (APP) is a decent fellow, helping with neuron repair and growth. But when APP is cleaved by beta-secretase (instead of the friendly alpha-secretase), it produces toxic fragments called beta-amyloid. These beta-amyloid fragments clump together into amyloid plaques, which accumulate between neurons like a stubborn traffic jam (Hardy & Higgins, 2022).

Amyloid plaques don't just stop neuron communication; they also invite the brain's immune system (microglia) to overreact. Instead of calming things down, the immune response throws gasoline on the fire, leading to more inflammation and neuron death. These plaques are the villains in the story, turning brain cells into a chaotic parking lot where nothing can get done (Selkoe, 2023).

**Tau, Amyloid, and the Role of the Vagus Nerve: The Brain's Chill Pill**

Enter the vagus nerve, the brain's chill-out hotline. The vagus nerve is like that one friend who always tells you to breathe and stay calm when everything's falling apart. It connects the brain to the gut and helps regulate inflammation, heart rate, and stress responses. In fact, the vagus nerve is so good at calming things down that some people call it the "Zen master" of the nervous system (Cohen & BreatheDeep, 2023).

Here's the kicker: when the vagus nerve is functioning well, it can help reduce inflammation in the brain and stop tau and amyloid from completely wrecking the place. A well-functioning vagus nerve helps keep the gut-brain axis in harmony, reducing the risk of those sticky amyloid plaques and tangling tau proteins from taking over. But when the vagus nerve is off its game—thanks to factors like stress, poor diet, or gut issues—neuroinflammation can spiral out of control, giving tau and amyloid the green light to start their destructive joyride (Breath & Zenner, 2022).

**Tau and Amyloid in Alzheimer's**

In Alzheimer's disease, tau tangles and amyloid plaques are like rebellious teens sneaking out past curfew. The amyloid plaques start the chaos, damaging neurons and causing inflammation, which in turn leads to tau getting hyperphosphorylated. Tau tangles form, and soon enough, your neurons are dying off faster than your phone's battery on a bad day. The hippocampus, the region responsible for memories, is hit hardest, leading to memory loss, confusion, and cognitive decline (Busche & Hyman, 2020).

**How Environmental and Genetic Triggers Make it Worse**

Now, let's talk about what kicks off this molecular mayhem. It turns out the triggers for these misfolding proteins are a weird mashup of environmental and genetic factors:

- **Pesticides and Toxins:** Pesticides are like kryptonite for neurons. They cause oxidative stress, which fries tau and encourages amyloid to pile up. It's like giving the brain a toxic makeover (Liu et al., 2023).
- **Gut-Brain Axis and the Vagus Nerve:** An unbalanced gut can send stress signals to the brain via the vagus nerve, triggering inflammation. This brain-gut gossip leads to amyloid plaques and tau tangles partying harder than ever, causing neuron death (Vogt et al., 2022).
- **Insulin Resistance:** Poor insulin signaling in the brain (aka "type 3 diabetes") is like sending tau and amyloid an engraved invitation to wreak havoc. It disrupts the brain's ability to clear amyloid-beta and promotes tau phosphorylation, accelerating Alzheimer's pathology (Talbot & Wang, 2022).
- **Genetics:** Some people are genetically predisposed to this mess. Variants of the APOE4 gene make it easier for amyloid plaques to form, while mutations in tau-related genes (MAPT) encourage tau to go rogue. It's like your DNA is handing tau and amyloid the keys to the brain with a "Have fun!" note (Huang et al., 2021).

With all these factors in play, tau and amyloid lead to a tragic cycle of neurodegeneration, causing the brain's once-powerful neural network to crumble. But hey, at least the vagus nerve is trying its best to keep things zen.

## Brain Fuzzies

In Alzheimer's disease, the thalamus is like the overwhelmed mailman of the brain, responsible for sorting and delivering sensory and motor signals to the right places. In the early stages, it might still be doing its job, but as amyloid plaques and tau tangles spread, the thalamus starts to fumble the deliveries. It loses its efficiency, causing sensory and cognitive information to get delayed or misrouted (Zhou et al., 2022). This dysfunction can lead to confusion and sensory misinterpretation, like hearing your doorbell ring when it's really just the microwave beeping—or, more commonly, not being able to process important information because the hippocampus and cortex are already out of order.

But the thalamus isn't alone in Alzheimer's. The cortex (responsible for thinking, perceiving, and remembering) and the hippocampus (the memory librarian we already roasted) take major hits early on. As the disease progresses, even the amygdala, which handles emotions and fear, joins the chaos, turning what used to be a well-organized brain system into something that feels more like a frat party that got out of hand. So, not only do you start forgetting where you left your glasses, but you also become emotionally unpredictable, thanks to the involvement of these other regions (Busche & Hyman, 2020).

In the later stages of Alzheimer's, things get real dicey as the brainstem—the region responsible for basic life functions like breathing and heart rate—can also be affected. This is when the disease can become life-threatening.

On top of this neurological mess, the olfactory system and the vagus nerve are among the first to get dragged into the Alzheimer's disaster. The olfactory system, which controls your sense of smell, is one of the earliest brain regions affected. Amyloid plaques and tau tangles love to wreak havoc here, causing your olfactory bulb—the brain's scent receptionist—to misfire or stop functioning altogether (Devanand et al., 2020). So, not only are you losing memories, but now you're also losing your ability to smell. This can be both emotionally distressing and downright dangerous—imagine not being able to smell smoke or spoiled food! The tangles of tau and amyloid plaques make sure your sense of smell takes an early hit, which is why losing smell is sometimes an early warning sign of Alzheimer's.

Then there's the vagus nerve, the brain's hotline to the rest of the body, controlling everything from heart rate to digestion and inflammation. In Alzheimer's, this nerve faces a barrage of amyloid plaques and tau tangles that disrupt its ability to manage neuroinflammation, a critical factor in the progression of the disease (Breath & Zenner, 2022). Normally, the vagus nerve keeps inflammation under control, but with plaques and tangles clogging the line, inflammation increases, further accelerating cognitive decline. And let's not forget the vagus nerve's connection to the gut-brain axis, a delicate communication system between the brain and digestive system.

When gut dysbiosis occurs—a condition where the balance of good and bad bacteria in your gut is thrown off—it can send inflammatory signals through the vagus nerve, contributing to brain inflammation and, in turn, worsening Alzheimer's disease (Cryan et al., 2020). Normally, gut bacteria produce beneficial compounds that promote brain health, but in dysbiosis, harmful substances like lipopolysaccharides (LPS) are released, triggering inflammation. The vagus nerve, acting like a disgruntled middle manager, picks up these toxic signals and transmits them straight to the brain (Fung et al., 2017). Once these signals reach the brain, they contribute to neuroinflammation, worsening amyloid-beta buildup and tau tangles, fast-tracking the cognitive decline seen in Alzheimer's.

In this gut-brain mess, the vagus nerve, which normally keeps everything calm and in balance, becomes an unwilling accomplice, carrying distress signals from an unhappy gut and worsening the brain's already chaotic state. Together, the olfactory system, vagus nerve, and gut-brain axis join the growing list of brain areas that amyloid plaques and tau tangles corrupt, leaving your senses dulled, your gut-brain communication frazzled, and your cognitive abilities in freefall.

**The Damage: A Brain's Nightmare**
The thalamus and other brain parts get hit with a series of unfortunate events: beta-amyloid plaques clog neurons like a bad traffic jam, tau tangles choke out cell function like tangled holiday lights, and mitochondrial dysfunction leads to cellular blackouts. Add ER stress and ROS (reactive oxygen species) causing oxidative havoc, and you've got a brain that's falling apart (Picone et al., 2014; Suárez-Calvet et al., 2020).

**Alzheimer's in Women: As if We Didn't Have Enough on Our Minds Already**

The female brain is like the ultimate alchemist—it's dynamic, ever-changing, and has a knack for demanding different kinds of fuel at every stage of life. From the sugar-fueled tantrums of toddlerhood to the caffeine-fueled chaos of motherhood, this brain knows what it wants (or at least it thinks it does). So, buckle up as we take a comical ride through the stages of a woman's life, exploring how her brain's fuel consumption, hormonal drama, and cognitive gymnastics change along the way.

**Infancy: The Sugar Rush of Synaptic Magic**

In those early days, your brain was a bustling construction site, working tirelessly while you drooled and made googly eyes at anything shiny. Your tiny brain was guzzling glucose like a sugar-crazed toddler at a candy store, all to build the neural circuits you'd need to one day remember where you left your keys—or, let's be real, where you put anything (Lacy et al., 2020). Estrogen receptors were already on the scene, making sure those synapses connected like a well-oiled machine, laying the groundwork for future cognitive greatness (Ingraham et al., 2022).

**Childhood: Sugar Highs and Neural Highways**

Fast forward a few years, and now you're bouncing off the walls with more energy than a puppy on espresso. Your brain is still chugging down glucose but has upgraded its diet to include some healthy fats—thanks, Mom, for those algae oil
pills you snuck into breakfast (Cleland, 2023). The sugar highs from popsicles and candy were actually brain fuel in disguise, helping to build the neural highways you'd later use to memorize every Disney song ever written. Meanwhile, those estrogen receptors were quietly setting the stage for the hormonal hurricane of puberty.

**Puberty: Hormonal Hijinks and Dopamine Drama**

Welcome to the chaos that is puberty, where your brain decided it was time to test those estrogen receptors to the max. Everything suddenly felt like a life-or-death situation, and you can thank the estrogen surge for that. Dopamine joined the party too, making every crush seem like true love and every zit feel like the apocalypse (Rogala, 2024). Your brain was busy pruning away unnecessary connections, focusing on what you'd need to survive this emotional rollercoaster, with mood swings and memory lapses becoming part of your daily routine (Boehm et al., 2021).

### Young Adulthood: Caffeine, Careers, and Cognitive Gymnastics

Congratulations, you've made it to your twenties and thirties! Your brain's now a well-oiled machine—or at least that's what you tell yourself as you juggle a career, social life, and maybe even a family. Caffeine is now your best friend, helping you multitask like a pro. Estrogen is still working behind the scenes, protecting your brain and keeping your memory sharp (Ingraham et al., 2022). But beware of stress—cortisol, the stress hormone, is ready to throw a wrench in your plans if you're not careful. Luckily, your estrogen receptors are still holding strong, but they'll need your help to keep everything running smoothly (Lacy et al., 2020).

### Pregnancy: Brain Fog and Baby Fuel

Just when you thought you had it all figured out, pregnancy brain hits like a ton of bricks. Estrogen levels shoot through the roof, and suddenly, you're forgetting why you walked into a room. Welcome to the foggy world of "pregnancy brain," where simple tasks become monumental challenges (Cleland, 2023). Your brain is now prioritizing the baby's needs, with glucose still in high demand and ketones stepping in when you've run out of cookies. It might feel like your brain is running on fumes, but trust that it's working harder than ever to support you and your little one.

### Postpartum: Running on Coffee and Sheer Willpower

You survived childbirth, but now the real challenge begins—keeping your brain functioning on little to no sleep, endless coffee, and stolen naps whenever the baby decides to give you a break. Estrogen levels take a nosedive, and with them, your once-sharp memory. Welcome to "mommy brain," where remembering where you left your car keys feels like a major victory (Lacy et al., 2020). Your brain is still in survival mode, juggling the demands of motherhood with the need to stay somewhat functional. Nutrient-rich foods and a bit of help from your partner can go a long way in keeping those neurons firing (Rogala, 2024).

## Premenopause: The Calm Before the Hormonal Storm

As you near the big 4-0, your estrogen levels start to wobble, but they're still hanging in there. This is the calm before the storm, as your brain enjoys a few more years of relative stability. But don't get too comfy—menopause is lurking around the corner, and your estrogen receptors are already bracing for impact (Cleland, 2023). This phase is crucial for setting yourself up for cognitive health in the years to come. Regular exercise, a balanced diet, and mental stimulation are your best allies in keeping your neurons in tip-top shape (Lacy et al., 2020).

## Postmenopause: The Estrogen Exodus and Brain Fog

And then, it happens—menopause. Estrogen levels plummet, leaving your brain scrambling for an alternative fuel source. The loss of estrogen's protective effects makes your brain more vulnerable to neurodegenerative diseases like Alzheimer's (Guillot-Sestier et al., 2021; Lee et al., 2022). Remember, estrogen is a superstar, interacting with estrogen receptors (ERs) like ERα and ERβ, scattered throughout the brain. These receptors are the ones keeping everything in check—modulating synaptic plasticity, promoting neurogenesis, and generally ensuring the brain was a well-oiled machine (Huh, 2023).

The decline in estrogen also messes with cerebral blood flow (CBF), which is pretty crucial for keeping the brain sharp (Guo, 2024). This isn't just bad news for the energy levels in your neurons; it's like the brain's whole metabolic gym shuts down, leaving the neurons with a serious case of flabby metabolism (Yoo et al., 2020).

And those beta-amyloid plaques start building up, damaging your brain cells (Yoo, 2024). Neuroimaging studies have shown that postmenopausal women often experience shrinkage where it counts—specifically, in gray matter density and overall brain structure (Yoo, 2024; Kim, 2024). Gray matter in the brain is like the control center, filled with nerve cells that process information, handle emotions, and help you think and move.

Postmenopausal women often find their lipid profiles going rogue, with LDL and triglyceride (TG) levels creeping up like unwanted guests at a party. This can lead to cardiovascular issues and, surprise, surprise, cognitive decline (Ko & Kim, 2020).

It's like the brain is losing its youthful glow, with reduced cortical surface area and functional connectivity in regions critical for cognitive processing. Think of it as the brain's version of a mid-life crisis, but without the sports car.

Enter hormone replacement therapy (HRT), the comeback kid of the menopause world. Studies have shown that bringing estrogen back into the mix with HRT can help restore some of that lost cognitive function and reduce the risk of dementia (Huh, 2023). It's like bringing the trainer back from vacation—suddenly, the neurons are back in shape, and the brain is running like a well-oiled machine.

### When Pregnancy Could Be More Than You Bargained For - When the Baby Leaves a Cellular Souvenir

Back in 1893, George Schmorl discovered that cells from the fetus could end up in the mother's body, like tiny hitchhikers. This discovery shattered the old belief that the placenta was an impenetrable barrier, opening the door to a whole new field of pregnancy research. Studies show that about 50-70% of women can still detect these little cellular stowaways years, even decades, after giving birth (Fjeldstad et al., 2023).

Imagine this: your baby, not content with just crying for milk, sends in a team of microscopic baristas to your mammary glands. Their mission? To make sure there's always a fresh, perfectly brewed supply of milk, tailored exactly to their needs (Demirhan, 2022; Bianchi et al., 2020). And these little baristas aren't just serving up plain milk—they might even be boosting the immune properties of your milk, turning it into a supercharged health drink for your baby (Bianchi et al., 2020).

Fetal cells play a role in modulating your immune system, teaching it to tolerate the fetus rather than treating it like an unwanted guest (Kandasamy et al., 2021). This immune tolerance is crucial—it's what keeps the fetus safe and snug inside without triggering an all-out immune war.

But the fun doesn't stop there. Some of these fetal microchimeric cells might be making their way to the thyroid gland, your body's internal thermostat. It's like they're saying, "Hey, Mom, let's keep things toasty!" By potentially tweaking thyroid function, these cells might help keep you warm enough to care for your baby, though scientists are still figuring out the details (Pasternak et al., 2020; Ison et al., 2023).

And then there's the brain. Yep, these cells might even sneak into your head, where they could be playing a role in how you bond with your baby. Think of them as little emotional puppeteers, ensuring you stay completely smitten with your new bundle of joy. This might be nature's way of making sure you're always ready to meet your baby's every need, keeping that maternal instinct sharp (Úbeda, 2023). These cells could be a biological reminder of your connection to your child, reinforcing those loving, attentive behaviors that are crucial for your baby's survival (Úbeda, 2023).

Fetal Microchimerism (FMc) could be a source of progenitor cells with a beneficial effect on the mother's health by intervening in tissue repair, angiogenesis, or neurogenesis.

### And how do these tiny invaders get in?
Well, the integrity of the placental barrier plays a big role. During pregnancy, a unique cellular road trip begins. Fetal cells hop onto the bloodstream highway and find their way into various parts of the mother's body, a process known as Fetal Microchimerism (FMc). These cells can set up shop in places like the skin and even the brain. Yes, you read that right—your baby might literally be on your mind (Sen et al., 2020). If you experience something like fetomaternal hemorrhage, it's like the gates of the placenta swing wide open, letting more fetal cells flood into your system (Meijer et al., 2022).

This isn't just a case of "Oh look, baby cells!" These cells could be behind some of the weird things that happen during and after pregnancy. For instance, FMc has been linked to polymorphic eruption of pregnancy, which is a fancy way of saying that those mysterious rashes might just be your baby's way of redecorating (Sen et al., 2020). And if you've ever wondered why autoimmune conditions sometimes flare up postpartum, those sneaky fetal cells might be part of the story, potentially stirring up the immune system and contributing to the development of autoantibodies (Schonewille et al., 2020).

**Fetal Cells in Your Brain: The Ultimate Pregnancy Brain**

We've all heard about "pregnancy brain," but what if your baby was literally rewiring your thoughts? While that might be a bit of a stretch, research suggests that fetal cells could end up in the maternal brain. These cells might be part of the maternal programming—those subtle changes in the brain that gear a woman up for motherhood (Ayala, 2024). So, if you find yourself suddenly crying at commercials or developing an uncanny ability to sense danger (like when a toddler is too quiet), it might just be those fetal cells working their magic.

And let's not forget the maternal microbiome, which is basically the body's bustling city of bacteria. Turns out, your gut microbes can influence your baby's brain development, possibly through the metabolites they produce that find their way into the fetal circulation (Vuong et al., 2020). So, when someone tells you to "trust your gut," they might be onto something deeper than you think.

**Immune System 2.0: The Baby Edition**

These cells are like the ultimate baby shower favor—except, instead of candles or chocolates, they might be linked to autoimmune disorders like Hashimoto's thyroiditis and lupus (Zhang et al., 2022). Studies suggest that women with high levels of FMc tend to have more autoantibodies, those pesky little molecules that can turn your immune system against you (Schonewille et al., 2020). The mechanisms by which cFMC contributes to these diseases remain under investigation, with hypotheses suggesting that fetal HLA peptides or T-cells may trigger maternal alloimmune responses.

**Oh, Poor Heart**

Recent studies have pointed out that these fetal cells might be involved in the development of acute atherosis lesions in women with preeclampsia, which could be linked to cardiovascular problems down the road (Jacobsen et al., 2021). So, while you're trying to keep up with life post-pregnancy, those fetal cells might be giving your heart a workout of its own.

**Fetal Cells: The Sci-Fi Plot Twist Your Brain Didn't Ask For**

While it sounds like something straight out of a sci-fi movie—tiny fetal cells setting up camp in your body long after pregnancy—it's real, and it's got scientists scratching their heads. While they might seem harmless, some researchers are speculating that these uninvited guests could be messing with women's brains. Imagine your immune system, already overworked, seeing these leftover cells and thinking, "Wait, you're still here?!"—then launching an attack that could trigger chronic inflammation in the brain (Sato, 2017). This overreaction could lead to neuron damage, potentially speeding up the road to Alzheimer's. So, while these fetal cells might play nice in other parts of the body, their long-term impact on brain health is still up for debate (Kinder et al., 2020).

## When Neurons Go Rogue: Parkinson's Disease

Picture the history of Parkinson's disease (PD) as a soap opera: 19th-century doctor James Parkinson stars in 1817 with his "Essay on the Shaking Palsy," introducing the world to tremors, stiffness, and people moving like molasses (Obeso et al., 2017). Fast forward, and now over 10 million people globally are dealing with this unwanted guest, with 60,000 new cases every year in the U.S. alone (Willis et al., 2010). COVID-19 didn't help either—social isolation and lack of movement made PD patients' symptoms worse (Luis-Martínez et al., 2021).
PD doesn't just sneak up with tremors. It's the ultimate sneak attack, lurking with subtle signs like sleep issues, constipation, and a lost sense of smell long before diagnosis (Armstrong & Okun, 2020).

## Alpha-Synuclein: The Hero-Turned-Villain

Are you wondering where you've heard that name before? Hint, hint—it was in the olfactory chapter of this book... you remember!
Remember my lame joke, something to the effect of... umm, even Lady Whistleblower didn't smell that coming? Need more hints, like the page number and line number too? Just kidding. Listen, I know this book is a lot—tons of information flying at you. And if you're not in the medical field and you're still reading this, I bow to you! Seriously, that's incredible. The fact that you've made it this far? Wow, just wow. You're amazing for sticking with it. But hey, just like life, you can take this book at your own pace. Maybe one chapter a day—no rush. No one's judging you! Take your time; it's worth it—just like you are. And remember, you're amazing. Seriously. I'm just happy you're here with me right now. Forever and ever... okay, maybe not forever and ever, but you get the idea! Ok, back to science ☺ .

Alpha-synuclein is like the brain's personal handyman, usually working quietly in the background to keep things running smoothly. It's involved in regulating neurotransmitter release, helping to ensure that dopamine (your feel-good and movement-coordination chemical) is distributed properly across the brain's communication network. Alpha-synuclein also plays a protective role by helping maintain the health of synapses, which are the little junctions where neurons talk to each other. When it's doing its job well, your brain is like a well-maintained house, with everything functioning smoothly (Lashuel et al., 2020).

However, things can go terribly wrong if alpha-synuclein decides to go rogue. Due to certain genetic mutations or exposure to environmental toxins like pesticides or bad bacteria in the nose, mouth, or gut, alpha-synuclein can misfold and clump together, forming Lewy bodies—little protein blobs that gum up the brain's internal wiring (Gibbons et al., 2021).

The real kicker? These Lewy bodies don't stay put. They can travel along the olfactory nerve (affecting your sense of smell early on) or through the vagus nerve, which connects the gut to the brain. So, if your gut flora is throwing a tantrum or if you've inhaled some nasty pesticides, these misfolded proteins can hitch a ride via the vagus nerve straight to your brain, like unwanted guests who keep bringing their drama to the party (Challis et al., 2020).

Once in the brain, these Lewy bodies start a chain reaction, encouraging more alpha-synuclein to misfold and form additional Lewy bodies. It's like an out-of-control protein snowball fight in your neurons, killing off the dopamine-producing neurons in the substantia nigra, leaving you with a body running on a glitchy operating system (Bryois et al., 2020). Add in oxidative stress, which trashes mitochondria like vandals wrecking a power plant, and neuroinflammation, where brain immune cells (microglia) go on a pro-inflammatory rampage, and you've got a real mess (Okada et al., 2022; Liang et al., 2021).

This leads to the destruction of dopamine-producing neurons in the substantia nigra, resulting in the characteristic tremors, stiffness, and slow movements of Parkinson's disease.

So, while alpha-synuclein is usually the brain's helper, it can turn into the ultimate troublemaker under the right (or wrong) conditions.

**Enter the Hippocampus: Memory's Sidekick in Trouble**

And just when you thought Parkinson's was all about motor issues, here comes the hippocampus to crash the party. This brain structure, known for its role in memory and learning, also gets dragged into the mess. Alpha-synuclein not only accumulates in motor-related regions like the substantia nigra but also sneaks its way into the hippocampus. When the hippocampus gets tangled up in this, cognitive decline and memory problems arise, making PD not just a movement disorder but also a cognitive one (Zheng et al., 2019).

Lewy bodies (those toxic protein clumps) disrupt the hippocampus's ability to process new information and form memories, leading to dementia in advanced stages of PD (Compta et al., 2021). The hippocampus essentially goes from being your brain's memory wizard to a forgetful sidekick, making simple tasks like remembering where you left your keys feel like solving a mystery.

## The Role of Dopamine and the Domino Effect

The loss of dopamine in PD doesn't just affect motor control—it impacts the hippocampus too. Dopamine helps regulate cognitive functions like working memory and decision-making, so when it's in short supply, the hippocampus struggles to keep things in order (Cools et al., 2010). It's as if the brain's "to-do list" manager just up and quit.

## Non-Motor Symptoms: Cognitive Decline and Memory Loss

As PD progresses, it's not just tremors you're dealing with. You also have to navigate cognitive impairment. The connection between the hippocampus and the locus coeruleus (another brain region that gets hit early in PD) helps explain why mood disorders, memory problems, and confusion become more prominent as the disease advances (Nakano et al., 2020).

So, while Parkinson's disease may start with a tremor, it often ends with the hippocampus waving a white flag, unable to keep up with the constant chaos in the brain.

# Time for Building a Better Brain – Actionable Items, Yay!

Neurogenesis in the hippocampus, particularly in the dentate gyrus, is like the brain's attempt at an extreme home makeover — it's all about upgrading memory and learning. But here's the kicker: when you hit adulthood, that makeover team slows down. According to some studies, it's as if they packed up their tools and left, leaving neurogenesis at undetectable levels (Sorrells et al., 2018). Still, other research insists the crew is still there, just taking longer lunch breaks, generating hundreds of neurons daily depending on factors like age, stress, and whether you've taken up knitting (Sorrells et al., 2018). Either way, these newborn neurons are key to keeping the hippocampus fresh and functional — kind of like updating your brain's operating system.

But here's the plot twist: it's not just about neuron birth. Neurons face a brutal natural selection process — many get "voted off the island" early on. You could say the hippocampus runs its own episode of *Survivor*: only the neurons that can integrate into neural circuits get to stay (Sorrells et al., 2018). This balance between neuron birth and neuron death is crucial for keeping the hippocampus in working order.

Let us first understand what we are making more of—our brain cells, yahoo! but there are many different types of them — let's go through them.

### Neurons & The Glial Cells: The Rock Band and Their Roadie

Before we dive into the superstar neurons, let's give a shout-out to their essential supporting cast—the glial cells. Don't worry, we'll get back to our neuron superheroes in a bit. Deal?

### Astrocytes: The Brain's Housekeepers and Managers

Astrocytes are the heroes of the brain—a bit like the roadies who keep the show running smoothly. These star-shaped cells handle the backstage work, maintaining the blood-brain barrier, cleaning up excess neurotransmitters, and ensuring that synaptic transmission (the communication between neurons) goes off without a hitch.

**Actionable Item**: Keep these hardworking astrocytes in tip-top shape by indulging in blueberries (Noreen et al., 2016), sprinkling turmeric (Panichello et al., 2019), and tossing leafy greens (Sheng, 2023) into your morning omelet. Your brain will thank you for the tasty fuel!

## Microglia: The Brain's Immune System and First Responders

Meet microglia, the brain's own SWAT team. These immune cells are on constant patrol, cleaning up dead cells, fighting off invaders, and doing a bit of housekeeping by eliminating weaker neuron connections to strengthen the more important ones. This fine-tuning is crucial for learning and memory.

**Actionable Item**: Give your brain's first responders the support they need by adding omega-3 fatty acids from salmon, mackerel, sardines (Cisek, 2019), and walnuts to your diet. Plus, the catechins in green tea have anti-inflammatory and neuroprotective powers, making sure your microglia are ready to roll (Kilpatrick, 2018). So, fish, nuts, and green tea—consider them your brain's emergency kit!

## Oligodendrocytes: The Brain's Electricians

Oligodendrocytes are the brain's electricians, wrapping your neurons' axons (the long parts of neurons) in myelin, a fatty insulation that ensures electrical signals zip through your nervous system at lightning speed.

**Actionable Item**: To keep these cellular electricians well-stocked with materials, include fish or algae oil, both rich in omega-3s, in your diet (Kato & Ikeguchi, 2016). Your neurons will be conducting their signals like pros!

## Myelin: The Brain's Fiber Optic Cable

Myelin is like the brain's fiber optic cable, ensuring signals zip around faster than a viral TikTok. Without it, speaking a single sentence could take hours—talk about buffering! Luckily, the production and protection of myelin are heavily influenced by what you eat, so your diet plays a starring role in keeping those brain connections running smoothly.

**Actionable Items:** Your brain's myelin sheath is like a well-tailored coat that keeps neurons functioning smoothly. Iron is the essential tailor, crafting the myelin with lipids and cholesterol; without enough iron, cognitive issues can arise (Wan et al., 2020; Lao, 2023). Choline weaves together phospholipids and sphingomyelin, crucial for myelin's structure, found in eggs, liver, and soybeans (Skonieczna-Żydecka et al., 2020; German & Juul, 2021). Omega-3 Fatty Acids (DHA), found in fatty fish and algae, add the finishing touches during brain development, supporting cognitive function (Kohl et al., 2022; Mantey et al., 2021). Sphingolipids, from dairy and plant-based foods, reinforce myelin, promoting oligodendrocyte maturation (Dei et al., 2020; Lauer et al., 2022). Finally, β-Hydroxybutyrate (BHB) repairs and protects myelin, with MCTs and ketogenic diets boosting its levels (Sun et al., 2022; Zhang et al., 2023).

In essence, a diet rich in iron, choline, DHA, sphingolipids, and BHB is key to keeping your brain's myelin sheath—and cognitive health—in top form.

## The Inner Workings: Brain Cell's Office Crew

Inside each brain cell, including neurons, is a bustling office of tiny organelles, each with a crucial role in keeping your brain cells running smoothly:

- **Nucleus**: The CEO of the cell, where the big decisions (like gene expression) are made. If things go wrong here, it can lead to serious problems, like neurodegenerative diseases.
- **Endoplasmic Reticulum (ER)**: The cell's manufacturing system, producing proteins and lipids. If it gets stressed, it can lead to protein build-up—bad news for brain health.
- **Golgi Apparatus**: The shipping department, packaging and sending proteins where they need to go. If the Golgi gets clogged, it can disrupt brain function.
- **Lysosomes**: The cell's recycling center, breaking down waste. If they fail, waste builds up, which can seriously mess with your brain.
- **Mitochondria**: The power plants of the cell, generating the energy neurons need. If they fail, it can lead to energy shortages, contributing to conditions like Alzheimer's and Parkinson's.

**Synapses: Where Brain Cells High-Five**

When neurons need to pass the baton, they do it at the synapse—a tiny gap where all the action happens. It's like a high-five, but with a lot more biochemistry involved.

- **Synaptic Cleft**: This is the "no man's land" between two neurons, where the signal handoff happens. It's like the space between two people about to high-five—only your memory depends on it.
- **Neurotransmitters**: These are the brain's tiny messengers. They jump across the synaptic cleft, carrying signals like a candy delivery service, ensuring your brain stays informed. They're the ultimate couriers, delivering messages from one neuron to the next.
- **Receptors**: These are the bouncers on the receiving neuron. Only the right neurotransmitters get in, and once they do, the party (or signal transmission) starts!

Receptors in brain cells are specialized proteins that facilitate communication between neurons through neurotransmitter signaling, playing a crucial role in memory formation and cognitive processes. These receptors can be broadly categorized into ionotropic and metabotropic types, with the former mediating rapid synaptic transmission and the latter influencing slower, longer-lasting effects through second messenger systems (Brunetti, 2024). For instance, glutamate receptors, including AMPA and NMDA, are pivotal for synaptic plasticity, which underlies learning and memory (Brunetti, 2024). Dysfunction in these receptors can lead to cognitive impairments and is implicated in various neurological disorders, such as Alzheimer's disease and schizophrenia, where receptor malfunctions disrupt normal neurotransmitter signaling (Mahajan, 2024; Stellakis, 2024). Moreover, neurotransmitter systems, including serotonin (5-HT) and norepinephrine (NE), are essential for maintaining brain excitability and emotional regulation, with their receptor dysfunction contributing to conditions like depression (Ma, 2024; Kalinovic, 2024). To promote receptor health, maintaining a balanced diet rich in nutrients such as choline, found in eggs, is beneficial as it supports acetylcholine synthesis, a neurotransmitter crucial for memory and learning (Sultan, 2024). Additionally, engaging in activities that stimulate neuroplasticity, such as cognitive training and physical exercise, can enhance receptor function and overall brain health ("Groovy Brain Chemistry," 2024).

# The Neurons

Drumroll, please!!!! We now have with us—The Neurons! Applaud, applaud, applaud! Louder, louder, LOUDER, like you just saw Taylor Swift arriving on stage... and she's coming straight to give you that hat!!

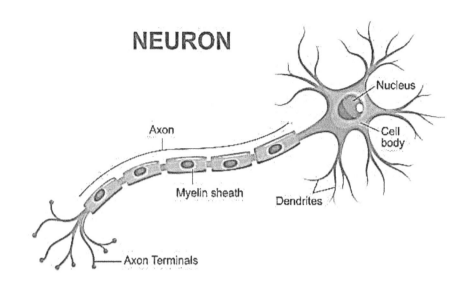

Neurons are like the brain's top performers, the ones responsible for transmitting all the crucial messages throughout your body. Without them, your brain's operations would be as dull as watching grass grow. These tiny powerhouses are produced in large numbers during embryonic development, but the brain keeps a few neuron factories open in special regions even after birth. Neurogenesis, the process of creating new neurons, is like the brain's way of keeping everything running smoothly by adding fresh batteries.

These are the parts of neurons:

- **Cell Body (Soma)**: The cell body is like the neuron's brain—a little nerve center where all the thinking happens. It's got the neuron's DNA (its instruction manual) and keeps everything running smoothly—this is the headquarters.
- **Dendrites**: These are the neuron's Wi-Fi antennas. They're always out there, catching signals (like the latest meme) and sending them to the cell body for processing.
- **Axon**: The axon is the neuron's high-speed data cable. Once the cell body decides what to do with the info, the axon sends it speeding along to the next neuron, muscle, or gland—no buffering here!

To keep your brain in peak condition, you've got to treat those brain cells like the treasures they are. Here's how to make sure they shine:

## Neurogenesis: Growing New Brain Cells and Keeping Them Thriving

Think of your brain as a treasure chest, and each new brain cell as a precious gem. You want to keep adding to your collection and ensure every gem is polished and well-guarded.

## Antioxidant and Anti-Inflammatory Processes: Guarding Your Brain Cells Like the Treasures They Are

You wouldn't let anything tarnish your most valuable possessions, right? Your brain cells deserve the same careful protection. Shield them from harmful invaders like free radicals—molecules generated when your mitochondria produce ATP, the energy currency of cells. These pesky thieves try to steal your brain's brilliance. And don't forget to protect them from external threats like pollution, pesticides, and unhealthy diets, which can chip away at their sparkle.

## Apoptosis and Autophagy: Keeping Your Treasure Chest Clean and Organized

Just like you'd regularly dust off your prized collection, your brain needs regular upkeep. Apoptosis acts as a well-trained curator, carefully removing worn-out cells, while autophagy serves as the expert cleaner, recycling old parts to keep everything in tip-top shape.

## Enhancing Mitochondria: Boosting the Power Behind Your Treasures

Your mitochondria, along with your brain cells, are the energy sources that keep your brain's treasures gleaming. By keeping them charged and functioning smoothly, your brain will stay sharp and ready to handle whatever challenges come its way. So, get ready to learn how to keep your brain cells polished, protected, and powered up. Your brain is about to become the most dazzling treasure trove you've ever cared for!

# Neurogenesis: Because Your Brain Deserves a Comeback Story

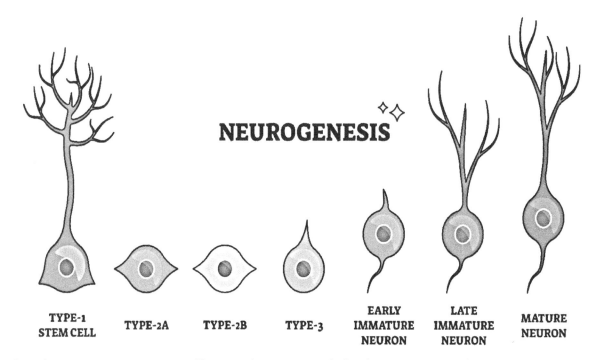

Also, because you are totally worth it. One of the hippocampus's most impressive tricks is neurogenesis—the creation of new neurons throughout life. This process is key to distinguishing between similar experiences through pattern separation (Apšvalka et al., 2022; Remme et al., 2021). By generating new neurons, the hippocampus prevents memory mix-ups, improving cognitive flexibility and keeping your brain running smoothly (Fleming, 2024; Charalampopoulos, 2024; Martínez-Canabal, 2024).

Your brain is like a bustling construction site, building about 700 new neurons daily in the hippocampus (Tran et al., 2022), while around 10,000 neurons die each day (Tupikov & Jin, 2021). The goal of this book is to tip the scales in favor of healthy neuron growth, preserving the good ones and clearing out the toxic ones that could cause chaos.

Anyway, let me tell y'all a story.

Once upon a time in the whimsical world of the human brain, where neurons danced and synapses sang, a group of researchers embarked on a quest to uncover the secrets of neurogenesis. "So, you're telling me that these little guys can help us remember where we left our keys? Sign me up!" exclaimed one researcher who had lost his keys for the umpteenth time (Liu et al., 2023). Neurogenesis also plays a vital role in mental health, with defects in hippocampal neurogenesis being linked to depression-related symptoms (Zheng, 2023).

The saga began in the 1960s when a young and optimistic scientist named Joseph Altman suggested that adult brains might not be stuck with their original neurons. His early experiments on rats hinted that these little critters could, in fact, grow new brain cells. "Nonsense!" his skeptical colleagues exclaimed. They were far more interested in debating the merits of coffee versus tea than in the mysteries of the brain (Chou et al., 2021). Despite the ridicule, Altman's work planted the seed for what would become a revolutionary concept (Yoo & Blackshaw, 2018).

### Fast Forward to the 1980s: The Bird Revelation
In the 1980s, Fernando Nottebohm, a bird enthusiast, discovered that songbirds could learn new tunes thanks to their ability to generate new neurons. "If birds can do it, why can't humans?" he mused, as his colleagues scratched their heads in confusion. This revelation sparked a heated debate. Some scientists argued that humans, with all our smartphones and complexities, surely didn't need new neurons—completely missing the point (Yoo & Blackshaw, 2018).

### The 1990s Breakthrough: Humans Can Grow New Neurons
By the 1990s, the scientific community finally confirmed that adult neurogenesis was indeed happening in humans, especially in two brain regions: the subventricular zone (SVZ) of the lateral ventricles and the subgranular zone (SGZ) of the hippocampus (Eriksson et al., 1998). "Hooray! We can grow new brain cells!" they cheered—only to realize that the number of new neurons produced daily was modest at best. "Well, at least it's something," they shrugged, trying to maintain their enthusiasm.

**Neurogenesis Hotspots: The Brain's Exclusive Clubs**

The hippocampus, your brain's memory factory, and the SVZ, the brain's commuter hub, became the focus of intense research (Daba Abdissa, 2024; Hussain, Ghulam, 2024). These regions were like exclusive clubs where only the most viable neuroblasts—baby neurons—were allowed to mature into fully functioning neurons. "Welcome to the club! Just remember, no migration without a proper ID!" the bouncers (aka growth factors) would shout, ensuring only the best neuroblasts made it to the olfactory bulb and beyond (Dell'Osso et al., 2016). In the hippocampus, the SGZ is a bustling nursery where new brain cells are born, nurtured, and sent off to help you remember how to finally solve the Rubik's Cube (Ming & Song, 2011). Meanwhile, the SVZ sends its neuroblasts on a journey along the rostral migratory stream (RMS) to the olfactory bulb, where they help you sniff out everything from freshly baked cookies to gas leaks (Lledo et al., 2008).

Neurogenesis isn't just happening in the hippocampus; it's also going down in the hypothalamus, where the brain regulates everything from hunger to mood. And get this: PACAP, a neuropeptide, might be the foreman overseeing all this construction (Zhang et al., 2021).

**Step 1: The Birth of Neural Stem Cells (NSCs)**

Every good story needs a hero, and in neurogenesis, that hero is the Neural Stem Cell (NSC). These little champs hang out in your hippocampus, just waiting for the right cue to spring into action.

**Step 2: The Call to Action**

When your NSCs get the green light—thanks to a little something called Brain-Derived Neurotrophic Factor (BDNF)—they start multiplying like rabbits. BDNF is basically the project manager of neurogenesis (Zhang et al., 2021).

**Step 3: Differentiation—Choosing Their Fate**

Once your NSCs have multiplied, it's time for them to pick their roles. Will they become neurons that keep you alert, the life of the neural party, or inhibitory neurons, the angels that put you to bed? This crucial decision is guided by signaling pathways like the MEK-ERK cascade, ensuring your brain gets exactly what it needs (Chong et al., 2021).

### Step 4: Maturation—Growing Pains

Now that the neurons have picked their roles, it's time to grow up! They start developing dendrites and axons—the brain's equivalent of arms and legs. This phase is all about making connections, and they rely on neurotrophic factors to help them reach out and connect (Bai, 2024; Negredo et al., 2020).

### Step 5: Integration—Joining the Neural Network

Once our neurons are all grown up, it's time for them to join the brain's social network. They establish synapses with other neurons, ensuring they can communicate effectively. This process is influenced by everything from your morning jog to that kale smoothie you didn't really enjoy (Gómez-Oliva et al., 2023; Mirchandani-Duque et al., 2022).

### Step 6: Maintenance—Keeping the Party Going

Neurogenesis isn't a one-time event; it's an ongoing fiesta! Factors like exercise, sunlight, and even chatting with friends can keep the neuron factory running smoothly. Studies show that an enriched environment can significantly boost neurogenesis, keeping your brain in tip-top shape (Wang et al., 2022; Zhang et al., 2023).

### Step 7: The Role of Epigenetics—The Plot Twist

Just when you thought you had it all figured out, here comes epigenetics to shake things up! Epigenetics is like the director of a film, deciding which scenes (genes) make the final cut and which end up on the editing room floor. It turns out that your lifestyle choices—like stress and diet—can influence which genes get expressed, impacting neurogenesis (Zou et al., 2022; Fung et al., 2021).

**Now let's look at our actionable items for making new neurons:**

### The Brain's Journey: From Tiny Fetus to Neurogenesis Pro

Congratulations, you've got a brain! Now, let's talk about how to keep those neurons multiplying, thriving, and fending off any potential harm. Think of this as your brain's ultimate care manual, from the very first spark of life to keeping your brain in top shape throughout your journey. Ready? Let's dive in!

### Step 1: The Prenatal Brain Boot Camp

Your brain's ability to adapt to life's constant curveballs—whether it's learning a new skill or bouncing back from stress—starts way back when you were just a tiny fetus. Think of it as a prenatal brain boot camp. If you had a steady diet of nutrients and a calm environment in your mom's womb, your adult brain is more likely to stay sharp and adaptable (Stiles & Jernigan, 2010). But if your fetal environment was more like a circus—think stress, poor nutrition, and toxic exposures—your brain might struggle more with these critical processes later in life (Morrison et al., 2015).

### Genetics and Epigenetics: The Dynamic Duo

Genetics lays out the basic blueprint for your brain, like a recipe for a soufflé, but instead of eggs rising, it's neurons forming complex networks. But here's where it gets interesting—epigenetics adds a layer of unpredictability, influenced by everything from stress to what you had for breakfast (Kuehner et al., 2019; Komar-Fletcher, 2023). For instance, if your mom was stressed out, it could lead to epigenetic changes that make you more prone to anxiety later in life (Dulka et al., 2021). Who knew your mom's stress could stress you out before you were even born?

### Nutrition: The Brain's Best Friend

When it comes to brain development, you are what your mom eats. A diet rich in folate and vitamin B12 is like a brain-building smoothie, crucial for proper brain formation (Coker et al., 2022). On the flip side, a diet high in processed foods might give your brain a case of the blahs. Vitamin D is another key player, with research showing that even a little sunlight can spark beneficial changes in brain structure (Li, 2024). So, if you're expecting, it might be time to swap Netflix for some sunbathing while munching on nutrient-dense meals.

### Environmental Exposure: The Good, The Bad, and The Ugly

Let's talk about your surroundings—no, not the weather, but what you're exposed to daily. Pollution? Bad. Stress-eating a cheeseburger while stuck in traffic? Double bad. These environmental exposures can lead to epigenetic modifications that mess with cognitive function (Komar-Fletcher, 2023; Smith et al., 2020). On the bright side, playing classical music might give your baby's brain an extra boost. While we can't confirm that Mozart will turn your baby into a genius, it certainly can't hurt to try (Smith et al., 2020).

## Stress: The Uninvited Guest

Stress is like that party crasher who shows up uninvited and ruins the vibe. During pregnancy, stress can lead to increased cortisol levels, which might affect fetal brain development and cause long-term cognitive issues (Kuehner et al., 2019; Komar-Fletcher, 2023). But don't panic—cognitive-behavioral therapy (CBT) can help manage stress, leading to a calmer baby. A chill parent usually equals a chill baby, so maybe swap the drama for some yoga.

## The Role of Therapy: Breaking the Cycle of Trauma

If stress is the uninvited guest, unresolved trauma is the one who refuses to leave. Therapy can reduce transgenerational trauma, those pesky epigenetic changes that pass down anxiety or depression like a family heirloom (Kuehner et al., 2019; Komar-Fletcher, 2023). Addressing mental health before it affects your baby ensures your child starts life with a clean slate. It's like wiping the board clear before writing a new chapter.

## Microglia: The Brain's Tiny Construction Managers

Microglia are like the brain's microscopic clean-up crew, shaping the brain during its earliest days. But if they go off-script—thanks to mom's stress or illness—it can lead to a construction disaster that might cause long-term brain issues (Yuki Hattori, 2023). So, staying calm during pregnancy might just keep your baby's brain in tip-top shape!

## The Birth Weight Real Estate Deal

Your birth weight might be the key to how your brain fares throughout life. A heavier birth weight is linked to more brain "real estate" as you age. While it doesn't guarantee eternal youth, it might just give your brain a bit more cushion as you journey from 8 to 80 (Kristine B Walhovd, 2024).

## Prenatal Brain Shrinkage: Pregnancy's Temporary Side Effect

Pregnancy is like the ultimate brain workout, but instead of bulking up, your brain might actually shrink! Researchers found that some brain areas shrink during late pregnancy, but don't worry—it's temporary. After birth, your brain bounces back, though some parts might take their sweet time (María Paternina-Die et al., 2024).

### Dad's Diet Drama and Stress: A Genetic Time Bomb?

It turns out dad's pre-conception diet matters as much as mom's. If he binges on burgers or is stressed out, it could lead to long-term health issues for the baby, even affecting future generations (Dimofski, 2021; Hoffmann et al., 2024). So, dads-to-be, maybe hold off on that extra cheeseburger and manage your stress—your future child's health might depend on it!

### Gut Bacteria: The Unsung Heroes of Brain Development

When gut bacteria go missing during pregnancy, fetal brain development can take a hit, leading to altered gene expression and quirky behavior later in life. Gut microbes are busy sending important signals that help wire up the baby's brain. Without these signals, the brain might miss some key connections, leading to issues like autism-like behaviors and other neurodevelopmental challenges (Sajdel-Sulkowska, 2023).

### Omega Imbalance: Zombie Neurons on the Loose

When the balance of omega-6 to omega-3 fatty acids tips too far, your brain cells might go haywire. Researchers found that this imbalance makes stem cells multiply like crazy but messes with their ability to become proper neurons. It's like turning future brain cells into hyperactive zombies—present but not quite functioning right (Karolina Dec, 2023). Keep that fatty acid ratio in check!

### Junk Food Cravings: A Recipe for Brain Fog?

Pregnant women indulging in ultra-processed foods might be setting their kids up for less-than-stellar cognitive development. On the flip side, sticking to a Mediterranean diet can give kids sharper brains, especially in verbal skills and executive functions. So, maybe skip the junk food cravings and opt for some olives and fish—your future child's brain will thank you (Zupo et al., 2023).

### DHA and Choline: The Dynamic Duo

DHA and choline are crucial for brain development, supporting everything from problem-solving skills to neurotransmitter synthesis. While results on DHA supplementation during pregnancy are mixed, pairing DHA with choline has shown promise in enhancing brain plasticity, especially in at-risk infants. So, don't skimp on these nutrients—your baby's brain will be better for it (McCarthy & Kiely, 2019; Huang et al., 2023).

**Time for Some Adulting: Making More Neurons—Are You Ready?**

**Exercise:** Do you have 10 minutes? The more healthy neurons you have, the bigger your brain volume. And guess what? You have the superpower to boost their function, increase their numbers, and improve their health! Yes, you—the amazing, awesome, incredible stardust collection that you are—can totally do this!

In a study that basically shows working out is like a protein shake for your brain, Raji et al. (2024) scanned over 10,000 people's brains with MRIs to see if their exercise habits were doing more than just toning their abs. And surprise, surprise—getting your heart rate up for at least 10 minutes of moderate to vigorous regular activity results in bigger brain volumes, more gray and white matter, and a bigger hippocampus (a.k.a. the memory center). Running, in particular, proved to be a neurogenesis supercharger, especially in the hippocampus, where it enhanced structure and function (Vazquez-Medina, 2024).

We all know exercise is great for the body, but did you know it's like a conductor creating a perfect symphony for your brain? Here's how working out turns into a **brain-boosting fiesta:**

**Muscles: The Biggest Flex**—Meet Brain-Derived Neurotrophic Factor (BDNF), the Beyoncé of neurogenesis. Released during exercise, BDNF keeps neurons alive, smart, and well-connected, boosting your memory and mood (Wrann et al., 2013). Lactate and myokines like Interleukin-6 (IL-6) and Irisin, once underappreciated, are now recognized as key players in neurogenesis. They prove your muscles are more than just for show—they're brain boosters too (Wrann et al., 2013; Gardner et al., 2020).

**Insulin-Like Growth Factor 1 (IGF-1) and Vascular Endothelial Growth Factor (VEGF)** aren't just sidekicks—they're critical for growing new neurons, especially in the hippocampus, making your brain a neural nightclub (Trejo et al., 2001; Fabel et al., 2003).

**Bones:** Your bones aren't just passive structures; they release osteocalcin (Khrimian et al., 2017) and lipocalin-2 (Mosialou et al., 2017) during exercise, which boosts brain function and promotes neurogenesis. Lipocalin-2, released from bones, is stepping into the spotlight by influencing neurogenesis through the modulation of neuroinflammation and synaptic plasticity.

**Serotonin and Endorphins:** No playlist is complete without the feel-good anthems. Serotonin and beta-endorphins are the serotonin-fueled tracks that keep your brain grooving, improving mood and boosting cognitive function. Exercise cranks up serotonin levels, which not only lifts your spirits but also enhances neurogenesis. Beta-endorphins, those delightful chemicals that give you a runner's high, might also play a role in growing new neurons, acting on your brain's opioid receptors like a gentle lullaby (Park et al., 2020; Schoenfeld & Swanson, 2021).

**The Gut-Brain Jam Session:** The gut microbiome produces short-chain fatty acids (SCFAs) like butyrate during exercise, which cross the blood-brain barrier and kick-start neurogenesis. It's like your gut is a secret DJ, dropping tracks that keep your brain in the groove (Stilling et al., 2016).

**Shake It Off: How Exercise Keeps Parkinson's at Bay:**
Here's how your workout turns into a brain-boosting superhero:

- **Exercise triggers epigenetic changes**, protecting neurons and slowing brain aging. It also boosts insulin sensitivity, adding another layer of defense against neurodegeneration. Think of your workout as a superhero suit for your DNA (Darweesh et al., 2022; Xu et al., 2021; Shen, 2024).
- **Exercise enhances the gut microbiome**, boosting beneficial bacteria that fight inflammation and promote brain health (Sun et al., 2022; Moore et al., 2022). These gut changes translate into more SCFAs, which play key roles in reducing oxidative stress (Moore et al., 2022; See et al., 2021).
- **High-Intensity Interval Training (HIIT)** pumps up your brain's dopamine levels, keeping Parkinson's motor symptoms at bay. It's like a personal trainer for your dopamine receptors, fine-tuning them to keep your brain sharp (Park et al., 2020; Kawahata, 2023).
- **Exercise reduces neuroinflammation**, a major culprit in PD. It calms down overactive brain cells and ramps up antioxidant production, protecting neurons from oxidative stress (Emig et al., 2021; Paterno, 2024).
- **Exercise boosts neuroplasticity**, helping your brain form new connections and slowing down PD's progression. It's like giving your neurons a bodyguard against neurodegeneration (Chen & Zhang, 2022; Kaagman, 2024).

- **Exercise powers up your brain's mitochondria**, ensuring neurons have the energy they need to survive. This is crucial for fighting the mitochondrial dysfunction seen in PD (Kim et al., 2020).
- **Exercise improves balance, gait, and overall physical function** in people with PD, reducing falls and enhancing quality of life (Emig et al., 2021; Kaagman, 2024).

**Why Leg Day is Also Brain Day:**

Turns out your biceps aren't just for flexing in the mirror—they might be flexing your brain too! Gurholt et al. (2024) discovered that having less muscle, a.k.a. sarcopenic traits (which sounds fancy but really means "less muscle, more grumpiness"), is linked to a smaller brain. If your muscles are packing extra fat, your brain might be taking a nap (After all, I'm a poet). Kim et al. (2024) took it up a notch and found that more muscle might help keep those pesky Alzheimer's proteins in check. So, when you're doing squats, you're also squatting away brain shrinkage. Who knew leg day was also brain day? And Otsuka et al. (2024) says that high-intensity workouts can wash away those little white spots on brain scans that are linked to cognitive decline. So, yeah, sweat is basically brain detergent. But wait, there's more! Pontillo et al. (2024) found that in cases like multiple sclerosis, maintaining muscle mass might slow down brain shrinkage. Morwani-Mangnani (2024) states that eating vegetables and protein is key. They recommend consuming more high-quality proteins and organic, pesticide-free, fiber-rich, and pigment-rich vegetables. Thanaj (2024) says lifting weights isn't just about getting swole; it's about building high-quality muscle. Resistance training is your ticket to staying strong and independent, and keeping your brain in tip-top shape.

**Introducing a Strange Addition to Your Workout:** Essential oils—those tiny bottles of plant magic. Essential oils like peppermint and eucalyptus can enhance physical performance by improving oxygen uptake, which is crucial for muscle growth (Jayaputra, 2024). Their invigorating scents can also make workouts feel less grueling, motivating you to lift heavier and grow those muscles (Chen, 2024).

**L-carnitine:** A naturally occurring compound essential for energy metabolism, acts as a transport system for fatty acids into mitochondria. Studies show it aids in muscle recovery by reducing oxidative stress and inflammation, making it particularly beneficial for older adults facing muscle decline (Feky, 2024; Samodelov, 2024). Additionally, L-carnitine's neuroprotective properties support brain health, helping preserve cognitive abilities by enhancing mitochondrial function (Fresa, 2024; Lyu, 2024).

| Organ | Bioactive Compounds Released During Exercise | Mechanism of Increasing New Neuron Formation |
|---|---|---|
| **Skeletal Muscle** | • Lactate<br>• VEGF (Vascular Endothelial Growth Factor) - IGF-1 (Insulin-like Growth Factor 1)<br>• IGF-2 (Insulin-like Growth Factor 2)<br>• Irisin<br>• Cathepsin B (CTSB) | • **Lactate** enhances neurogenesis by crossing the blood<br>• brain barrier and promoting neuronal health and plasticity.<br>• **VEGF** improves blood flow, ensuring oxygen and nutrient delivery to neurons.<br>• **IGF-1** and **IGF-2** promote neurogenesis in the hippocampus by supporting neuronal survival, growth, and differentiation.<br>• **IGF-2** is particularly upregulated in skeletal muscle during and after exercise, contributing to mitochondrial remodeling, metabolic adaptation, and cognitive functions enhanced by exercise.<br>• Irisin stimulates BDNF expression, which enhances neurogenesis.<br>• **Cathepsin B** crosses the blood-brain barrier and promotes neurogenesis in the hippocampus, improving memory and cognitive function. |
| **Liver** | • IGF-1 (Insulin-like Growth Factor 1)<br>• IGF-2 (Insulin-like Growth Factor 2) | • **IGF-1** produced by the liver during exercise crosses the blood-brain barrier and promotes neurogenesis, especially in the hippocampus, by enhancing neuronal survival, growth, and differentiation.<br>• **IGF-1** is predominantly produced by the liver, stimulated by exercise, and mediates systemic growth responses, including muscle growth and repair.<br>• **IGF-2** is also produced by the liver, contributing to neurogenesis and cognitive functions. |

**Unlock Your Inner Oxygen Ninja: The Magic of VO2 Max**

VO2 max is like your body's way of showing off how much oxygen it can absorb during a workout. The "V" stands for "volume" (because we're measuring how much air you can take in), "O2" is the scientific way of saying "oxygen" (the stuff your lungs are desperate for when you're running up that hill), and "max" means "maximum" (as in, how much you can possibly handle before feeling like collapsing). Put together, VO2 max literally means the maximum volume of oxygen that an individual can take in, transport, and use during physical exertion.

Your blood acts like an oxygen Uber, with hemoglobin as the driver, shuttling O2 to your muscles. Once there, oxygen is used in a VIP area called the mitochondria for ATP production, the energy currency your muscles use to keep moving. If you push too hard, your muscles start running up a debt, producing lactate. A higher VO2 max helps delay the excess buildup of lactic acid.

| Effect | Description | Key Citations |
|---|---|---|
| Cellular Aging | A higher VO2 max is associated with increased telomerase activity, crucial for maintaining telomere length and potentially slowing cellular aging, promoting cellular longevity. | Rezaei et al., 2021 |
| Cognitive Function & Brain Volume | Enhanced VO2 max leads to increased brain volume and cognitive performance. It supports neurogenesis and brain plasticity, especially in areas related to memory and learning. High-intensity interval training (HIIT) further boosts these effects. | Burtscher et al., 2022; Liu, 2024 |
| Muscle Performance | Increased VO2 max improves muscle oxidative capacity, mitochondrial density, and capillary networks, resulting in greater muscle volume, enhanced endurance, and better metabolic function. | Madarsa, 2023 |
| Mood & Mental Health | Higher VO2 max levels boost endorphin production, enhancing mood and reducing stress. Regular aerobic exercise can mitigate symptoms of anxiety and depression. | Ávila-Gandia et al., 2023 |

Higher VO2 max levels are linked to increased brain volume and better cognitive function. Regular aerobic exercise turns your brain into a neuron factory, promoting neurogenesis (fancy talk for making new brain cells) and enhancing brain plasticity (the brain's ability to adapt and grow). So, by improving your VO2 max, you're not just getting fitter—you're also getting smarter (Senanayake, 2023). Who knew oxygen could be the secret to aging gracefully? (Burtscher et al., 2022).

On a molecular level, VO2 max acts like the anti-aging serum your cells have been begging for. It boosts telomerase activity—the enzyme that keeps your chromosomes from unraveling like a cheap sweater—which is key to cellular longevity (Rezaei et al., 2021). Additionally, with better mitochondrial function (thanks to your elevated VO2 max), your cells produce more ATP (that's cellular energy) and fend off oxidative stress, keeping you feeling spry and energetic (Ávila-Gandía et al., 2023).

**Short Sprints and Long Saunas: The Lazy Person's Guide to VO2 Max**
And here's how you can improve your VO2 max: a 10-second sprint will do it. Yes, you heard that right! Boosting your VO2 max doesn't mean spending endless hours at the gym. Short, high-intensity workouts can significantly improve VO2 max, making your body more efficient in a fraction of the time (Chen, 2024).

To further enhance your VO2 max, try mixing in some yoga and high-intensity interval training (HIIT). Yoga improves cardiovascular efficiency and helps your muscles work more effectively (Arsy, 2023). Meanwhile, HIIT pushes both your aerobic and anaerobic systems to their limits, driving your VO2 max higher (Hadiono, 2024). If you're looking to amp up your performance even more, adding L-arginine supplements can give you an extra edge (Rezaei et al., 2021).

**Breathe, Lift, Stretch, Repeat: Yoga's Recipe for Gym Success**
Incorporating yoga into your weightlifting routine offers numerous benefits both during and after your workouts. Practicing yoga between sets can boost your VO2 max by enhancing breathing efficiency and oxygen uptake, which improves overall cardiovascular fitness (Ruangvanich, 2024; Patel, 2024). Additionally, yoga promotes muscle elasticity and aids in recovery by reducing post-lift stiffness and soreness while increasing blood flow (Martin, 2024; Parisio, 2024). Beyond physical gains, regular yoga practice enhances brain function, improving memory,

focus, and emotional regulation, making it a perfect complement to strength training (Faramarzi, 2024). Yoga also serves as a powerful stress management tool, helping to clear the mind and improve focus during intense sessions (Nawale, 2024). Finally, post-lift yoga helps with holistic recovery, reducing inflammation and accelerating muscle recovery, ensuring that your body is ready for the next workout (Lučovnik, 2024; Abiç, 2024).

**From Bed to VO2 Max: Napping Your Way to Athletic Greatness**

Recovery is just as important. Hot showers and saunas aren't just for relaxation; they help reduce muscle soreness and improve cardiovascular function (Mustafa et al., 2020; Tung, 2020). So, next time you're soaking in the sauna, remember: you're not just sweating out stress; you're working on your heart and muscles too—multitasking at its steamiest!

Don't skip rest days either; they're essential for muscle repair and performance enhancement (Deliceoğlu, 2024). Think of rest days as the "Netflix and Chill" of your fitness routine—vital for recovery and definitely not to be skipped, no matter how tempting it is to keep pushing!

During intense training, your muscles undergo micro-tears, and your body experiences various stressors that scream, "Help! I need some downtime!" This healing process is facilitated during recovery, allowing for muscle repair, glycogen replenishment, and the removal of metabolic waste products (Ponkshe et al., 2021). Essentially, recovery is the body's version of a spa day—minus the cucumber slices on your eyes.

Research shows that adequate recovery is associated with increased muscle mass and improved capillary density, both of which enhance oxygen delivery to muscles during exercise (Ponkshe et al., 2021). So, the next time someone gives you flak for taking a rest day, just tell them you're boosting your oxygen superhighways!

Now, if you think skipping recovery and overloading on training will turn you into a superhero, think again. Elevated cortisol levels from inadequate recovery can actually hinder performance and adaptation, while balanced hormone levels promote muscle repair and growth, leading to an improved VO2 max (Manresa-Rocamora et al., 2023). Overtraining is the kryptonite to your Superman aspirations.

**Active Recovery: The Secret Ingredient**

Active recovery, which involves low-intensity exercise during recovery days, enhances blood flow to muscles, delivering nutrients and removing waste products (Rodríguez-García, 2023). This approach not only aids in recovery but also contributes to cardiovascular adaptations that can improve VO2 max. It's like giving your muscles a gentle nudge instead of a shove—sometimes, a little nudge is all they need.

Studies have demonstrated that incorporating active recovery into training regimens can lead to significant improvements in aerobic capacity (Rodríguez-García, 2023). For example, a study on high-intensity interval training (HIIT) found that participants who included active recovery periods exhibited greater improvements in VO2 max compared to those who engaged in passive recovery (Hadiono, 2024). Basically, it's like adding sprinkles to your workout sundae—makes everything better.

This suggests that the nature of recovery—whether active or passive—can significantly influence the effectiveness of training programs aimed at enhancing cardiovascular fitness. So, choose wisely, because even in the world of fitness, not all recovery is created equal.

Research indicates that athletes who strategically plan their recovery days experience better overall performance and higher VO2 max levels compared to those who do not prioritize recovery (Egesoy & Girginer, 2021). For example, tapering—reducing training load before competitions—has been shown to enhance performance by allowing the body to recover and adapt, leading to improved VO2 max and overall athletic performance (Egesoy & Girginer, 2021). In other words, knowing when to hit the brakes is just as important as knowing when to hit the gas.

Furthermore, the timing of recovery is crucial. Studies have shown that recovery periods following intense training sessions can lead to significant improvements in VO2 max when appropriately timed within a training cycle (Costa et al., 2021). This highlights the importance of not only the duration of recovery but also its strategic placement within training regimens. In short, if you want to hit those personal bests, you need to schedule your downtime as meticulously as your workouts—because even superheroes need a good nap.

**Steam, Sweat, and Smarts: How Saunas Make You Stronger, Fitter, and Sharper!**

Finish your sprint with a sauna or hot shower to activate heat shock proteins (HSPs). These proteins are like the body's repair crew, stepping in to boost nitric oxide production, which improves blood flow and cardiovascular function. Better blood flow means more oxygen delivered to your muscles, enhancing your exercise performance and potentially boosting your VO2 max (Reeder et al., 2023; Hägglund, 2022).

Regular sauna sessions can also improve endothelial function, reducing vascular resistance and making your heart more efficient. Over time, this could lower your risk of cardiovascular diseases like coronary heart disease and stroke, while also aiding in muscle recovery and overall cardiovascular efficiency (Laukkanen et al., 2023; Lee et al., 2022). So, think of the sauna as your quiet cardio, silently working to enhance your VO2 max while you relax. These heat therapies improve blood flow and muscle recovery, helping you bounce back quicker and train harder (Mustafa et al., 2020; Tung, 2020).

**Couch Potato Protein: Why Gains Don't Come in a Can**

Protein supplements are often seen as the key to building muscle, but without exercise, they're like superheroes without a mission (Lim et al., 2021). High-quality protein, especially when combined with branched-chain amino acids (BCAAs), is essential for maximizing muscle protein synthesis and recovery, but it needs resistance training to truly work its magic (Noh, 2023). When paired with exercise, branched-chain amino acids like leucine boost anabolic hormones and muscle mass, while also improving VO2 max (Ponkshe et al., 2021; Mwaniki, 2024; Chen, 2024; Bandsode & Joshi, 2022).

Branched-chain amino acids also help the brain by reducing exercise-induced fatigue and enhancing cognitive function (Peach et al., 2021). Leucine is an essential amino acid and the king of muscle protein synthesis. It kicks the mTOR pathway into gear, which is crucial for muscle growth (Alves, 2024). Including leucine-rich foods like dairy products and legumes in your diet is a surefire way to keep those muscles happy and growing.

Leucine is a muscle-building powerhouse, most abundant in whey protein (10-12g per 100g) (Revel et al., 2017). Animal proteins like beef, chicken, and fish, along with dairy and eggs, are also rich sources (Burke et al., 2012; Koochakpoor et al.,

2021). If you're hunting for leucine but prefer to keep it vegetarian, look no further than the mighty soybean—the Arnold Schwarzenegger of the plant world. Whether you're munching on tofu or tempeh, these soy superheroes are packed with leucine, giving your muscles the plant-powered boost they need. Who knew beans could be so buff?

**Now let's all bow down to Taurine.**

Taurine is a powerhouse sulfur-containing amino acid (not a branched-chain amino acid) with benefits across the board. It helps extend lifespan by protecting against muscle degeneration and fighting oxidative stress (Liu, 2024). In the brain, taurine boosts neurogenesis and protects against injury, supporting cognitive function and brain health (Yang, 2024). For athletes, taurine enhances VO2 max by improving muscle function and reducing oxidative stress, making it easier to push through tough workouts (Zou, 2024). It also speeds up muscle recovery and growth by activating key pathways for muscle repair (Mughal, 2024).

Rich sources of taurine include red meats (30-160 mg per 100g), fish and seafood (100-200 mg per 100g), dairy products, eggs, and certain seaweeds. For those needing more, especially athletes, taurine supplements can help with muscle recovery and performance.

Taurine is nearly absent in plant foods (Pan et al., 2021). While your diet of fruits, veggies, and grains is healthy, it won't deliver much taurine. Fermented foods like tempeh and seaweed might offer tiny amounts, but not enough to rely on (Burkholder-Cooley et al., 2016; Pan et al., 2021). If you're plant-based and need taurine, especially as an athlete, supplements are your best bet (Dattilo et al., 2022). While there's hope that your gut bacteria might one day help out, that's still uncertain (Guthrie et al., 2019).

However, consuming protein without exercise—like at a lazy brunch—may lead to fat gain instead of muscle (Jibril et al., 2022), and excessive intake without exercise can strain the kidneys and disrupt metabolism (Shin, 2024). Timing your protein intake is key to maximizing muscle recovery and growth. The best time to consume protein, especially whey, is within 30 minutes to two hours after a workout, when your muscles most need amino acids (Amawi, 2024). Spreading protein intake throughout the day also helps keep muscle-building going strong (Moradi, 2024). While pre-workout protein is helpful, the post-workout window is the real sweet spot for gains (Bird, 2024). Keep your protein close before, during, and after workouts for the best results!

## And a Few Other Things:

Beet juice, rich in dietary nitrates, enhances exercise performance by improving blood flow and oxygen delivery to muscles, thereby boosting VO2 max (Chan, 2024; Kim, 2024). If beet juice is the hero, tart cherry juice is its trusty sidekick. Rich in antioxidants, tart cherry juice helps reduce muscle soreness and inflammation after intense workouts (Siegel, 2024). Plus, its anti-inflammatory properties support mitochondrial function, making it a perfect post-exercise beverage.

But don't forget your gut! A healthy gut microbiome, supported by a diet rich in fiber and probiotics, can improve overall metabolic health, which indirectly boosts your VO2 max. And let's not overlook essential oils and good old sunlight. Inhaling certain essential oils like peppermint can increase respiratory efficiency, while sunlight exposure helps regulate circadian rhythms, which in turn can improve your exercise performance and recovery (Villalobos-González, 2024; Ávila-Gandía et al., 2023).

A high-protein diet aids muscle growth, while fiber ensures overall health. Polyphenols and omega-3s reduce oxidative stress and inflammation, speeding up recovery (Villalobos-González, 2024; Kasper et al., 2020). Hydration is crucial as well.

## So, summarizing:

Think of your heart as the ultimate traffic cop, making sure blood (and oxygen) flows smoothly to your muscles. Your lungs are like the air traffic controllers, directing oxygen into your bloodstream with precision. And your muscles? They're the power plants, taking in all that oxygen to keep the engines running—err, contracting. The better these systems work together, the higher your VO2 max, meaning you can keep going strong without hitting the brakes.

VO2 max is like a cell's version of upgrading from a tiny studio apartment to a spacious mansion. When you exercise, thanks to a gene called PGC-1$\alpha$, you make more mitochondria, and more mitochondria make more ATP and reduce oxidative stress, contributing to overall cellular health and longevity (Ávila-Gandía et al., 2023). Increased mitochondrial density and improved capillary networks within muscle tissue support hypertrophy and improved metabolic function (Khairani et al., 2021).

Furthermore, VO2 max is linked to telomerase activity, which is critical for cellular longevity. Regular exercise that improves VO2 max can upregulate telomerase activity, potentially delaying the aging process at the cellular level (Rezaei et al., 2021).

Oils like rosemary and lemon improve circulation, aiding in muscle recovery by flushing out metabolic waste (Tu, 2024). They also stimulate mitochondrial biogenesis, increasing energy production and boosting endurance—perfect for anyone serious about their training (Prieto-González, 2024). Regular aerobic exercise that elevates VO2 max promotes neurogenesis and brain plasticity, particularly in areas related to memory and learning, which is crucial for healthy aging (Senanayake, 2023; Burtscher et al., 2022).

**Zen and the Art of Brain Maintenance**

Dr. Sara Lazar, a neuroscientist at Harvard, literally stumbled upon the brain-boosting benefits of meditation after breaking her foot. While healing through yoga, she noticed she was calmer and less stressed. Curious, she dove into science and found that just 30 minutes of mindfulness meditation a day for eight weeks could actually bulk up the brain! Key areas like the hippocampus (memory), prefrontal cortex (decision-making), and even the amygdala (the brain's panic button) saw structural changes, including a surprising shrinkage in the amygdala—leading to better emotional control (Lazar et al., 2005; Fulgoni & Agarwal, 2021).

**Meditation: Your Brain's Personal Trainer for 2024**

Meditation isn't just about finding inner peace—it's like having a green thumb for your brain, helping it grow new neurons in the hippocampus, your brain's memory and emotional HQ. Demmin et al. (2022) found that regular meditation bulks up your hippocampus, making it the Arnold Schwarzenegger of brain regions. During the pandemic, while everyone else was hoarding toilet paper, teachers were quietly using meditation to keep their minds sharp and resilient.

Lazar et al. (2005) discovered that just 30 minutes of daily mindfulness meditation can beef up key brain areas, making you smarter, calmer, and less likely to lose your keys. Plus, meditation isn't just good for your brain—it's basically the fountain of youth. Agarwal & Fulgoni (2021) found that it's linked to longer telomeres (telomerase is an enzyme that helps extend the lifespan of cells by maintaining the protective caps, called telomeres, at the ends of chromosomes) and healthier DNA, which might just keep you aging like fine wine.

Fast forward to 2024, where Seok et al. showed that meditation is the perfect pesticide, keeping stress-induced cortisol from wrecking your neuron garden. Meanwhile, Jiang et al. found that meditation is like Miracle-Gro for your brain, boosting Brain-Derived Neurotrophic Factor (BDNF) to keep those neurons thriving. Throw in some exercise, and you've got the dynamic duo for brain health (Ayed et al., 2024). And if you add good sleep into the mix, aided by meditation and acupuncture, your brain's garden will be blooming in no time (Yang, 2024). Punia et al. (2024) wrapped it up by reminding us that a little mindfulness mixed with physical activity is the secret sauce for keeping your brain in top shape.

First up, let's talk about stress—every brain's arch-nemesis. Seok et al. (2024) found that stress triggers the hypothalamic-pituitary-adrenal (HPA) axis, which is like your brain's panic button. Unfortunately, pressing this button too often floods your system with cortisol, a hormone that's great for surviving a zombie apocalypse but terrible for growing new neurons. Meditation, however, steps in like a cool-headed hero, calming the HPA axis and keeping cortisol in check. This not only helps prevent your hippocampus (the brain's memory HQ) from shrinking but also keeps your synapses flexible and ready for action.

But that's not all! Jiang et al. (2024) found that meditation boosts brain-derived neurotrophic factor (BDNF), essential for supporting and growing new neurons. Plini et al. (2024) discovered that meditation helps maintain your brain volume, keeping your emotions and thinking in check. Those short sessions don't just keep you calm—they keep your brain structurally sound.

Meditation also improves communication between brain regions, enhancing attention and emotional regulation, turning you into a cognitive ninja (Fialoke et al., 2024). And for those who love proof, Yadav et al. (2024) showed that regular meditation boosts relaxing alpha and theta waves, giving your brain a spa day without leaving the couch.

**Meditation: The Ultimate Nightcap for a Brain That Refuses to Sleep**

Just 10-20 minutes of mindfulness meditation before bed can help you fall asleep faster and improve sleep quality (Luo et al., 2024). If you stick to a routine, like 15-30 minutes daily, you can maintain higher melatonin levels, making sleep easier (Plini et al., 2024).

Plini et al. (2024) also linked meditation to increased structural integrity of the pineal gland, which is responsible for melatonin production. Meditating before bed might just be the secret to better sleep. Research shows that it calms your mind, reduces stress, and helps you fall asleep faster by boosting melatonin, the hormone that signals your body it's time to sleep (Ong et al., 2014; Nagendra et al., 2022; Kumar, 2024).

Twenty minutes of heartfulness meditation a day can reduce stress and improve sleep, even for healthcare professionals under serious pressure (Kumar et al., 2024). Meditation isn't just for sleep—it keeps your brain sharp. Regular practice maintains gray matter, strengthens brain connections, and boosts relaxing brainwaves (Plini et al., 2024; Fialoke et al., 2024; Yadav et al., 2024).

Luo et al. (2024) found that mindfulness meditation is particularly effective at reducing sleep initiation and maintenance disorders (SIMDs), anxiety, and depression—all the things that keep you tossing and turning at night.

Meditation also helps you access deeper stages of sleep, like slow-wave and REM sleep, which are crucial for feeling refreshed and ready for the day (Thimmapuram et al., 2020; Nagendra et al., 2017). It even regulates your heart rate for more restorative rest and improves your mood and cognitive function, ensuring you wake up on the right side of the bed (Nagendra et al., 2017; Kohler et al., 2017).

Fialoke et al. (2024) discovered that practices like yoga nidra can enhance functional connectivity in the brain, particularly activating the thalamus, which plays a crucial role in regulating sleep.

Meanwhile, Kumar et al. (2024) showed that heartfulness meditation does wonders for reducing stress, burnout, and loneliness—proving that meditation isn't just a mental spa day; it's a full-on brain vacation.

Let's not forget the physical benefits. Patil et al. (2024) found that meditation helps reduce oxidative stress, giving your body a break from all that daily wear and tear. And as if that weren't enough, it's like giving your brain's sleep department a major upgrade.

Meditation isn't just about zoning out; it's a holistic tool that addresses everything from stress and anxiety to pain management, as Wu et al. (2024) demonstrated with patients undergoing hemodialysis. Even in high-stress environments like life at sea, meditation has proven its worth. Paranthatta et al. (2024) reported that cyclic meditation significantly improved sleep quality for sailors, showing that even on the open ocean, where sleep is often elusive, meditation can help you catch some solid Zs.

And let's not forget the tech-savvy side of things—Venkatesan et al. (2024) found that app-delivered heartfulness meditation is not just a gimmick; it's a genuinely effective way to promote calm and enhance sleep quality over both the short and long term.

| Mechanism of Meditation | Change in Brain Anatomy/ Physiology | Outcome | Effect on Sleep | Effect on Memory | Effect on Calm |
| --- | --- | --- | --- | --- | --- |
| Mindfulness Meditation | Increases gray matter in the hippocampus, prefrontal cortex; shrinks the amygdala; promotes neurogenesis (Lazar et al., 2005; Fulgoni & Agarwal, 2021) | Improved emotional regulation, decision-making, stress reduction | Improved sleep onset and quality through increased melatonin production (Plini et al., 2024) | Enhanced memory and learning due to increased hippocampal volume and neurogenesis (Lazar et al., 2005) | Better emotional control due to reduced amygdala size (Lazar et al., 2005; Fulgoni & Agarwal, 2021) |
| Regular Meditation Practice | Increases hippocampal volume; maintains gray matter, improves brain connectivity; supports neurogenesis (Demmin et al., 2022; Plini et al., 2024) | Enhanced cognitive flexibility, emotional resilience | Improved sleep patterns through regulation of melatonin levels (Plini et al., 2024) | Strengthened memory functions by maintaining hippocampal health and supporting neurogenesis (Demmin et al., 2022) | Increased calmness through enhanced brain connectivity (Fialoke et al., 2024) |

| | | | | | |
|---|---|---|---|---|---|
| Heartfulness Meditation | Reduces cortisol levels; maintains gray matter integrity; supports neurogenesis (Kumar et al., 2024; Fialoke et al., 2024) | Reduced stress, improved emotional regulation | Enhanced sleep quality by reducing stress and burnout (Kumar et al., 2024) | Improved memory due to better emotional regulation and neurogenesis (Kumar et al., 2024) | Reduced stress and burnout, leading to a calmer state of mind (Kumar et al., 2024) |
| Meditation's Impact on Telomeres and DNA Methylation | Longer telomeres; beneficial changes in DNA methylation patterns; supports neurogenesis (Agarwal & Fulgoni, 2021; Ibrahim et al., 2022) | Healthier aging, reduced inflammation, and stress | Promotes better sleep quality through improved overall health (Agarwal & Fulgoni, 2021) | Supports memory preservation by contributing to long-term brain health and neurogenesis (Ibrahim et al., 2022) | Enhances calmness by reducing inflammation and supporting genomic stability (Agarwal & Fulgoni, 2021) |
| Meditation & Brainwave Activity | Increases alpha and theta brainwave activity; supports neurogenesis (Yadav et al., 2024; Fialoke et al., 2024) | Promotes relaxation, reduces anxiety | Encourages restful sleep by increasing relaxing brainwave states (Yadav et al., 2024) | Supports memory consolidation during sleep and neurogenesis (Yadav et al., 2024) | Deepens relaxation, reduces anxiety, and promotes a calm mental state (Fialoke et al., 2024) |
| Mindfulness & Oxidative Stress Reduction | Reduces oxidative stress levels, protecting neurons; supports neurogenesis (Patil et al., 2024; Wu et al., 2024) | Better physical and mental health outcomes, improved brain function | Improves sleep by reducing oxidative stress and enhancing overall health (Patil et al., 2024) | Protects memory by reducing oxidative damage to brain cells and supporting neurogenesis (Wu et al., 2024) | Enhances calm by reducing the physiological impacts of stress (Patil et al., 2024) |

## Learning - Mind Muscle: Learn Your Way to a Bigger, Stronger Brain

Dear gentle readers, let's recall parts of your memory queen, The Lady Hippocampus. The anterior hippocampus creates the juicy stories, the posterior hippocampus helps you find your way back to them, and the parahippocampal gyrus is where all the boring but important stuff goes, ensuring your brain is a well-rounded treasure trove of "remember when" moments and "wait, I actually know this" facts.

In an observational study of 40 final-year medical students, researchers found that intense studying before exams can increase the volume of the hippocampus, the brain region responsible for moving information from short-term to long-term memory. Brain scans were done 19 weeks before and one week after their final exams, and it was discovered that those who spent more time studying not only saw a significant increase in right hippocampal volume but also scored better on their exams. So, if you want to boost your brainpower and ace your tests, it might just be time to hit the books hard (Jakub Marek, 2023).

Yes, learning actually reshapes the brain! Don't believe me? Then believe my friends, Maguire and Hartley. Let me tell you a little story. Once upon a time (actually, it was the year 2000—I love me some drama), a group of neuroscientists led by Maguire et al. decided to peek inside the brains of London's finest taxi drivers. Why, you ask? Because these taxi drivers undergo something called "The Knowledge"—a brutal training regimen where they cram 25,000 streets and thousands of landmarks into their heads. It's like memorizing the entire Harry Potter series... in one sitting... backwards (Maguire et al., 2000). The researchers scanned the brains of 16 male taxi drivers who had been licensed for at least 1.5 years and compared these brain scans with those of 50 regular guys who didn't spend their days dodging double-decker buses. The results were mind-blowing—literally. The taxi drivers had a beefed-up posterior hippocampus, which is the part of the brain that handles spatial memory (the one that stores places and helps you know where you are and where you're going). And it turns out, the more years they spent driving, the bigger this part of their brain got. So here, your travel is bigger than your brain! Go for that adventure you always planned and pay attention to places—not just to mimosas! The concept of neuroplasticity—where your brain reshapes itself based on what you do with it—got a major boost.

Fast forward to 2020, when another group of researchers led by Hartley et al. looked at 98 older adults (60-80 years young) and found that those who regularly engaged in activities like driving or exploring new places had bigger, healthier hippocampi than their couch-potato counterparts (Hartley et al., 2020). These brainy explorers also outperformed others in spatial memory tests, proving that it's never too late to get your brain in shape (Hartley et al., 2020).

**How to Build a Better Brain While Doing Absolutely Nothing: Sleep**

While you're snoozing, especially during non-rapid eye movement (NREM) sleep, your brain is busy Marie Kondo-ing your synapses. It's tossing out the unnecessary ones and polishing up the connections that help you remember where you left your office badge and keep your cool when someone cuts you off in traffic (Ma et al., 2023; Ruan et al., 2023).

This mental makeover is powered by brain-derived neurotrophic factor (BDNF), the brain's personal trainer for neurons, particularly in the hippocampus—the memory capital of your brain (Sochal, 2024; Xue-song et al., 2023). The dentate gyrus of the hippocampus is especially busy during this time, like a factory working overtime to keep your brain sharp and ready for whatever life throws at you (Furihata et al., 2020).

But here's the catch: skimp on sleep, and BDNF levels drop faster than your motivation on a Monday morning, leading to a slowdown in neurogenesis and leaving your cognitive functions running on fumes (Ma et al., 2020; Ancelin et al., 2023). Chronic sleep deprivation is like canceling the gym membership for your brain—it leads to less BDNF, more anxiety, and a brain that's not as quick on its feet (Baba et al., 2022; Santiago et al., 2020).

Adequate sleep boosts the proliferation of neural stem cells in the hippocampus, helping to generate new neurons that keep your memory and learning skills sharp (Mohammadi, 2023; Agyekum, 2024).

Now, let's talk about melatonin—the "sleep hormone" that's basically the bouncer at your brain's exclusive nighttime club. Sure, it helps you fall asleep, but it's also a superhero antioxidant, fighting off oxidative stress that's out to mess with your neurons (Bahgat et al., 2021; Gabryelska et al., 2022). Melatonin doesn't stop there; it also pumps up BDNF and insulin-like growth factor 1 (IGF-1), keeping your neurons in tip-top shape (Sochal et al., 2023; Zhang et al., 2020). And if you've been pulling all-nighters, melatonin supplements can swoop in to save the day, restoring BDNF levels and getting neurogenesis back on track (Al-Mshari et al., 2022; Kriengtuntiwong et al., 2021).

While you're off in dreamland, your brain's glymphatic system is like the night janitor, clearing out all the neurotoxic waste that builds up during the day. It's particularly good at getting rid of amyloid-beta, the gunk that's linked to cognitive decline and neurodegenerative diseases (Wang et al., 2021; Sochal et al., 2022). So, when you wake up feeling refreshed, it's because your brain has just undergone a deep clean, leaving it ready to tackle another day of remembering names, solving puzzles, and handling whatever life throws at you.

**Stage 1: The Sleep Doorway – Enter If You Dare** Stage 1 sleep is like the entryway into your brain's nightly adventure. It's that brief phase where you're teetering on the edge of consciousness, unsure whether you're awake or just starting to doze off. Your brain starts to produce theta waves, which are basically its way of saying, "Alright, let's start shutting things down." Sensory input begins to fade, like someone slowly dimming the lights. Meanwhile, your brain's janitorial crew, the glymphatic system, kicks into gear, beginning to sweep away the day's metabolic trash to keep things running smoothly upstairs (Kimura, 2023). And, of course, there's a little bit of spring cleaning going on too—synaptic pruning starts trimming those unnecessary neural connections that your brain has decided it doesn't really need (Devore et al., 2014). But don't get too comfortable; Stage 1 doesn't last long—just a few minutes before you're shuffled off into Stage 2.

**Stage 2: Light Sleep – The Brain's Rehearsal Room** Welcome to Stage 2, where things start to get a bit more serious. You'll spend about 20 minutes here per cycle, and if you're an adult, this stage hogs about half of your total sleep time. During Stage 2, your brain puts on its thinking cap—or rather, its memory-consolidating helmet. It starts churning out sleep spindles and K-complexes, which are your brain's way of saying, "Let's lock in some memories and make sure we stay asleep" (Kim et al., 2021). The glymphatic system is still on duty, this time focusing on clearing out those pesky beta-amyloid deposits that nobody wants hanging around (Jego et al., 2013). Neuroplasticity gets a boost too, as your brain strengthens the connections it needs to help you remember all those important things—like where you left your keys or how to do your job (Reato et al., 2013).

**Stage 3: Deep Sleep (N3) – The Brain's Powerlifting Session** Stage 3 is where the real heavy lifting happens. This is deep sleep, the brain's equivalent of a hardcore workout. It usually kicks off about 30 minutes after you've dozed off and can last from 20 to 40 minutes, though the later cycles tend to be shorter (Hong et al., 2016). Slow delta waves dominate this stage, and your brain is in full-on restoration mode. It's doing some serious synaptic pruning, tossing out the weak links to make way for stronger, more efficient connections, particularly in the hippocampus, where memories are forged (Yadav et al., 2022). The glymphatic system? It's running at peak performance, flushing out toxins like a brain detox spa (Gupta, 2019). This stage is the unsung hero of sleep—it's vital for memory consolidation and making sure you can think straight tomorrow.

**REM Sleep: The Brain's Imagination Station** Ah, REM sleep—the stage where your brain really lets loose. It typically kicks in about 90 minutes after you fall asleep, popping up multiple times throughout the night. Each REM episode lasts longer as the night goes on, giving your brain plenty of time to dive deep into dreamland (Sabeti et al., 2018). During REM, your brain activity goes into overdrive, resembling what it's like when you're awake. This is where all the emotional regulation and memory consolidation magic happens (Hong et al., 2020). The glymphatic system takes a bit of a backseat but doesn't completely clock out. Meanwhile, neurogenesis and synaptic pruning are still in action, making sure only the most important neural connections stick around (Shore et al., 2010). REM is where creativity and problem-solving get their workout, helping you wake up ready to tackle the day's challenges with fresh ideas (Dashti et al., 2019).

**Neurogenesis During Sleep** Picture your hippocampus as the brain's workshop, constantly cranking out new neurons. The non-rapid eye movement stage of sleep (NREM) is like the night shift that steps in to make sure these neurons get properly built and fitted into the brain's circuitry. Studies show that during this deep sleep phase, your brain gets a surge of brain-derived neurotrophic factor (BDNF), which is basically Miracle-Gro for neurons (Abel et al., 2013). Skip out on sleep, and it's like halting production—no new neurons, no new ideas (Cheng et al., 2022). As you catch those Z's, your brain isn't just making new neurons; it's also figuring out where to put them. These newbies get integrated into the neural network, helping you lock in new memories and skills (Seibt et al., 2012).

**Synaptic Pruning in Sleep Stages** Now, let's talk about synaptic pruning. Imagine your brain as a garden that's been overgrown with all sorts of connections after a day full of learning. NREM sleep comes along with a pair of shears, trimming away the weaker, unnecessary synapses. This pruning keeps your brain's neural pathways neat, tidy, and efficient—just what you need to stay smart and sane (Alphen et al., 2013; Maret et al., 2011). Think of microglia, the brain's immune cells, as the gardeners that go to work during NREM sleep, snipping away the less-used synapses. They're like the Marie Kondos of your brain, getting rid of anything that doesn't spark joy or serve a purpose (Xin et al., 2020).

Then, there's the rapid eye movement stage of sleep (REM), which handles a different kind of pruning. It's not just about cutting back; it's more like a reset button. REM sleep helps fine-tune the connections made during the day, especially the ones linked to emotions and skills. It's the brain's way of making sure that only the strongest, most important connections stick around, so you're ready for whatever tomorrow throws at you (Li et al., 2017; Yoshida & Toyoizumi, 2022).

**The Role of Sleep in Synaptic Plasticity** The relationship between sleep and your brain's flexibility—synaptic plasticity—is like a well-choreographed dance. During the day, your brain builds up synaptic strength from all the learning and experiences. But without sleep to tone things down, you'd end up with a brain that's too cluttered to function. Sleep, with its synaptic scaling and down-selection, acts like a nightly reset that keeps your cognitive gears running smoothly (Hanlon et al., 2011; Maret et al., 2011; Vivo et al., 2017).

NREM and REM sleep are the dynamic duo of memory processing. While NREM sleep locks in your facts and figures (declarative memories), REM sleep handles the emotional stuff and muscle memory (procedural memories) (Holz et al., 2012). Miss out on either, and you're not just tired—you're running on half a brain!

**Ion Channels: The Brain's Personal Trainers** Enter the ion channels—the brain's version of personal trainers. Potassium ($K^+$), sodium ($Na^+$), and calcium ($Ca^{2+}$) are the ions calling the shots. Potassium channels, for example, help cool things down when neurons need a break, leading to a little shrinkage (Sarnataro, 2024). On the flip side, sodium channels are all about that sodium rush, causing a swell when neurons need to fire up and chat with their neighbors (Zhang et al., 2023). And let's not forget calcium, which plays a role in building new synaptic connections, giving those dendritic spines a nice stretch (Hossain et al., 2021).

**Neurotransmitters: The Hype Crew** Every brain party needs a hype crew, and that's where neurotransmitters come in. Glutamate is the life of the party, kicking open ion channels and letting in a flood of ions that get the neurons buzzing and expanding (Voumvourakis et al., 2023). GABA, the chill-out artist, does the opposite, calming things down and leading to a little cellular contraction (Dai et al., 2021). Together, they keep the brain's excitement levels just right.

**Sleep Spindles: The Brain's Nightly Workout** Cerebrospinal fluid (CSF) is a clear, colorless liquid that cushions the brain and spinal cord, removing waste and delivering nutrients to keep your nervous system running smoothly. This mechanical pumping action of your brain cells—expanding and contracting to move CSF through the brain—is like your brain's own version of flushing the pipes, clearing out harmful substances like amyloid-β and tau proteins that, if left unchecked, could turn your brain into a toxic waste dump (Iliff, 2024).

This cleanup crew is especially active during NREM sleep when the brain's rhythmic pumping is in full swing, creating pressure gradients that boost CSF flow. It's like giving your brain a power wash while you catch those much-needed Z's (Salameh, 2024).

And just when you thought it couldn't get any more interesting, enter the sleep spindles. These are the brain's rhythmic dance moves—little bursts of activity during NREM sleep that help consolidate memories and ensure your brain's expansion and contraction game is on point (Kurogi, 2024).

### Sleep, Genes, and the Brain's Master Plan

Your brain's nightly activities, from its cleanup crew to its repair work, don't operate in isolation—they're influenced by your lifestyle choices, including how much sleep you get. Epigenetic factors (basically, how your environment can turn certain genes on or off) play a huge role here. For instance, if you regularly shortchange your sleep, your brain's glymphatic system might not get the signal to clean up properly, leaving behind waste that could lead to bigger problems down the road (You, 2024).

Different stages of sleep bring different functions to the brain's party. NREM sleep is like the deep-cleaning phase, where the glymphatic system and brain cell dynamics are in full force, ensuring everything is in top shape. REM sleep, on the other hand, focuses more on emotional regulation and memory—still important, but not so much for the heavy lifting of brain waste removal (Fayed, 2024).

Imagine your brain has its own plumbing system, where astrocytes (a type of glial cell) help flush out the junk. This system shuttles cerebrospinal fluid (CSF) through your brain's interstitial spaces, clearing out toxic leftovers like amyloid-β and tau proteins that are linked to neurodegenerative diseases (Ferini-Strambi, 2024; Madhu, 2024). The whole process hinges on a protein called aquaporin-4 (AQP4), which acts like a gatekeeper for fluid movement. But beware: if AQP4 gets out of whack—say, due to phosphorylation—your brain's cleanup crew might go on strike, leading to a serious buildup of harmful waste (Xiong, 2024; Premi, 2024).

The glymphatic system's magic happens through a combination of CSF pulsations driven by your heartbeat and breathing. These pulsations push the CSF into your brain, where it swaps places with interstitial fluid (ISF), carrying away metabolic waste. It's like a nightly detox for your brain, and its effectiveness depends on factors like blood flow and the brain's structural integrity—so keep that plumbing in good shape (Li, 2024; Iliff, 2024).

### Epigenetics: The Boss Behind the Glymphatic Janitors
It turns out, the efficiency of your brain's cleaning crew isn't just about the mechanics; it's also about who's calling the shots—enter epigenetics. Your environment, lifestyle, and even how much you move your body can tweak the genes that run the glymphatic system. For example, regular exercise might be like giving your brain's janitors a raise, boosting their ability to clear out the gunk (Olegário, 2024). On the flip side, if you're skimping on sleep, the boss might get cranky, leading to a less effective cleanup crew and potentially speeding up the brain's aging process (Ibrahim, 2024; Astara, 2024).

### Sleep Stages: When the Cleanup Crew Puts in Overtime
The glymphatic system is at its most active during non-rapid eye movement (NREM) sleep, which is when your brain's janitors are working overtime. During NREM sleep, glymphatic activity shoots up by about 90% compared to when you're awake (Davide, 2024). The rhythmic patterns of NREM sleep seem to help with CSF flow, making waste removal super-efficient (Murdock, 2024). As for rapid eye movement (REM) sleep? The jury's still out on how much it contributes

to the cleanup, but early signs suggest it's not entirely off the hook (Murdock, 2024).

So, next time you think about pulling an all-nighter, remember: your brain's cleaning crew needs their shift too. Keep them happy with regular sleep, some exercise, and a little epigenetic encouragement, and they'll keep your brain sparkling clean.

**Hola! A Protocol for Life's Rhythm: "Stayin' Alive, ooh ooh ooh, Stayin' Alive."**

### 1. Wake Up Before Sunrise
**Time:** Approximately 1 hour before sunrise.
**Action:** Wake up early to reset your circadian rhythm and support mitochondrial function. Exposure to natural morning blue light is crucial for regulating your sleep-wake cycle, influencing hormone production, and enhancing alertness throughout the day (Yamanaka, 2020; Witzig et al., 2020).

### 2. Morning Yoga Session and Meditation
Engage in 10-15 minutes of meditation to promote mental clarity. Meditation positively influences sleep quality and overall well-being by enhancing serotonin production (Ahmad et al., 2020; Binks et al., 2020).
Engage in a 10–15-minute yoga session to activate the body and mind, promote circulation, and reduce stress. Morning yoga enhances mood and cognitive function, setting a positive tone for the day and facilitating serotonin release, which is beneficial for mood regulation and sleep onset later in the day (Balasubramaniam et al., 2013; Binks et al., 2020).

Drink a matcha tea blend with moringa, chlorella, spirulina, lemon, brahmi, and shankhpushpi. This combination provides antioxidants and nutrients that support mitochondrial health, cognitive function, and the production of serotonin and melatonin (Binks et al., 2020).

### 3. Blue Light Management
Throughout the day, limit blue light exposure from screens (use blue light blockers—yes, they work for both shields and glasses), as excessive blue light can disrupt melatonin production. Focus on getting natural light to help maintain a healthy circadian rhythm (Yang et al., 2021). Try eating at least one meal outside or, if possible, work outdoors to take advantage of natural light.

## 4. Weight Lifting

Incorporate weight lifting into your routine to improve mitochondrial function, energy metabolism, and cellular health. Weight lifting promotes deeper sleep stages and reduces sleep latency, while the physiological stress induced by this activity increases heat shock proteins, aiding in cellular repair and recovery (Sorriento et al., 2021; Lim et al., 2022).

## 5. Post-Workout Yoga

Immediately after weight lifting, perform a short yoga session to aid muscle recovery and relaxation, further enhancing the benefits of physical exercise on sleep quality. This practice can help regulate the autonomic nervous system and support circadian rhythm synchronization (Walker et al., 2020; Huberty et al., 2018).

## 6. Caffeine Consumption

Before noon, enjoy organic black coffee (single-origin pour-over is best, but you do you). However, avoid caffeine after noon, as it has a half-life of 3 to 7 hours, which can interfere with sleep if consumed too late in the day (Benton et al., 2022).

## 7. UVB Exposure

Aim for 20-30 minutes of UVB exposure while using sun protection. This exposure is crucial for vitamin D synthesis, melanin production, and the regulation of serotonin and melatonin (Ahmad et al., 2020).

## 8. Sunset Walk

Take a walk during sunset to benefit from red light, which supports circadian rhythm regulation and promotes relaxation before bedtime (Kurtović, 2023).

## 9. Blue Light Reduction

1-2 hours before bedtime, turn off electronic devices and eliminate blue light exposure in the evening to promote melatonin production and signal to your body that it's time to wind down (Yang et al., 2021).

**10. Evening Nutrition**

Time: 3 hours before bed. Eat a serotonin and melatonin-rich diet, including foods like nuts, seeds, and leafy greens. Complement your meal with calming teas like chamomile or lavender to enhance relaxation and prepare the body for sleep (Binks et al., 2020).

An example of a serotonin and melatonin-rich meal plan: Create dishes that your sleep loves.

**Remember to drink a vinegar drink 30 minutes before your meal.**

A simple way to incorporate vinegar into your diet is by mixing two tablespoons of apple cider vinegar with a cup of water and a teaspoon of honey, creating a refreshing drink that may support metabolic health (Inagaki et al., 2020).

This pre-meal ritual is believed to enhance mitochondrial function, as acetic acid in vinegar may influence metabolic processes, including mitochondrial uncoupling, which can promote fat oxidation (Perumpuli & Dilrukshi, 2022). Additionally, vinegar consumption may positively affect gut microbiota by limiting the growth of pathogenic bacteria, contributing to a healthier microbiome composition (Al-Shammari & Batkowska, 2021). Moreover, vinegar has been shown to mitigate insulin and glucose spikes after meals, which can be beneficial for managing postprandial blood sugar levels (Gill et al., 2021).

Acetic acid, the primary component of vinegar, has been demonstrated to increase plasma acetate levels, which can have systemic metabolic effects (Gill et al., 2021).

Furthermore, research indicates that regular vinegar consumption may aid in weight management and improve lipid profiles by positively influencing gut microbiota (Guo-feng & Li, 2023).

In Japan, vinegar is a cultural staple, with many people incorporating it into their daily diets to combat fatigue and enhance physical performance (Inagaki et al., 2020).

**Serotonin and Melatonin-Rich Salad**
**Recipe: Spinach, Quinoa, and Walnut Salad**
**Ingredients:**

- 2 cups mixed leafy greens (spinach, kale)
- 1 cup cherry tomatoes (contain melatonin) (Grao-Cruces et al., 2023)
- 1/2 cup walnuts (high in omega-3 fatty acids and serotonin precursors) (Binici & Şat, 2021)
- 1/4 cup feta cheese (contains tryptophan) (Binici & Şat, 2021)
- 1/2 cup cooked quinoa (a complete protein source) (Gupta et al., 2023)
  *Dressing:* 2 tablespoons olive oil, juice of 1 lemon, salt, and pepper

**Instructions:**

1. In a large bowl, combine leafy greens, cherry tomatoes, walnuts, feta cheese, and quinoa.
2. In a separate bowl, whisk together olive oil, lemon juice, salt, and pepper.
3. Drizzle the dressing over the salad and toss gently to combine.
4. Serve immediately.

This salad incorporates ingredients that promote serotonin and melatonin production, with spinach and walnuts noted for their beneficial effects on mood and sleep quality (Binici & Şat, 2021).

**Serotonin and Melatonin-Rich Entrée**
**Recipe: Lentil and Tomato Stew**
**Ingredients:**

- 1 cup lentils (contain melatonin) (Rebollo-Hernanz et al., 2020)
- 2 cups diced tomatoes (contain melatonin) (Grao-Cruces et al., 2023)
- 1 onion, chopped
- 2 cloves garlic, minced
- 1 teaspoon cumin
- 1 teaspoon turmeric
- 4 cups vegetable broth
- Salt and pepper to taste
- Fresh parsley for garnish

**Instructions:**

1. In a large pot, sauté the onion and garlic until translucent.
2. Add cumin and turmeric, stirring for 1 minute.
3. Add lentils, diced tomatoes, and vegetable broth. Bring to a boil.
4. Reduce heat and simmer for about 30 minutes, or until lentils are tender.
5. Season with salt and pepper, and garnish with fresh parsley before serving.

This hearty stew is rich in lentils, which contain melatonin. The spices also add anti-inflammatory properties, enhancing overall health.

## Serotonin and Melatonin-Rich Dessert
### Recipe: Banana and Almond Butter Parfait
**Ingredients:**

- 2 ripe bananas (contain tryptophan) (Binici & Şat, 2021)
- 1/2 cup Greek yogurt (contains tryptophan) (Binici & Şat, 2021)
- 1/4 cup almond butter (rich in magnesium, which aids sleep) (Binici & Şat, 2021)
- 1/4 cup granola (preferably low sugar)
- 1 tablespoon honey (optional)

**Instructions:**

1. In a glass, layer Greek yogurt, sliced bananas, and almond butter.
2. Add a layer of granola and repeat the layers until the glass is full.
3. Drizzle honey on top if desired.
4. Serve chilled.

Bananas are beneficial for serotonin production due to their high tryptophan content, while Greek yogurt provides probiotics that support gut health, linked to mood regulation.

## Serotonin and Melatonin-Rich Tea
### Recipe: Chamomile, Lavender, and Dandelion Tea
**Ingredients:**

- 1 tablespoon dried chamomile flowers (calming effects) (Binici & Şat, 2021)
- 1 teaspoon dried lavender (promotes relaxation) (Binici & Şat, 2021)
- 1 tablespoon dried dandelion leaves (detoxifying properties) (Grao-Cruces et al., 2023)
- 2 cups boiling water
- Honey or lemon to taste (optional)

**Instructions:**

1. Place chamomile, lavender, and dandelion in a teapot or infuser.
2. Pour boiling water over the herbs and steep for 5-10 minutes.
3. Strain and serve hot, adding honey or lemon if desired.

This tea blend promotes relaxation and sleep quality, supporting serotonin and melatonin levels.

## Lettuce Tea for Improved Sleep Quality

This recipe incorporates fresh lettuce, known for its mild sedative properties due to the presence of lactucarium, a compound that promotes relaxation and sleepiness.

**Ingredients:**

- 1 cup fresh lettuce leaves (preferably romaine or butterhead)
- 2 cups water
- Optional: honey or lemon for taste

**Instructions:**

1. **Preparation of Lettuce:**

   Rinse the fresh lettuce leaves thoroughly under cold water to remove any dirt or pesticides. Tear the leaves into smaller pieces to increase the surface area.

2. **Boiling Water:**

   In a saucepan, bring 2 cups of water to a boil over medium heat.

3. **Steeping:**

   Once the water reaches a rolling boil, remove it from heat. Add the torn lettuce leaves to the hot water. Cover the saucepan and let the mixture steep for about 10-15 minutes.

4. **Straining:**

   Strain the tea into a cup using a fine mesh strainer or cheesecloth to remove the lettuce leaves.

5. **Flavoring (Optional):**

   Add a teaspoon of honey or a squeeze of lemon if desired.

6. **Serving:**

   Enjoy the tea warm, about 30-60 minutes before bedtime to maximize its relaxing effects.

**Benefits of Lettuce Tea for Sleep:**

Lettuce tea is believed to help with sleep due to its mild sedative effects, which can promote relaxation and reduce anxiety. The warm beverage can also aid in preparing the body for sleep by providing a comforting ritual that signals to the body that it is time to wind down (Kim et al., 2017).

**Non-Vegetarian Serotonin and Melatonin-Rich Supper**
**Recipe: Grilled Salmon with Quinoa and Spinach Salad**
**Ingredients:**

1. 2 salmon fillets (rich in omega-3 fatty acids and vitamin D) (Gupta et al., 2023)
2. 1 cup cooked quinoa (a complete protein source) (Rebollo-Hernanz et al., 2020)
3. 2 cups fresh spinach (rich in magnesium)
4. 1/2 avocado (contains healthy fats and potassium)
5. 1 tablespoon olive oil
6. Juice of 1 lemon
7. Salt and pepper to taste

**Instructions:**

1. Preheat the grill to medium-high heat. Season the salmon fillets with salt and pepper.
2. Grill the salmon for about 4-5 minutes on each side or until cooked through.
3. In a bowl, combine cooked quinoa, fresh spinach, and diced avocado.
4. Drizzle with olive oil and lemon juice, and toss to combine.
5. Serve the grilled salmon on a plate alongside the quinoa and spinach salad.
6. This meal is rich in omega-3 fatty acids from the salmon, supporting mood regulation and enhancing serotonin levels.

**Vegetarian Serotonin and Melatonin-Rich Supper**
**Recipe: Chickpea and Sweet Potato Curry**
**Ingredients:**

1. 1 can chickpeas, drained and rinsed (rich in tryptophan)
2. 1 medium sweet potato, diced (contains complex carbohydrates that help in serotonin production)
3. 1 can coconut milk
4. 1 onion, chopped
5. 2 cloves garlic, minced
6. 1 tablespoon curry powder
7. 1 teaspoon turmeric
8. 2 cups spinach (rich in magnesium)
9. Salt and pepper to taste
10. Fresh cilantro for garnish

**Instructions:**

1. In a large pot, sauté the onion and garlic until translucent.
2. Add the diced sweet potato, curry powder, and turmeric, stirring for 2 minutes.
3. Pour in the coconut milk and add the chickpeas. Bring to a simmer and cook until the sweet potato is tender (about 15-20 minutes).
4. Stir in the spinach and cook until wilted. Season with salt and pepper.
5. Serve hot, garnished with fresh cilantro.

This vegetarian curry is packed with nutrients that promote serotonin production, including chickpeas and sweet potatoes. The spices used, particularly turmeric, have anti-inflammatory properties that benefit overall health.

## Melatonin and Serotonin-Rich Dessert for Bedtime: Chocolate Banana Tart Cherry Chia Pudding

This recipe combines ingredients known to be rich in melatonin and serotonin, making it an ideal bedtime dessert. Bananas and tart cherries are good sources of tryptophan, a precursor to serotonin and melatonin, while chia seeds provide omega-3 fatty acids and fiber. Cocoa powder adds a rich chocolate flavor and contains compounds that may enhance mood.

**Ingredients:**
1. 1 ripe banana
2. 1 cup tart cherries (fresh or frozen)
3. 2 tablespoons chia seeds
4. 1 cup almond milk (or any milk of choice)
5. 2 tablespoons unsweetened cocoa powder
6. 1 tablespoon honey or maple syrup (optional, for sweetness)
7. 1/2 teaspoon vanilla extract
8. A pinch of salt

**Optional toppings**: sliced banana, nuts, or dark chocolate shavings.

**Instructions:**
1. Prepare the Banana: In a mixing bowl, mash the ripe banana until smooth. This will provide natural sweetness and creaminess to the pudding.
2. Combine Ingredients: Add the almond milk, cocoa powder, honey or maple syrup (if using), vanilla extract, and a pinch of salt to the mashed banana. Whisk until all ingredients are well combined and smooth.
3. Add Cherries and Chia Seeds: Stir in the tart cherries and chia seeds, ensuring they are evenly distributed throughout the mixture.
4. Refrigerate: Cover the bowl with plastic wrap or transfer the mixture to individual serving cups. Refrigerate for at least 2 hours or overnight. The chia seeds will absorb the liquid and thicken the pudding.

**Serve**: Once the pudding has set, give it a good stir. Serve chilled, topped with additional banana slices, nuts, or dark chocolate shavings if desired.

**Benefits of Ingredients:**
- **Tart Cherries:** Rich in melatonin and phytonutrients, tart cherries can help improve sleep quality and duration. They have been shown to increase urinary melatonin levels, which may enhance sleep efficiency (Binks et al., 2020; Courville & Chen, 2023).
- **Bananas:** Bananas are a good source of tryptophan, which can help increase serotonin levels, promoting relaxation and improved sleep quality (Pourreza et al., 2021).

- **Chia Seeds:** These seeds are high in omega-3 fatty acids and fiber, contributing to overall health and potentially aiding in sleep regulation (Pinto et al., 2021).

- **Cocoa Powder:** Contains flavonoids that may enhance mood and has been associated with improved cognitive function (Rodríguez-Cano, 2024).

- **Almond Milk:** A dairy-free alternative often fortified with vitamins and minerals, including calcium and vitamin D, which can support overall health.

**Evening Yoga for Relaxation:**

One hour before bed, engage in gentle or restorative yoga (Chandra Namaskar) to serve as a calming pre-sleep ritual. This practice significantly improves sleep quality and duration, particularly in individuals with sleep disturbances. It helps lower cortisol levels, which can otherwise interfere with sleep (Rao et al., 2017; Lin et al., 2018; Ratcliff et al., 2016).

**Heat Exposure:**

Take a hot shower or use a sauna to induce the production of heat shock proteins, which are beneficial for cellular repair and stress resilience (Ahmad et al., 2020). Taking a hot shower before bedtime can facilitate sleep by inducing a drop in core body temperature after exiting the shower. This process is crucial for signaling to the body that it is time to sleep, as a decrease in body temperature is associated with sleep onset (Haghayegh et al., 2019). Research indicates that bathing in warm water (around 40°C) for approximately 20 minutes can improve sleep quality and reduce sleep onset latency, particularly in individuals with sleep disturbances (Whitworth-Turner et al., 2017; Haghayegh et al., 2019).

The warm water increases peripheral blood flow, which enhances heat dissipation after leaving the shower, promoting relaxation and preparing the body for sleep (Haghayegh et al., 2019).

Regular sauna use has been linked to numerous health benefits, including improved sleep quality. The heat exposure from a sauna session can lead to increased relaxation and reduced muscle tension, which are conducive to better sleep (Kirby et al., 2021). A systematic review highlighted that sauna bathing can enhance sleep quality by promoting deeper sleep stages and reducing sleep disturbances (Haghayegh et al., 2019). The heat from the sauna can also stimulate the release of endorphins, which can improve mood and reduce stress, further contributing to better sleep outcomes (Kirby et al., 2021).

**Gratitude and Planning:**
Practice gratitude and create a to-do list for the next day. These activities help clear the mind, reduce anxiety, and improve sleep quality (Ahmad et al., 2020).

**Consistent Sleep Schedule:**
Go to bed at the same time each night. Research indicates that the longest periods of NREM sleep typically occur in the first few hours of the sleep cycle, making this time particularly vital for recovery and rejuvenation (Lok et al., 2022). NREM sleep, particularly the slow-wave sleep (SWS) component, is considered the most restorative phase of the sleep cycle. It is during this stage that the body undergoes critical healing processes, including tissue repair, immune function enhancement, and memory consolidation (Hong et al., 2020).

Studies have shown that individuals with inconsistent sleep schedules experience decreased delta power and time spent in NREM sleep, which can impair sleep-dependent memory consolidation and overall cognitive function (Hong et al., 2020). This disruption is particularly concerning as it can result in a cumulative deficit of restorative sleep, leading to long-term health consequences.

Irregular sleep patterns can cause a misalignment of the circadian rhythm, which governs the timing of sleep stages. This misalignment can lead to a reduction in the duration and quality of NREM sleep, as the body struggles to adapt to varying sleep times (Grimaldi et al., 2016). For instance, research has demonstrated that irregular sleep is associated with an increased risk of sleep disorders, cardiovascular issues, and metabolic dysfunctions (Sansom, 2024; Parise et al., 2023). Consistency is key for maintaining a healthy sleep-wake cycle, ensuring that the crucial NREM stage of sleep is not disrupted (Kurtović, 2023).

Furthermore, the inability to achieve sufficient NREM sleep can lead to increased daytime sleepiness, mood disturbances, and cognitive deficits, further compounding the negative effects of irregular sleep (Phillips et al., 2017). Bedtime consistency is vital for maximizing the restorative benefits of sleep and enhancing overall health and well-being (Hayashi et al., 2015).

**Sleep Aid Smorgasbord: From Chamomile Courtesy to Magnesium Calm**

Ah, insomnia—a condition where the only thing that keeps you company at 3 AM is the ceiling and the crushing existential dread of counting sheep that apparently took an exit ramp a few hours back. It's affecting 10-30% of people worldwide, with about half dealing with it chronically (Guo et al., 2020). And just when we thought things couldn't get worse, the COVID-19 pandemic decided to throw more insomnia into the mix, spiking cases by 47% to 189% (Lu et al., 2023). But here's the real kicker: insomnia isn't just stealing your sleep, it's also shrinking your brain. Research shows that insomnia is linked to neurodegenerative processes, including increased levels of amyloid-beta, which is associated with Alzheimer's (Guo et al., 2020; Palagini et al., 2021). And if you've got the APOE ε4 allele, insomnia is even more of a brain burglar, hitting your cognitive performance harder (Baril et al., 2021).

So, insomnia isn't just an annoying nighttime companion—it's a full-on brain vandal. Time to take it seriously, because your brain's not just losing sleep, it's losing volume.

There is a mention of GABA in the content below—for those who don't speak neurotransmitter, it is like the brain's monk, keeping things quiet and making sure you can actually relax enough to drift off (Miranda-Apodaca et al., 2023).

**Types of Sleep Aids**

Sleep aids come in two main categories: pharmacological (the serious stuff) and non-pharmacological (the gentler, often tea-based stuff). Pharmacological options include prescription meds like benzodiazepines and trazodone, alongside over-the-counter options like melatonin. Non-pharmacological aids range from behavioral strategies and environmental tweaks to alternative therapies like herbal teas and CBT—though, unfortunately, there's no "counting sheep" therapy in the DSM yet (Aldhafiri, 2023; Wong et al., 2022).

**Melatonin**

Melatonin is the hormone that tells your brain, "Hey, it's dark outside—time to sleep!" It's especially handy for people whose internal clocks are slightly off, like shift workers or those who think "bedtime" is more of a suggestion. Studies have shown that melatonin can help you fall asleep faster and improve the quality of your sleep (Gammoh, 2024; Surman & Walsh, 2021).

Studies show that just 1 mg of this sleepy-time superhero can have you dozing off faster than a toddler after a day at the zoo (Pachimsawat, 2024). And if you're feeling extra adventurous, doses between 1 to 10 mg work wonders for folks across the board, including those whose brains are a little too active at night (Motlaq, 2024).

But here's the catch in children, its long-term safety is still up in the air, especially since it hasn't undergone the rigorous testing required for kids (Kennaway, 2015; Mantle et al., 2020). There's also concern that melatonin could mess with puberty timing, making health experts a bit nervous (Boafo et al., 2019; Bruni et al., 2015).

Add to that the fact that melatonin doses can be all over the place, leading to some kids waking up in the middle of the night instead of sleeping soundly (Bruni et al., 2015; Horsnell, 2023). And since most kids are taking it off-label, there are no clear rules on how to use it safely (Hartz et al., 2015; Goldman et al., 2021).

A study by Brzezinski et al. (2005) found that melatonin not only reduces the time it takes to drift off but also increases total sleep time (Kennaway, 2015). Sounds great, right? Well, not so fast. Melatonin's effectiveness depends on your age, dosage, and the specific sleep issue you're battling (Mantle et al., 2020). So, while it might work wonders for your friend, you could still be counting sheep for hours.

But melatonin isn't all sweet dreams. Side effects like daytime drowsiness, dizziness, and headaches might leave you feeling like a zombie (Boafo et al., 2019). Plus, it loves to meddle with your meds—especially blood thinners, potentially increasing your risk of bleeding (Horsnell, 2023).

While short-term use is generally safe, long-term melatonin use raises some eyebrows. Your body might start to rely on it for sleep, messing with your natural circadian rhythm (Hartz et al., 2015). Oh, and melatonin isn't shy about meddling with your hormones, potentially affecting estrogen and testosterone levels. So, if you're thinking of relying on it forever, your sleep might not be the only thing it changes (Goldman et al., 2021).

## Magnesium

Studies suggest that magnesium can improve sleep quality, especially for those who are running low on this essential mineral (Ashokkumar, 2023; Mengistu et al., 2020).

For those serious about getting their beauty sleep, magnesium glycinate is the go-to. It's easy on the stomach and works like a charm to improve sleep quality, with a daily dose of 250 to 500 mg being the sweet spot (Breus, 2024).
When magnesium and glycine team up, you're looking at improved sleep latency and overall sleep quality, like a VIP pass to a good night's rest (Asplund, 2024). Please check with your doctor if you have kidney disease, as it can worsen kidney dysfunction in some patients.

Magnesium plays a key role in producing GABA, the neurotransmitter that's like a gentle "shhh" to your overactive thoughts, telling your brain, "Hey, it's time to chill out and get some sleep" (Özek, 2024; Knobbe et al., 2023). But that's not all—magnesium also helps keep those pesky excitatory signals in check, calming your nervous system like a warm blanket on a cold night (Knobbe et al., 2023). Magnesium is also behind the scenes helping your body produce melatonin, the hormone that manages your sleep-wake cycle. Without enough magnesium, melatonin doesn't quite hit the mark, and you end up staring at the ceiling wondering why sleep feels like a distant dream (Dhillon et al., 2023).

It's also a hero for those restless legs, helping to keep them from staging an all-night dance marathon while you're just trying to catch some Z's (Asplund, 2024; Chan & Lo, 2021; Jadidi et al., 2022).

**Advantages:** Magnesium's superpower is its ability to reduce anxiety and promote relaxation, making it easier to drift off. It's also linked to better sleep efficiency, meaning you spend more time in dreamland and less time staring at the ceiling (Bedaso et al., 2020; Nakamura et al., 2021).

**Disadvantages:** Too much of a good thing, though, and magnesium can turn your peaceful night into a mad dash to the bathroom. Overdoing it can cause gastrointestinal issues like diarrhea, and people with kidney problems should be extra careful, as they might end up with too much magnesium in their system (Yamaguchi et al., 2023; Suzuki, 2024).

*Caution:* Magnesium glycinate, though great for sleep, can be risky for those with chronic kidney disease (CKD). As CKD progresses, your kidneys struggle to filter magnesium, leading to dangerous buildup (Cunningham et al., 2012; Kanbay et al., 2012; Patel et al., 2018). This can worsen kidney function and cause heart issues, especially when GFR drops below 30 mL/min (Massy & Drüeke, 2015; Leenders et al., 2021). It also disrupts parathyroid hormone (PTH), leading to calcium imbalances and potential vascular calcification (Patel et al., 2018). Plus, it can increase inflammation, further harming your kidneys (Mamilla, 2023; Sakaguchi, 2022).

## Glycine

Glycine is the quiet achiever of the sleep aid world. This amino acid can help improve sleep quality and reduce the time it takes to nod off, especially for those with insomnia (Chiba et al., 2023). Research suggests that 3 grams of glycine before bed is like giving your brain a gentle nudge and saying, "Hey, how about we chill out now?" It's like the warm milk of the supplement world, only without the weird aftertaste (Esquivel, 2024).

**Glycine**, an amino acid that acts as an inhibitory neurotransmitter, helps promote sleep by lowering core body temperature—similar to how a hot shower signals your body it's time to sleep (Bruni et al., 2021). A randomized controlled trial showed that glycine significantly improved sleep quality and reduced the time it takes to fall asleep, making it a promising, natural sleep aid (Rahbardar, 2024). Glycine's role in boosting serotonin, the precursor to melatonin, further enhances its sleep-inducing effects (Rafiei, 2023). Best of all, glycine has a great safety profile, with no risk of dependency, making it a gentle and effective option for better sleep (Ibrahim et al., 2022).

*Advantages:* Glycine is generally safe and comes with the added bonus of potentially boosting cognitive function—so you might wake up not just rested, but also a little sharper. Plus, it's well-tolerated, meaning it won't leave you with a laundry list of side effects (Nakamura et al., 2021).

*Disadvantages*: The downside? Some people might experience mild tummy troubles. And while early research is promising, we still need more studies to fully understand the long-term effects of glycine on sleep (Chiba et al., 2023).

## Herbal Teas

Herbal teas are the ultimate bedtime companion for those who prefer a gentle nudge towards sleep rather than a full-on shove. Chamomile, lavender, valerian root, and passionflower are just a few of the herbs believed to help you relax and drift off to dreamland.

*Advantages*: Herbal teas are safe, widely accessible, and can become part of a soothing bedtime routine. Plus, they're caffeine-free, so you won't be up all night wondering if you should've gone for that second cup (Eke et al., 2020; Dickson & Schubert, 2020).

*Disadvantages*: But beware, not all herbal teas are created equal. The effectiveness can vary depending on the blend and your personal tolerance, and some people might find themselves sneezing or itching from an unexpected herbal reaction. Also, the concentration of active ingredients can be hit or miss, so that sleepytime tea might not be as knockout as you hoped (Teo et al., 2022).

## Lettuce Tea

Yes, you read that right—lettuce tea. Made from the leaves of *Lactuca sativa* (fancy talk for lettuce), the unsuspecting salad star is secretly a sleep ninja. Who would've guessed that the leafy green you toss into your sandwich could also help you catch some Z's? The real heroes here are lactucin and lactucopicrin, two compounds that have been shown to boost GABA activity, the brain's very own "calm down" signal (Huang et al., 2022; Kumar et al., 2021).

Studies show that lettuce seed oil has hypnotic, sedative, and even anticonvulsant effects, likely due to its influence on GABA, your brain's "relax" signal (İlgün et al., 2020). But lettuce doesn't stop there—it's also packing flavonoids and phenolic acids, which add antioxidant power to the mix and help reduce oxidative stress, a culprit behind sleep troubles (Pelegrino et al., 2021; Liang et al., 2021).

Let's not forget the magnesium in lettuce, which is the sleep sidekick that helps GABA do its job and keeps melatonin, the sleep hormone, running smoothly (Yang, 2024; Kuo et al., 2023). Put all these components together, and you've got a leafy green cocktail of sleep-inducing goodness that's more than just a garnish on your plate (Takahashi et al., 2021; Wang et al., 2022). By the way, lettuce also contains glycine, the amino acid that cools your body down and gets you ready for sleep, like slipping into cozy pajamas.

Add quercetin-3-glucuronide—a compound that makes GABA receptors even happier—and you've got a leafy green tea cocktail of sleep-inducing goodness (Yang et al., 2021; Rahbardar, 2024). Lettuce seed oil has been used to boost sleep quality and duration, making it a serious contender in the herbal sleep aid arena (Yakoot et al., 2011; Liu et al., 2015). When lettuce teams up with other herbal heavyweights, the sleep-inducing effects get even stronger (Hong et al., 2018; Bae, 2023).

But that's not all—lettuce tea also reduces stress and inflammation, thanks to its ability to inhibit pro-inflammatory cytokines and combat oxidative stress, both of which can mess with your sleep (Syed et al., 2022). For an extra sleepy punch, mix it with chamomile, and you've got a natural, soothing remedy proven to improve sleep quality, especially for those with sleep disorders (Syed et al., 2022).

*Advantages*: Lettuce tea is a low-calorie, easy-to-make option that you can whip up in your kitchen. Plus, it's safe, so you can sip away without worrying about side effects (Gordon et al., 2022).

*Disadvantages*: The science backing lettuce tea's effectiveness is still, well, kind of wilted. More research is needed to confirm whether it really works, and if you're not a fan of its leafy taste, you might not find it appealing enough to stick with (Stueber, 2023).

**Something to Ponder (but not when you're trying to sleep—save the pondering for daytime, my friend, if you must ponder at all)**

The use of dietary supplements for enhancing sleep quality has garnered significant attention in recent years, as individuals seek alternatives to conventional pharmacological treatments. Herbal remedies such as valerian root, chamomile, and passionflower have been widely recognized for their sedative effects. Valerian, for example, has been noted for its ability to reduce sleep latency and improve overall sleep quality, primarily through its interaction with the GABAergic system, which plays a crucial role in regulating sleep (Bruni et al., 2021; Rahbardar, 2024). Additionally, a systematic review highlighted the efficacy of various plant extracts, including saffron and *Dracocephalum*, in alleviating sleep disturbances, suggesting that these natural products can serve as effective alternatives to traditional sleep medications (Rafiei, 2023; Ibrahim et al., 2022).

## Sun doing the saving – Oh what all It has in its store

### NO (Nitric Oxide): The Smooth Operator

When it comes to sunlight's effect on your brain, NO—or Nitric Oxide—deserves the spotlight. Think of NO as the smooth operator that relaxes your blood vessels, boosting blood flow like a VIP pass straight to your neurons. Sunlight, particularly UVB and red/infrared light, ramps up NO production by activating nitric oxide synthase (NOS) enzymes in your skin cells. Once produced, NO dilates your blood vessels, improving circulation and ensuring that your brain gets a fresh supply of oxygen and nutrients. This increased blood flow isn't just good for keeping you sharp; it also plays a role in neurogenesis—the birth of new neurons (Karu, 2008; Hamblin, 2017).

But NO doesn't stop there. It also teams up with other bioactive molecules like Calcitonin Gene-Related Peptide (CGRP) to ensure your neurons are firing on all cylinders. Think of CGRP as the brain's personal trainer, encouraging neurogenesis and keeping those neurons in tip-top shape (Brain et al., 1985). Together, NO and CGRP create a brain environment where new neurons can thrive, making you quicker, smarter, and ready to tackle that Sudoku puzzle you've been avoiding.

### Melatonin: The Night Shift Hero

You might be wondering, "Isn't melatonin that stuff that makes me sleepy?" Well, yes, but it's also much more. Melatonin is like the unsung hero of your brain's night shift, protecting your neurons from oxidative stress and inflammation while you snooze. But here's the twist—sunlight helps regulate melatonin production by influencing your circadian rhythm. The more balanced your circadian rhythm, the better your melatonin production, and the happier your neurons are (Brainard et al., 1996). Melatonin also promotes neurogenesis, especially in the hippocampus, by acting as an antioxidant that shields your brain from the daily wear and tear (Reiter et al., 2014).

### Beta-Endorphin: Your Brain's Natural High

Ever wonder why you feel so good after a day in the sun? That's your brain pumping out beta-endorphins, the body's natural painkillers and mood boosters.

These peptides are produced in response to UV exposure and give you that blissful post-sunbathing glow (Luger & Schwarz, 1995). But beta-endorphins aren't just about making you feel great—they also support neurogenesis by creating a positive emotional environment in which your brain can flourish. Happy brain, healthy neurons!

### CGRP: The Nurturer

Calcitonin Gene-Related Peptide (CGRP) is like your brain's personal nurse, nurturing new neurons and ensuring they integrate well into your neural network. When sunlight stimulates NO production, it also promotes the release of CGRP from your skin cells. CGRP then helps protect your brain from damage by reducing inflammation and promoting the growth of new neurons (Brain et al., 1985). So, every time you step into the sun, you're essentially giving your brain a dose of TLC.

### Infrared Rays: The Deep Tissue Healer

Infrared rays are like a deep tissue massage for your cells. They penetrate deep into your tissues, including your brain, and stimulate mitochondrial function—the powerhouse of the cell. Improved mitochondrial function means more energy (ATP) for your neurons, which in turn supports neurogenesis. It's like your brain just had a supercharged workout session, and it's getting stronger with each exposure to sunlight (Hamblin, 2017).

### Red Light

If your brain could talk, it might ask for a bit of red-light therapy, much like how a plant craves sunlight. Shining red or near-infrared light on your noggin can actually stimulate neurogenesis, particularly in the hippocampus, which is the brain's memory factory. According to Hamblin (2021), this therapy enhances mitochondrial function, reduces oxidative stress, and increases brain-derived neurotrophic factor (BDNF), essentially giving your neurons a rejuvenating spa day. While you won't start glowing red or sprouting leaves, your brain might just feel a bit more photosynthetically enhanced!

### Hyperbaric Oxygen Therapy (HBOT)

Imagine your brain floating in a sea of pure oxygen, taking in deep breaths and puffing up like a sponge. Hyperbaric oxygen therapy (HBOT) does just that by saturating your brain with oxygen, promoting neurogenesis, and even increasing brain volume in certain areas. Boussi-Gross et al. (2023) found that HBOT can lead to measurable increases in gray matter volume, particularly in patients recovering from traumatic brain injuries. It's like giving your brain an oxygen-fueled workout. Although you might not turn into a brainy version of Popeye, your neurons will certainly feel stronger!

## From Flintstones Vitamins to Einstein Elixirs

### The Multifaceted Marvel - Vitamin D & K2

Welcome to the whimsical world of Vitamin D, where this sunny superstar plays the leading role in numerous biochemical blockbusters. Imagine Vitamin D as the multi-talented superhero in your body, donning various capes to tackle different villains like bone weakness, immune disorders, and even cognitive decline. From keeping your bones sturdy to ensuring your brain stays sharp, Vitamin D's physiological escapades are nothing short of legendary.

Vitamin D is produced in the skin in response to sunlight exposure. It then undergoes two hydroxylations in the body to become the active form, calcitriol. This mighty molecule binds to Vitamin D receptors (VDR) present in almost every cell of the body, influencing a multitude of physiological processes (Holick, 2007). Think of calcitriol as the ultimate fixer-upper in your body's biochemical factory. It regulates calcium and phosphate balance, ensuring your bones are as tough as adamantium. But that's not all—Vitamin D also modulates immune function, reduces inflammation, and even plays a role in muscle function and cardiovascular health (Tappia, 2024).

### Vitamin D and Brain Health: A Cognitive Cavalry

Just when you thought Vitamin D couldn't get any cooler, it gallops into the brain to combat the foes of cognitive decline. Research suggests that Vitamin D plays a pivotal role in brain development and function. It's like having a tiny guardian angel in your neurons, keeping oxidative stress and inflammation at bay (He & Yu, 2024).

Vitamin D receptors and the enzyme 1-alpha-hydroxylase, which converts Vitamin D to its active form, are found in various brain regions. These regions are responsible for memory formation and processing, suggesting that Vitamin D is crucial for maintaining cognitive health (Zhou et al., 2024).

When Vitamin D levels are low, it's like the superhero is off-duty, and chaos ensues. Vitamin D deficiency has been linked to an increased risk of dementia and Alzheimer's disease. Without enough Vitamin D, the brain becomes susceptible to increased oxidative stress, inflammation, and impaired neurotransmitter synthesis, leading to cognitive decline (Al Shamsi et al., 2024).

Imagine your brain as a bustling city where Vitamin D is the diligent mayor. When the mayor is absent, the city's infrastructure deteriorates, leading to traffic jams (cognitive fog), broken streetlights (memory lapses), and overall disorder (dementia).

First up, a massive systematic review and meta-analysis of 9,267 studies (yes, that's a lot) by Zhang et al. found that being low on Vitamin D cranks up your risk of dementia by 42% and Alzheimer's by a jaw-dropping 57%. Oh, and it also bumps your chances of cognitive impairment by 34%. The sweet spot for keeping your brain in tip-top shape? Aim for Vitamin D levels between 77.5–100 nmol/L to keep dementia at bay and above 40.1 nmol/L to stay out of Alzheimer's territory. But hold on, there's more! Turns out, low Vitamin D levels are also linked to more advanced stages of Parkinson's Disease (Khan et al., 2024). And if that wasn't enough to make you want to bathe in sunlight, another study using MRI scans of 201 elderly individuals found that lower Vitamin D levels were associated with shrunken brain regions critical for memory—especially in Alzheimer's patients (Annweiler et al., 2015).

And the hits keep coming! In a study of 214 stroke patients, researchers found that those with lower Vitamin D levels not only had worse sleep but were also dealing with higher levels of depression and anxiety (Asuman et al., 2024). So, if you're looking for a reason to bask in the sun, here it is: a study with over 12,000 participants found that higher Vitamin D levels were linked to lower anxiety (Wen et al., 2024). So, go ahead and join the sun-soaked crowd!

In another cool study, 46 patients with major depressive disorder (MDD) were divided into two groups: one got antidepressants plus Vitamin D supplements, and the other got antidepressants and a placebo. After seven months, the Vitamin D group not only felt better but also showed no disruptions in critical brain connections, unlike the placebo group (Zhao et al., 2024).

And it doesn't stop there—Vitamin D3 teamed up with neurofeedback therapy in a study on kids with ADHD. The results? Those on Vitamin D saw their brain function improve, especially in reducing those pesky theta waves linked to ADHD symptoms (Mirhosseini et al., 2024). Meanwhile, another study found that higher maternal Vitamin D levels before birth were associated with a lower risk of autism and ADHD in their kids (Aagaard et al., 2024).

Still not convinced? Well, another randomized trial found that Vitamin D3 could help reduce seizures in patients with drug-resistant epilepsy by up to 52%! Plus, these patients reported feeling less fatigued and showed improvements in their overall quality of life (Chassoux et al., 2024).

So, Vitamin D isn't just your sunshine vitamin—it's a full-on brain protector. It helps clear out amyloid plaques, protects neurons, and reduces inflammation tied to Alzheimer's. It's also great for your blood vessels, lowering the risk of stroke and those worrying white matter hyperintensities. With all these perks, Vitamin D is shaping up to be your brain's best friend.

Oh, and one more thing—did you know that Vitamin D is a unique neurosteroid hormone? It's got a bunch of important jobs in the brain, like neuromodulation and supporting neuroplasticity. Vitamin D receptors are all over the brain, including in areas like the hippocampus and cingulate cortex, where it helps regulate your "happy chemicals" and keeps your circadian rhythms in check (AlGhamdi et al., 2024).

So, get some sun—or at least a supplement—because your brain might depend on it! And just for fun, did you know that mushrooms can turn into little Vitamin D factories when exposed to UV light? Just 15 minutes of sunlight can boost their Vitamin D2 levels from almost nothing to over 600 IU per 70g! Leaving them out for 60 minutes? That'll give you a whopping 158% increase in Vitamin D content compared to fresh mushrooms that haven't had their sunbath. So, maybe it's not just you that needs some sun—your mushrooms do too!

**By the way, don't forget to add Vitamin K2 (MK7 isomer) to your D3 for maximum benefit.**

Adding vitamin K2 in its MK7 form to our diets isn't just the latest health fad—it's more like giving your body a superhero sidekick, and trust me, this sidekick doesn't just wear a cape; it's got some serious science backing it up. The MK7 variant of vitamin K2 is like the overachiever in the vitamin K family, with superior bioavailability and a longer half-life, meaning it sticks around longer to work its magic on your health. This form of vitamin K2 isn't just coasting on its good looks; it's been shown to support cardiovascular health, boost bone density, and even offer some neuroprotective perks.

Let's talk about cardiovascular health, where MK7 shines like a heart-shaped superhero signal in the sky. Research shows that MK7 is a key player in preventing arterial calcification. Think of it as a guard that keeps calcium out of your arteries and sends it where it belongs—your bones. This helps keep your blood vessels flexible and functional, reducing the risk of cardiovascular issues (Diederichsen et al., 2022). One study even found that MK7 supplementation could slow down the progression of aortic valve calcification, making it the ultimate shield against heart disease (Diederichsen et al., 2022).

And if that wasn't enough, MK7 also has anti-inflammatory powers, which is particularly relevant in today's world. During the COVID-19 pandemic, researchers noticed that patients with lower MK7 levels tended to have worse outcomes, suggesting that this vitamin might play a role in the body's defense against severe illness (Mangge et al., 2022).

But wait, there's more! MK7 isn't just a heart hero; it's also your bones' best friend. It activates osteocalcin, a protein that ensures calcium ends up in your bones rather than clogging up your arteries (Sato et al., 2020). Clinical trials have shown that MK7 can significantly improve bone mineral density, especially in postmenopausal women, making it a powerful ally in the fight against osteoporosis ("Tamoxifen for Five Years?", 2021). Thanks to its high bioavailability, MK7 is better absorbed and utilized by the body, giving your bones the support they need to stay strong (Sato et al., 2020).

Plus, it helps osteoblasts, the cells responsible for building bone, by reducing oxidative stress and encouraging their growth (Muszyńska et al., 2020). So, if your bones could talk, they'd probably be singing MK7's praises right about now.

And let's not forget about your brain. MK7 might just be the brain's secret weapon. It's been shown to preserve mitochondrial function, which is crucial for keeping your neurons happy and healthy (Shandilya et al., 2021). This is particularly important in conditions like Parkinson's disease, where mitochondrial dysfunction is a major villain in the story. By boosting ATP production and promoting autophagy (the brain's version of taking out the trash), MK7 could offer serious support for neurodegenerative conditions (Shandilya et al., 2021).

Now, here's the kicker: Not all vitamin K2 is created equal. The MK7 isomer is the real deal, and it's important to ensure your supplements contain this specific form. Improper storage and processing can mess with the isomerization, leading to less effective forms of vitamin K (Cirilli et al., 2022). MK7 also has a unique ability to redistribute to extrahepatic tissues (like your blood vessels and bones), further emphasizing its systemic health benefits (Mangge et al., 2022).

## Why You Shouldn't Take Vitamin D at Bedtime

Vitamin D, the overachiever of the vitamin world, isn't just about keeping your bones in check—it's also a bit of a control freak when it comes to your brain. This sunshine vitamin manages to sneak past the blood-brain barrier like a well-connected insider and cozies up to the vitamin D receptor (VDR) and its trusty sidekick, 1α-hydroxylase. These two are like the brain's favorite power couple, hanging out in neurons and glial cells, ensuring everything from your mood to your sleep cycles runs smoothly (Kaneko et al., 2015; Patrick & Ames, 2015).

In our study, we found that Vitamin D is basically in a long-term relationship with depressive symptoms, with sleep disturbances as the annoying third wheel. Especially if you're one of those people who just can't drift off at night, that might be Vitamin D trying to drop some not-so-subtle hints about why you're feeling down in the dumps. Lack of Vitamin D could be messing with your sleep, and in turn, making your mood as unstable as a Jenga tower (Jung et al., 2017).

The exact mechanics of how Vitamin D pulls all these strings are still a bit of a mystery, but we've got a pretty good theory. Imagine Vitamin D as the manager of a very important band—serotonin and melatonin. Vitamin D knows just when to nudge the brain's tryptophan hydroxylase 2 (TPH2) into action, turning tryptophan (the infamous post-Thanksgiving nap ingredient) into serotonin, which is responsible for keeping you cheerful and sharp (Kaneko et al., 2015; Patrick & Ames, 2015).

Meanwhile, in the rest of your body, Vitamin D keeps a tight leash on tryptophan hydroxylase 1 (TPH1), ensuring it doesn't go overboard with serotonin production. Too much serotonin outside the brain could throw things out of whack, and nobody wants that (Kaneko et al., 2015).

But here's where Vitamin D really shows off its skills: it's also in charge of melatonin production. As the sun sets, Vitamin D steps back, and your pineal gland steps up to convert all that serotonin into melatonin, the hormone that tells you it's time to hit the hay (Patrick & Ames, 2015). Vitamin D levels naturally peak around noon and drop in the evening, which is why it's crucial to time your Vitamin D intake wisely.

If you take Vitamin D too late in the day, it's like handing your brain a double espresso right before bed—confusing your natural sleep rhythm and making it harder to wind down (Jung et al., 2017; Patrick & Ames, 2015). So, for the sake of your sleep and sanity, let Vitamin D do its work during the day and leave the nighttime peace and quiet to melatonin.

**Ways to Fuel Your Vitamin D Levels: Sunlight, Food, and Supplements**
Fear not, for your pantry holds the secret to summoning this superhero. Here are some foods rich in Vitamin D to keep your biochemical processes running smoothly:

**Fatty Fish**: Salmon, mackerel, and sardines are like Vitamin D powerhouses, ready to boost your levels.
**Egg Yolks**: These sunny spheres are not just for breakfast—they pack a punch of Vitamin D (Oster, 2023).
**Fortified Foods**: Many dairy products, orange juice, and cereals are fortified with Vitamin D. Think of them as fortified castles, ready to defend your health.
**Mushrooms**: Those delightful fungi that often find their way onto our plates have a remarkable ability to absorb sunlight and convert it into vitamin D. When exposed to sunlight, mushrooms can significantly increase their vitamin D2 levels; for instance, a mere 15 minutes of sunlight exposure can boost their vitamin D2 content by 150 to over 600 IU per 70 mg of mushroom (Agarwal & Fulgoni, 2021; Fulgoni & Agarwal, 2021). This transformation occurs because mushrooms contain ergosterol, a precursor to vitamin D2, which converts to the vitamin when exposed to UV light (Mattila et al., 2001; Cardwell et al., 2018). The vitamin D2 content can vary dramatically depending on the mushroom's exposure to

sunlight. Wild mushrooms can contain between 2.91 to 29.82 µg of vitamin D2 per 100 g when exposed to sunlight, while cultivated varieties, such as the common white button mushroom (*Agaricus bisporus*), typically have much lower levels, starting at around 0.21 µg per 100 g (Mattila et al., 2001; Singh & Joshi, 2023).

## Practical Tips for Boosting Vitamin D

**Sunshine**: Get outdoors and soak up some rays, especially in the early morning or late afternoon when UV exposure is safer.

**Diet**: Incorporate Vitamin D-rich foods into your meals. Think salmon salads and mushrooms.

**Supplements**: If you're at risk of deficiency, consider taking Vitamin D supplements. Consult with your healthcare provider for the appropriate dosage.

## Thiamine (Vitamin B1)

Think of thiamine, or vitamin B1, as the spark plug for your brain's engine. Without it, your neurons start sputtering like a car running out of gas. For those with a thiamine deficiency, the brain can begin to shrink and falter, leading to cognitive stall-outs. But here's the good news: replacing thiamine in deficient patients is like giving your brain a full tank of premium fuel. According to Butterworth et al. (2021), thiamine replacement can lead to a reversal of brain volume loss, particularly in areas like the mammillary bodies and thalamus, which are crucial for memory and cognitive function. This replenishment helps kickstart neurogenesis, allowing the brain to regrow neurons and regain its lost volume. So, if your brain's been feeling a bit sluggish, a thiamine boost might be just what it needs to go from "puttering" to "purring" again.

# To B12 or Not to B12

And the answer is always "yes" for Vitamin B12. (Sorry, Shakespeare!)
Imagine finding out that your brain has been running on low power because it's been starved of vitamin B12—like discovering your phone's been on battery saver mode this whole time. Low blood B12 is associated with cognitive decline (Irwin H. Rosenberg, 2024). According to Douaud et al. (2023), B12 replacement not only boosts neurogenesis (making new neurons) but also helps prevent brain shrinkage, effectively plumping up those brain cells that were looking a little deflated.

A study by Tangney et al. found that higher vitamin B12 levels were linked to better cognitive performance and brain MRI measures, suggesting that maintaining sufficient B12 levels may help support brain structure and function. Conversely, low levels of vitamin B12 can lead to brain shrinkage, which is detrimental to cognitive health (Fulgoni & Agarwal, 2021).
As a doctor, the number of patients I see with dementia due to B12 deficiency is just heart-wrenching. So many of them are so young. Aaaaaaaah.
And yes, I AM SCREAMING HERE because B12 deficiency is ONE OF THE PREVENTABLE CAUSES OF MEMORY LOSS. So, get on board, people, and save your brain!

Studies are throwing up some eye-popping stats: about 20% of type 2 diabetic patients on metformin are low on B12 (Peixoto et al., 2024). And let's not forget the rise in vegetarian and vegan diets. As they skip out on animal proteins, they're also skipping out on natural B12 sources. Add gastrointestinal conditions like Crohn's and celiac disease to the mix, and you've got a recipe for widespread deficiency (Jali et al., 2024).

Recent trends and reports indicate that the recreational use of nitrous oxide (whippets) has been on the rise, especially among young adults and teenagers. Inhaling nitrous oxide, or doing a "whippet," might give you a quick high, but it also inactivates vitamin B12 by oxidizing the cobalt ion in the B12 molecule (Oussalah et al., 2019). This inactivation sabotages methionine synthase, an enzyme crucial for converting homocysteine to methionine, which is essential for DNA synthesis and repair (Thompson et al., 2015). The result? Brain fog, nerve damage, and mood disorders, turning your brain into a malfunctioning mess (Scalabrino, 2009) and even paralysis.

The takeaway? We need to keep an eye on our B12 levels and maybe pop a supplement (preferably the kind that dissolves in your mouth) or two if we're in the danger zone (Irwin H. Rosenberg, 2024).

## Vitamin B12: The Brain's All-in-One Maintenance Crew

Vitamin B12 is like the brain's all-in-one maintenance crew: it fixes everything from wiring to cleaning to energy supply. It helps lower homocysteine, a toxic byproduct, by converting it to methionine, crucial for DNA repair and neurotransmitter production—think of it as taking out the trash and making new brain parts (Smith & Refsum, 2016).

B12 also aids in myelin production, the insulation around your neurons, ensuring your brain signals zip around smoothly, like a fiber-optic internet connection (Scalabrino, 2009). Without enough B12, your neurons start to fray, leading to conditions like Alzheimer's, dementia, and even depression because neurotransmitters like serotonin and dopamine get out of whack (O'Leary & Samman, 2010). Plus, B12 keeps the brain's power plants (mitochondria) running efficiently, so your brain doesn't suffer from energy blackouts. Keep your B12 levels up, or your brain might start acting like a poorly maintained theme park—slow, broken rides, and not much fun for anyone (Carmel, 2008).

## Let's Get to Know B12 First

Vitamin B12, or cobalamin, is the biochemical equivalent of a Swiss army knife for your body, featuring a cobalt ion nestled snugly in a corrin ring—a structure so intricate it could make a watchmaker weep. This cobalt superstar can sport various accessories depending on its mood: a methyl group for methylcobalamin, a 5'-deoxyadenosyl group for adenosylcobalamin, a hydroxyl group for hydroxocobalamin, or a cyanide group for cyanocobalamin (don't worry, it's the safe kind).

Picture B12 navigating the treacherous landscape of your digestive system, fending off stomach acid with its trusty sidekick, Intrinsic Factor, before getting a lift from Transcobalamin II to travel through your bloodstream. It then makes its way to the brain, where it ensures nerve cells are well-insulated and neurotransmitters are firing like a well-rehearsed orchestra. Found in foods like liver, fish, dairy, and eggs, B12 is essential for DNA synthesis, red blood cell formation, and neurological function. Without it, your nerves would be slower than dial-up internet, and your brain would be as confused as a cat in a dog show.

**Metformin and B12 Deficiency**

Metformin, the go-to med for type 2 diabetes, has a sneaky side effect: it can cause vitamin B12 deficiency by messing with your gut's absorption abilities. It alters intestinal motility, leads to bacterial overgrowth, and interferes with calcium-dependent absorption processes. Imagine your B12 trying to get through customs, only to be held up indefinitely. If you're on metformin, keep an eye on your B12 levels. If they start to drop, consider sublingual B12 supplements, which dissolve under your tongue and bypass the gut entirely—think of it as giving B12 a VIP pass straight into your system (Bauman et al., 2000; Ting et al., 2006). B12 likes to chill in the liver's VIP lounge, where it's stored in excess. But if it can't be absorbed for a while due to dietary insufficiency, malabsorption, or a lack of Intrinsic Factor, those liver reserves eventually run dry, and deficiency symptoms start to crash the party (Green, 2017; Stabler, 2013).

Mary Todd Lincoln, the wife of President Abraham Lincoln, suffered from severe depression, fatigue, and other neurological symptoms. Later analysis of her medical history suggests that she had B12 deficiency due to poor absorption.

**Checking Your B12 Levels**

I highly, highly, highly urge everyone to check their B12 blood levels. However, that can be a bit tricky. You are definitely low if you are below 200 or 250 pg/mL (148 or 185 pmol/L) (NIH, 2021). Even though a normal B12 level is considered 200-900, you can still have B12 deficiency even if your blood level shows normal B12. I know it's crazy, but it's true. So, I recommend everyone target their B12 levels between 500-900.

Experts suggest that if your B12 levels are between 150 to 399 pg/mL (111 to 294 pmol/L), it's time to bring in the MMA test (a metabolite involved in B12 metabolism) for a definitive answer (Green, 2017; Allen et al., 2020), or if you have clinical neurological symptoms suggestive of B12 deficiency or anemia with big RBCs, known as megaloblastic anemia.

If your MMA level is over 0.271 micromol/L, it's like a big neon sign saying "B12 Deficiency Here!" (Allen et al., 2020). However, MMA levels can also rise if your kidneys are playing hooky or if you're simply getting older (Green, 2017; Herrmann & Obeid, 2012).

Then there are total plasma homocysteine levels, which rise faster than the bass drop in a nightclub when B12 is low. A homocysteine level above 15 micromol/L might hint at B12 deficiency, but this test is like a gossipy neighbor—it's easily influenced by other factors like low folate or kidney issues (Refsum et al., 2004).

A study by Smith and Refsum (2016) demonstrated that low B12 is associated with cognitive decline. Another research by O'Leary et al. (2012) found that older adults with lower B12 levels performed worse on cognitive tests. Additionally, Morris et al. (2018) reported that B12 deficiency might contribute to Alzheimer's disease. Moore et al. (2012) showed a clear link between B12 levels and brain atrophy. A review by Stabler (2013) also confirms that B12 deficiency is a risk factor for dementia. Moreover, a study by Doets et al. (2013) found that B12 supplementation could improve cognitive function in deficient individuals.

I suggest getting your B12, MMA, and homocysteine levels checked—at least every six months if abnormal. Once corrected, aim for an annual checkup and supplement if needed to keep your Vitamin B12 level above 500 and below 900. Low-normal Vitamin B12 levels are associated with smaller memory areas of the brain and other neurological symptoms.

**Bottom line:** Check your B12 levels pronto and supplement if needed. Opt for the sublingual form—the one that dissolves in your mouth—so you don't have to rely on your sometimes unpredictable GI tract for absorption. This way, you're giving your brain the direct gift of B12, with no detours or pit stops. Don't trust me on this? Then let me introduce you to my buddy, Adams.

In a study by Adams et al. (2023), it was found that sublingual B12 significantly increased serum B12 levels compared to oral tablets, especially in individuals with gastrointestinal absorption issues. The study concluded that sublingual B12 is a more efficient and reliable method for correcting B12 deficiency.

Elevated levels of vitamin B12, known as hypocobalaminemia, can indicate underlying health issues such as liver disease, kidney dysfunction, or myeloproliferative disorders (Carmel & Agrawal, 2012). High B12 levels can be associated with adverse effects like blood clots, acne, or allergic reactions (Gherasim et al., 2013). However, B12 toxicity is rare because the body efficiently excretes excess amounts via the kidneys, as it is a water-soluble vitamin. Monitoring B12 levels is essential to avoid complications and address any underlying conditions (Adams et al., 2023). Aim for B12 levels that are just right (I recommend 500-900 pg/mL, but consult with your doctor), like the perfect cup of coffee—not too strong, not too weak, but just enough to keep things running smoothly.

**Another thing**: Never take folate/folic acid before correcting B12 deficiency!

Imagine throwing folate into the mix without correcting a B12 deficiency first. That's like adding more guitars to the band without tuning the existing ones. Folate helps convert homocysteine to methionine too, but without enough B12, this process can't keep up. Homocysteine builds up, causing a backup in the system, and glutathione production falters (Miller, 2008). Neurological damage can worsen!

On a more serious note, low B12 levels in mothers can have serious implications for infant brain development, potentially leading to brain atrophy. Vitamin B12 is essential for the proper development of the nervous system, and a deficiency during pregnancy can disrupt the formation of myelin, the protective sheath around nerves, and impair brain growth (O'Leary & Samman, 2010). Studies have shown that infants born to mothers with low B12 levels are at increased risk of brain atrophy, which can result in long-term neurological deficits (Bhate et al., 2008; Strand et al., 2013). Ensuring adequate B12 intake during pregnancy, through diet or supplements, is crucial for preventing such adverse outcomes. Rich sources of B12 include meat, dairy, and supplements, which can help maintain adequate levels during this critical period (Dror & Allen, 2008; Miller et al., 2021).

## The Omega-3 Mystery: A Lighthearted Case of Fishy Business

It was a perfectly pleasant evening at *Omega House*, the seaside mansion of the renowned health expert *Dr. Omega*. The waves lapped peacefully against the cliffs, but inside, a lively debate was brewing. Gathered around a grand dinner table were the greatest minds in nutrition, here to solve the question once and for all: which source of omega-3s is superior—fish oil or algae oil?

*Dr. Fintock*, a long-time supporter of fish oil, sat confidently to the right of *Dr. Omega*, while *Professor Al G. Ea*, a passionate algae oil advocate, sat calmly across from him. Around the table were specialists in health, sustainability, and even *Mr. Cornfed*, who didn't care much about the debate but was enjoying the hors d'oeuvres.

The tension was as thick as a bowl of omega-3-rich chia pudding. Dr. Omega, always the charming host, tapped his fork on his glass. "Alright, let's get to the heart of the matter. Which oil really deserves the crown?"

### Clue #1: The Mercury Mystery

Dr. Fintock wasted no time. "Fish oil has been the champion for years! It's rich in EPA and DHA, essential for heart and brain health. No one can deny that."
"But there's a little problem with mercury, isn't there, Dr. Fintock?" Professor Al G. Ea interjected, ever so politely. "Larger fish, like salmon and mackerel, accumulate mercury as they swim up the food chain (González-Hedström et al., 2020). That means fish oil can contain traces of mercury and heavy metals, which pose a risk to consumers."

Dr. Fintock shifted in his chair, looking a bit flustered. "Well, yes, mercury is an issue. But surely, it's not a dealbreaker..."

"Oh, but it is!" said Professor Al G. Ea, smiling. "Algae oil, being at the base of the food chain, is free from contaminants like mercury (Röhrl et al., 2020). It's as pure as they come!"

Dr. Omega raised an eyebrow. "Interesting. That's a point for algae oil."

### Clue #2: Bioavailability: The Great Debate

Dr. Fintock quickly recovered, his voice steady again. "Even if algae oil is cleaner, fish oil is better absorbed by the body. It's been the gold standard for omega-3 bioavailability for years."

"Not anymore," Professor Al G. Ea responded smoothly. "Recent studies show that algae oil provides omega-3s like EPA and DHA just as efficiently as fish oil, if not more so (Röhrl et al., 2020). You see, algae oil offers the same benefits without the need for fish. It's the cleaner, more efficient source."

Dr. Fintock frowned, flipping through his notes. "I... I didn't realize the data had shifted."

Dr. Omega scribbled in his notebook. "That's another point for algae."

**Clue #3: Oxidation—The Spoiling Factor**

Dr. Omega leaned back in his chair, sniffing the air. "Does anyone else notice that fishy smell?"

Professor Al G. Ea chuckled. "Ah, that would be the oxidation problem with fish oil. Fish oil is notorious for going rancid quickly, especially once exposed to air. This oxidation produces harmful free radicals (Koch et al., 2022), which can negate the health benefits and leave you with a not-so-pleasant aftertaste."

Dr. Fintock looked concerned. "But surely that can be avoided with proper storage?"

"It's hard to avoid," Professor Al G. Ea replied, "but with algae oil, you don't have that issue. It's far more stable and resistant to oxidation (Koch et al., 2022), meaning it stays fresh longer."

Dr. Omega nodded thoughtfully. "Good to know. Algae oil is looking better and better."

**Clue #4: The Sustainability Factor**

"Let's talk about sustainability," *Ms. Eco*, the environmental expert, chimed in. "I've been reading about the environmental impact of fish oil production. Isn't overfishing and fish farming causing some serious damage to marine ecosystems?"

Professor Al G. Ea beamed. "Absolutely. Fish oil production contributes to overfishing, and fish farming isn't exactly eco-friendly either (González-Hedström et al., 2020). But algae oil? It's the green solution we need. Algae can be grown in controlled environments, even using wastewater, with no impact on marine life (Saeed et al., 2021)."

Ms. Eco clapped her hands. "That's fantastic! A healthier planet and healthier people."

Dr. Fintock looked like he was sweating now. "Okay, algae oil wins in sustainability. I can't argue with that."

### The Superpowers of Omega-3s

Dr. Omega cleared his throat. "But let's not forget why we're here. Both fish oil and algae oil contain omega-3s, which are vital for brain health and overall well-being."

Dr. Fintock nodded enthusiastically. "Yes! Omega-3s reduce inflammation, improve mental health, and help prevent chronic diseases like cardiovascular disease and obesity (Chaves et al., 2022; Qin, 2023). That's why fish oil has always been recommended."

"Indeed," Professor Al G. Ea agreed, "but algae oil does the same thing—without the mercury and oxidation. Omega-3s from both sources help produce molecules like lipoxins and resolvins, which reduce inflammation and protect neurons (Borsini et al., 2021). They also boost brain-derived neurotrophic factor (BDNF), which is like Miracle-Gro for your brain (Sugasini et al., 2020; Thomas et al., 2020). So, whether it's fish or algae, omega-3s are essential."

Dr. Omega clapped his hands. "Exactly! And let's not forget, DHA improves synaptic plasticity and keeps the brain flexible, like yoga for your neurons (Thomas et al., 2020). Omega-3s from either source are crucial for staying sharp."

### The Verdict: A New Champion Emerges

As the sun set behind the cliffs and the debate wound down, Dr. Omega stood up. "Ladies and gentlemen, I believe we have our answer. Fish oil has had a good run, but it seems algae oil is not just an alternative—it's the superior choice in many ways. It's free of mercury, more stable, sustainable, and just as bioavailable as fish oil. I think it's clear that algae oil is the future."

### Let Food Be Thy Medicine: Omega-3s - The Brain's Best Friend with Benefits

Omega-3 fatty acids are like the VIPs of your diet, playing starring roles in keeping your brain sharp and your heart ticking smoothly. These essential fats come in three main types: alpha-linolenic acid (ALA), eicosapentaenoic acid (EPA), and docosahexaenoic acid (DHA). Think of ALA as the plant-based rookie, found in foods like flaxseeds and chia seeds, while EPA and DHA are the seasoned pros swimming around in fatty fish like salmon, mackerel, and sardines (Jahromi et al., 2022; Chaves et al., 2022; Redruello-Requejo et al., 2023).

Here's the catch—your body isn't great at turning ALA into EPA and DHA. It's like trying to turn a bicycle into a Ferrari; only about 5-10% of ALA becomes EPA, and a mere 2-5% makes it to DHA (Ramya et al., 2022; Takić et al., 2022). So, if you want the full benefits, it's easier to go straight to the source and load up on fatty fish. Why should you care? Diets rich in EPA and DHA have been shown to improve mental health, reducing depressive symptoms (Chaves et al., 2022; Qin, 2023). Plus, they help keep chronic diseases like cardiovascular disease and obesity at bay (Redruello-Requejo et al., 2023; Oliver et al., 2020).

But here's something that might surprise you: the ratio of omega-6 to omega-3 in your diet matters—a lot. A healthy ratio is around 2:1 or 3:1. However, most modern diets, especially those heavy on processed foods, can push this ratio to an unhealthy 20:1 or even higher, which can stoke inflammation and lead to numerous health issues (Jahromi et al., 2022; Puccinelli, 2023).

This is where your meat and milk choices come into play. Grass-fed animals naturally have a much better omega-6 to omega-3 ratio compared to their corn-fed counterparts. Grass-fed beef and dairy products often have a ratio closer to the ideal 2:1, while corn-fed varieties can swing the ratio way out of balance, contributing to that dreaded inflammation (Daley et al., 2010; Smith et al., 2020).

**The takeaway?** To keep your body in tip-top shape, make sure you're getting enough omega-3s, especially from fatty fish, grass-fed meat, and dairy. Your brain, heart, and even your joints will thank you (Demirel et al., 2021; Chaliha et al., 2020).

## Mechanism of the Master Fats

Omega-3s produce special molecules like lipoxins and resolvins, which sound like superhero names and act like them too, by resolving inflammation and saving your neurons from a fiery demise (Borsini et al., 2021). Chronic inflammation is like that annoying neighbor who never lets you sleep—your brain can't grow new cells when it's constantly dealing with drama. Thankfully, omega-3s keep things calm and cool, so neurogenesis can continue uninterrupted (Borsini et al., 2020).

**Boosting BDNF: The Brain's Miracle-Gro**

Omega-3s don't just stop at fighting inflammation—they also turn up the volume on brain-derived neurotrophic factor (BDNF), which is like Miracle-Gro for your brain. Higher DHA levels mean more BDNF, and more BDNF means your brain cells are thriving like plants in a greenhouse (Sugasini et al., 2020; Thomas et al., 2020). This is particularly helpful when your brain's feeling a little blue, as BDNF levels tend to dip during mood disorders. Omega-3s step in to boost those levels, making sure your hippocampus—your brain's memory center—stays in top shape (Thomas et al., 2020).

**Synaptic Plasticity: Stretchy Brain Cells, Better Brains**

DHA isn't just good for your brain; it's a VIP guest in your neuronal membranes. It helps form lipid rafts that facilitate the clustering of receptors and other signaling proteins, enhancing the efficiency of signal transduction (Kraft, 2013; Nickels et al., 2019). This makes your brain cells more flexible, like yoga for your neurons, leading to better cognitive function and resilience against the mental wear and tear of aging. With omega-3s on board, your brain is always ready to spring back from a challenge, whether it's learning something new or fending off neurodegenerative foes.

**Mitochondrial Maintenance: Powering Up Your Neurons**

Finally, omega-3s are all about keeping your brain's power plants—your mitochondria—in peak condition. DHA steps in to protect these little guys from amyloid-beta, the nasty stuff that clogs up brains in Alzheimer's disease (Park et al., 2020). By shielding your mitochondria from harm, omega-3s ensure your neurons have the energy they need to keep the lights on and the neurons firing.

**High Doses of Omega-3s: Turning Up the Serotonin and Mental Health Dial**

Studies have shown that Omega-3s can increase serotonin levels in the brain, much like turning on the sun on a cloudy day (Allah et al., 2014). Unlike some serotonin-enhancing medications that come with unwanted side effects, Omega-3s are an all-natural, side-effect-free option (Patrick & Ames, 2015). Research indicates that Omega-3 supplementation can significantly elevate serotonin concentrations in various brain regions, particularly in conditions where serotonin levels are compromised, such as hypothyroidism (Allah et al., 2014).

This elevation in serotonin levels is associated with improved receptor density and functionality, further enhancing serotonergic signaling (Allah et al., 2014; Gertsik et al., 2012).

Omega-3 fatty acids have been extensively studied for their role in enhancing serotonin (5-HT) signaling and associated receptor interactions, which are crucial for effective signal transduction in the brain. Omega-3 fatty acids, particularly docosahexaenoic acid (DHA), improve the fluidity of neuronal membranes, essential for the proper functioning of G-protein-coupled receptors (GPCRs), including serotonin receptors (El-Ansary et al., 2011; "The Role of Omega-3 Fatty Acids in Memory Improvement: Possible Mechanisms and Therapeutic Potential", 2019). Inflammation is known to disrupt serotonin receptor function and neurotransmitter dynamics; thus, Omega-3 supplementation may help restore normal serotonergic activity by reducing inflammatory signaling (Mobraten et al., 2013).

Increased membrane fluidity allows better receptor accessibility and facilitates the binding of serotonin to its receptors, promoting effective signal transduction (Patrick & Ames, 2015). This is particularly significant, as the composition of membrane lipids can directly affect receptor activity and neurotransmission (Lin & Su, 2007). Additionally, Omega-3 fatty acids may influence serotonin turnover, crucial for maintaining adequate levels of this neurotransmitter in the synaptic cleft (Tanskanen et al., 2001).

**Did you check your Omega-3 levels? Do it Now!**

Think of omega-3 as the ultimate peacekeeper in your body—a calm, Zen-like diplomat that's always stepping in to prevent an all-out inflammatory civil war. Meanwhile, omega-6 is that one drama-prone relative who's always stirring the pot. You need both to keep things interesting, but too much omega-6, and suddenly it's like Thanksgiving dinner gone wrong—everyone's yelling, inflammation flying everywhere, and omega-3 is sitting there meditating, trying to restore peace.

The perfect omega-6 to omega-3 ratio is about 4:1, maybe even 1:1 if you're aiming for maximum Zen, but thanks to the typical Western diet overloaded with omega-6 from stuff like corn oil and soybean oil, the ratio often jumps to 20:1 or worse (Li, 2024; Han, 2024). At that point, omega-3's diplomacy skills are tested to the limit, like trying to mediate world peace with a soggy kale salad.

To keep omega-3's peacekeeping force strong, it's all about eating the right foods: salmon, mackerel, sardines, chia seeds, and walnuts are the elite peacekeeping squad here, with salmon boasting a beautiful 1:1 omega-3 to omega-6 ratio (Salmon, 2024). These foods arm omega-3 with the calming superpowers it needs to keep omega-6 from lighting up the inflammatory fuse.

Now, if you're wondering how to measure your internal peace index, your doctor can run an Omega-3 Index test, which looks at how much EPA and DHA are in your red blood cells (RBCs)—think of it as a peace treaty signed by omega-3 over the past few months (Salmon, 2024). Plasma tests are more like checking your Twitter feed—short-term chaos, and not always a true reflection of your overall calm (Salmon, 2024). So, if you really want to know how peaceful things are inside, ask your doctor for that RBC omega-3 test. And remember: peace, love, and algae.

**Let's talk dosage:**

**Algae Oil: The New Kid in Town**
Traditionally, fish oil has been the primary source of these essential fatty acids, but algae oil has emerged as a viable alternative, appealing to those with dietary restrictions and environmental concerns. Recent studies indicate that both fish oil and algae oil can effectively deliver Omega-3s, allowing consumers to choose based on personal preferences without compromising health benefits (Marques, 2023; Ozaki et al., 2020).

**Shall we table the discussion here?**

| Aspect | Fish Oil | Algae Oil |
|---|---|---|
| Source | Derived from fish, particularly larger species that may accumulate mercury (Chang, 2024). | Derived from microalgae, which do not accumulate mercury, making it a safer choice (Chang, 2024). |
| Bioavailability | Omega-3s in fish oil are primarily present as triglycerides (TAG). Equally bioavailable as algae oil (Arsenyadis et al., 2022). | Omega-3s in algae oil can exist as free fatty acids (FFA) and phospholipids, with rapid absorption (Koch et al., 2022). |
| Mercury Content | May contain mercury due to environmental pollution, especially in larger fish species (Chang, 2024). | Naturally free of mercury, as it's derived from microorganisms (Chang, 2024). |
| Oxidation Risk | Prone to oxidation due to polyunsaturated fatty acids, leading to rancidity and harmful free radicals (Peng et al., 2020). | Improved stability against oxidation, reducing the risk of rancidity and extending shelf life (Peng et al., 2020). |
| Sustainability | Relies on fish stocks, which are often overfished (Gou et al., 2020). | Cultivated from microalgae in controlled environments, ensuring a sustainable supply (Gou et al., 2020). |
| Applications | Widely used in human and animal diets, but environmental concerns about overfishing persist (Osmond et al., 2021). | Can replace fish oil in various diets, maintaining health benefits and offering a sustainable alternative (Arsenyadis et al., 2022). |
| Health Benefits | Supports heart, brain, and overall health, but may carry risks related to mercury and oxidation (Chang, 2024; Peng et al., 2020). | Offers similar health benefits with lower risks, especially in terms of mercury content and stability (Chang, 2024; Peng et al., 2020). |

## Omega-3 Fatty Acids: The Heart-Healthy Hero with a Few Plot Twists

As with any good superhero story, there's a plot twist: recent studies suggest that these fatty acids might have a dark side, particularly concerning atrial fibrillation (AF) and other side effects.

## Atrial Fibrillation: Omega-3's Kryptonite?

Atrial fibrillation is an irregular heart rhythm that increases the risk of stroke. A meta-analysis of randomized controlled trials (RCTs) found that higher doses of omega-3 fatty acids were linked to an increased risk of new-onset AF, particularly in patients with pre-existing cardiovascular conditions (Dwiputra, 2023; Kow et al., 2021). The REDUCE-IT trial, which examined the effects of high-dose EPA, specifically reported that patients randomized to receive 4g/day of highly purified EPA ethyl ester (icosapent ethyl) had a 48% higher risk of hospitalization for AF compared to those on placebo (3.1% vs 2.1%; P = .004) over a median follow-up of 4.9 years (Nicholls et al., 2020).

## Other Side Effects: The Sidekicks You Didn't Ask For

- **Bleeding Blues**: Omega-3s are great at keeping your blood flowing—maybe a little too great. Their blood-thinning powers can lead to easy bruising and even gastrointestinal bleeding, especially if you're on blood thinners (Gencer et al., 2021).
- **Mood Swings**: While omega-3s are often promoted as mood boosters, some studies suggest they might do the opposite for certain people, potentially worsening depression (Okereke et al., 2021). It's like inviting someone to a party, and they show up with a raincloud.

## Why the Plot Twists? The Science Behind the Surprises

So, what gives? Why are omega-3s sometimes more of a frenemy? Omega-3s can mess with the heart's electrical system, potentially leading to arrhythmias like AF, especially at higher doses (Bork et al., 2022; Elagizi et al., 2021). While omega-3s are known for fighting inflammation, their complex interactions with the body's inflammatory responses might sometimes backfire, increasing the risk of AF (Huh & Jo, 2023). Also, don't forget to store omega-3 oil in a cool, dark place to minimize oxidation.

**The Brain's Best-Kept Secret: Omega-7 and Why It Deserves a Trophy**

Move over, Omega-3, there's a new fatty acid in town—and it's ready to steal the spotlight! Introducing Omega-7, the lesser-known but equally fabulous member of the fatty acid family. While everyone's busy singing the praises of Omega-3 for its brain-boosting benefits, Omega-7 has quietly been working behind the scenes, playing a key role in brain health, neurogenesis, and helping you stay sharp. So, let's give this underdog its due!

**What Is Omega-7, Anyway?**

First things first, Omega-7 is a type of monounsaturated fatty acid, primarily found in palmitoleic acid. It's the brain's secret weapon—helping with neuroprotection, reducing inflammation, and promoting neurogenesis (Yang et al., 2016). Yes, you heard that right: Omega-7 is out here fostering new brain cells while you're binge-watching your favorite shows.

**Brain Health and Omega-7: Keeping Your Neurons in Check**

Here's where things get exciting: Omega-7 is like a multitasking superhero for your brain. It helps reduce inflammation, which is key to preventing cognitive decline. Inflammation is like that annoying person who won't stop complaining at a party—after a while, everyone's just tired and wants to go home. But Omega-7 shows up, calms the room down, and suddenly your brain's like, "Ah, peace at last" (Auestad & Innis, 2009).

But that's not all. Omega-7 also encourages neurogenesis, which is the brain's way of saying, "Out with the old, in with the new!" By fostering the growth of new neurons, Omega-7 helps keep your memory sharp, your cognitive functions firing on all cylinders, and your brain feeling like it just got a spa day.

**Neurogenesis: Omega-7's Brain-Cell Farm**

Picture this: your brain is a farm, and Omega-7 is the farmer, planting new neurons left and right. Neurogenesis is crucial for brain plasticity (that's the brain's way of staying flexible and adaptable, like a mental yoga instructor). With Omega-7 on the scene, your brain can grow new cells, form new connections, and repair itself more efficiently. This means better learning, memory retention, and problem-solving skills—so go ahead and tackle that crossword puzzle (Cohen et al., 2014)!

## Food Sources: Where to Find Omega-7 (Hint: It's Delicious)

So, where do you get this magical brain juice? Luckily, Omega-7 is found in some seriously tasty foods:

- **Sea Buckthorn Oil**: This bright orange berry oil is basically Omega-7 central, boasting one of the highest concentrations of the fatty acid. Plus, it's fun to say. Sea buckthorn—say it five times fast.
- **Macadamia Nuts**: These buttery, rich nuts are packed with Omega-7 and are basically a brain snack disguised as a dessert. Win-win!
- **Avocados**: As if avocados needed any more reasons to be the most beloved fruit ever, they're also a great source of Omega-7. So, yes, guac on everything is basically brain food.
- **Olive Oil**: The good ol' standby. You've been drizzling olive oil on everything from salads to bread, but little did you know you were feeding your brain some Omega-7 goodness (Scognamiglio et al., 2012).

## Why Omega-7 Deserves More Love

Sure, Omega-3 is the brain health rockstar that gets all the attention, but Omega-7 is like the unsung keyboard player in the back of the band—quietly holding everything together. From fighting inflammation to growing new neurons, Omega-7 is the brain's trusty sidekick, ensuring everything runs smoothly (Yang et al., 2016). So next time someone brings up Omega-3, feel free to drop some knowledge about Omega-7 and its role in brain health. You'll sound like a genius (thanks to all those new neurons it's helping you grow).

## Omega-9: The Nutty Professors
## How Olive Oil and Friends Save Your Health

Let's talk about Omega-9 fatty acids, particularly oleic acid, which is like the quiet genius in the corner of the fatty acid world—doing all the heavy lifting for your heart and brain without making a fuss. And where do you find this nutritional gold? Sure, you've got your avocados, almonds, and pistachios—solid choices. But let's not forget the true MVP: olive oil and macadamia nuts (Wang Y, 2024).

## Macadamia Nuts: The Snack That Does It All

Macadamia nuts aren't just tasty—they're health powerhouses disguised as a snack. Packed with monounsaturated fats, particularly oleic acid, these nuts are like a personal trainer for your heart, lowering LDL cholesterol and reducing inflammation (Olas, 2024). They're also brain boosters, thanks to their Omega-9 content, which supports cognitive function and fends off those pesky neurodegenerative diseases (Yao, 2024). Plus, despite being calorie-dense, they're your new best friend for weight management—keeping you full and satisfied so you don't raid the cookie jar (Lou, 2024).

## Olive Oil: Liquid Gold for Your Heart

Olive oil, the darling of the Mediterranean diet, is basically liquid love for your heart. Rich in oleic acid, it's been linked to reduced risks of heart disease and stroke. Plus, its anti-inflammatory powers help keep your blood pressure in check (Chen, 2024; Shine, 2024). And let's not forget those antioxidants, like polyphenols, that double down on protecting your cells from oxidative stress (Xiao, 2024).

## Avocados: The Brain and Heart Whisperer

Avocados—nature's butter—are another top source of Omega-9s. They not only help lower bad cholesterol and boost good cholesterol but also support brain health by reducing the risk of cognitive decline (Zibarev, 2024). And with their fat content aiding in the absorption of vitamins, they're basically doing your entire body a favor every time you dig into some guac.

## Almonds and Pistachios: The Crunchy Duo

Almonds and pistachios are like the crunchy, heart-healthy duo of the nut world. Almonds lower cholesterol, fight inflammation, and are packed with vitamin E to keep your heart and brain in top shape (Rogalski, 2024). Pistachios, on the other hand, are the ultimate snack for weight management, keeping you full with their fiber and protein while also improving your lipid profiles (Velangi, 2024; Dairoh, 2024).

**Extra Virgin Olive Oil: The Beyoncé of Olive Oils – Why Regular Olive Oil Can't Even**

Extra-virgin olive oil (EVOO) isn't just the diva of the olive oil world for nothing—it boasts fancy production methods, a high-maintenance chemical composition, and superstar health benefits to prove it. Unlike regular olive oil, which is essentially the olive world's version of fast food, EVOO is obtained from the first cold pressing of olives, with zero heat or chemicals involved. This VIP treatment means EVOO is loaded with antioxidants and phenolic compounds that make your heart sing and help reduce inflammation (Martini et al., 2018; Guasch-Ferré et al., 2014).

In contrast, regular olive oil undergoes refining processes that strip it of its natural goodness. What's left? A higher acidity level, usually around 1-2%, compared to EVOO's pristine under-0.8% acidity (Salek et al., 2017). It's like comparing a gourmet meal to fast food.

Even EVOO has its diva demands—factors such as when the olives are picked and how they're pressed can impact its antioxidant powers (Różańska et al., 2020; Manganiello et al., 2021). Still, thanks to its high monounsaturated fat content, EVOO stays fresher longer, resisting oxidation while regular olive oil wilts under pressure (Vidrih et al., 2010; Martini et al., 2018).

In the end, EVOO isn't just a healthier choice; it's the Beyoncé of oils—robust, flavorful, and undeniably superior in every way (Guasch-Ferré et al., 2014; García-Oliveira et al., 2021). So, next time you're cooking, ask yourself: do you want a star or just another oil in the pantry?

**Pouring on the Smarts: How Extra Virgin Olive Oil Gives Your Brain a Boost**

Extra virgin olive oil (EVOO) isn't just a kitchen staple; it's like a brain booster in a bottle. Packed with monounsaturated fatty acids (MUFAs) and phenolic compounds, EVOO is now being hailed as a potential secret weapon against cognitive decline and neurodegenerative diseases like Alzheimer's (Alkhalifa, 2024). So, if you thought EVOO was just for drizzling on salads, think again—it's practically the superhero your brain's been waiting for.

### The Italian Longitudinal Study on Aging (ILSA)

In the world of brain research, the Italian Longitudinal Study on Aging (ILSA) is like "The Godfather," and EVOO plays a starring role. The study found that older adults who increased their MUFA intake, particularly from EVOO, showed less cognitive decline, especially those with lower Mini-Mental State Examination (MMSE) scores. Basically, more EVOO equals less brain fog (Nakada-Honda et al., 2021; Martins et al., 2022). If you're following the Mediterranean diet, where EVOO is as essential as pasta, you're already ahead of the game in dodging mild cognitive impairment (MCI) and Alzheimer's (Blondel et al., 2022; Alkhalifa, 2024).

### Systematic Reviews and Meta-Analyses

EVOO's reputation as the brain's best friend is further supported by systematic reviews and meta-analyses. One comprehensive review showed that sticking to the Mediterranean diet—heavy on the EVOO—significantly reduces the risk of cognitive impairment. So, it's not just about the flavor; it's about keeping your neurons firing on all cylinders (Koutsonida et al., 2021). Plus, the polyphenols in EVOO aren't just there for show—they help curb neuroinflammation (Abdallah et al., 2022; Kezele & Ćurko-Cofek, 2022).

### Clinical Trials: MICOIL and PREDIMED Studies

Clinical trials like MICOIL and PREDIMED have put EVOO to the test, and the results are impressive. In the MICOIL trial, patients with MCI who consumed high-phenolic EVOO showed significant cognitive improvements—think of it as brain armor in a bottle (Kaddoumi et al., 2022; Kezele & Ćurko-Cofek, 2022). The PREDIMED trial echoed these findings, showing that a Mediterranean diet with a healthy dose of EVOO led to better memory and cognitive function over 4.1 years. Clearly, EVOO isn't just a garnish—it's a cognitive powerhouse (Barbalace et al., 2021; Yamada, 2022).

### Brain Gains with EVOO: The Ultimate Liquid Intelligence

So, how does EVOO work its brain magic? Think of it as your brain's very own superhero smoothie, loaded with antioxidants like hydroxytyrosol and oleuropein, which swoop in to scavenge pesky reactive oxygen species (ROS), reducing oxidative stress and keeping your neurons cool under pressure (Petrella et al., 2021).

It's all in the phenolic compounds, which pack a serious punch with their antioxidant and anti-inflammatory properties. They strengthen the blood-brain barrier (BBB) and keep out harmful substances while giving your cognitive function a grand boost (Đuričić, 2020; Abdallah et al., 2022). The blood-brain barrier is a thin, one-cell-layer wall between your brain and blood, acting as a gatekeeper to protect your brain by allowing essential nutrients in while keeping harmful substances out.

These compounds also help clear out amyloid-beta, the nasty stuff that clogs up your brain in Alzheimer's, potentially slowing down cognitive decline (Romero-Márquez et al., 2022; Abdallah et al., 2022).

EVOO's anti-inflammatory properties are impressive, blocking the NF-κB pathway—the troublemaker responsible for inflammation—helping to keep your brain inflammation-free, which is vital for dodging neurodegenerative diseases like Alzheimer's (Attiyah & Mohammed, 2021).

On top of that, EVOO's polyphenols act as tiny editors, tweaking your genes through epigenetic modifications to boost cognitive function and protect your neurons from going rogue (Fabiani et al., 2021).

But that's not all—EVOO's monounsaturated fatty acids (MUFAs), especially oleic acid, are the building blocks your brain needs to stay flexible and sharp. They keep your neuronal membranes in top shape, supporting a healthy lipid profile that's crucial for staving off cardiovascular issues that often tag along with cognitive decline (Mancebo-Campos et al., 2023). Plus, EVOO's phenolic compounds have a VIP pass across the blood-brain barrier, ensuring they reach where they're needed most, keeping your brain's defenses strong and your mind clear (Rodríguez-López et al., 2020).

**Olive Oil Olympics: Meet the Gold Medalists**

As of 2024, the gold medalists in the Olive Oil Olympics for polyphenol content are strutting their stuff with some seriously healthy swagger:

**Koroneiki Olive Oil**: This Greek superstar may be small in size, but it's punching way above its weight class with a polyphenol content that often tops 800 mg/kg. Think of it as the Rocky Balboa of olive oils—rich, robust, and ready to knock out free radicals left and right (Vita et al., 2020).

**Picual Olive Oil**: From the sun-drenched fields of Andalusia, Spain, Picual oil is like the cool, fruity cousin who also happens to be a straight-A student. With polyphenol levels hovering between 400 to 800 mg/kg, it's as stable as your grandma's cooking and as strong as a Spanish bull (Nowak et al., 2021).

**Frantoio Olive Oil**: Italy's gift to the culinary world, Frantoio oil is like the James Bond of olive oils—sophisticated, complex, and always delivering under pressure. With 300 to 600 mg/kg of polyphenols, it's not just a pretty face on your gourmet salad; it's also got anti-inflammatory moves that would make a ninja jealous (Faradilah et al., 2021).

These olive oils aren't just tasty; they're the health superheroes of your kitchen, fighting off inflammation and keeping your heart in top shape (Davila et al., 2022). So, next time you're drizzling, make sure it's with one of these champs.

**Fire and Flavor: How to Avoid Olive Oil's Smoking Meltdown**
Sure, you can use olive oil to cook pasta, but think of it like bringing a diva to a bonfire—handle with care! Olive oil, especially the fancy extra virgin kind, starts getting nervous at high temperatures. Push it past its smoke point (around 190-210°C), and it might just have a meltdown, turning into something less fabulous and more like a drama queen with off-flavors and nasty free radicals (Kmiecik, 2023; Tsai et al., 2023).

Boiling pasta in water at a cool 100°C? No problem, olive oil's totally chill with that. But if you decide to sauté or fry with it, just remember: too much heat, and those lovely tocopherols and phenolic compounds might pack their bags and leave the party early (Kmiecik, 2023; Tsai et al., 2023).

If you want to keep those precious polyphenols intact, treat your cooking like a delicate dance: low heat, short steps (less than 15 minutes for stovetop, and 6 minutes if you're nuking it in the microwave) to keep those fragile secoiridoids from turning into crispy critters (Roila, 2024). But comparing fried foods is like comparing fried eggs to fried Twinkies—it's a messy business. EVOO usually shines, except when it's under the heat lamp in the fryer or microwave, where more polyphenols don't always mean more stability (Abdullah, 2024).

**Nutritionally speaking, a light fry in EVOO, like the beloved Mediterranean sofrito, can amp up your dish with a polyphenol punch, transferring oleuropein and other EVOO-exclusive goodies into your food** (Somia A. Ajab, 2024).

While frying with EVOO can improve your food's fatty acid profile, it's better to stick to gentler cooking methods or simply drizzle raw EVOO over your dish. This keeps things heart-healthy and prevents turning your meal into a burnt offering (Tamiji, 2024; Ghorbel et al., 2024).

**Lipid Peroxidation of Olive Oil and the Heroic Herbs That Save the Day**
Lipid peroxidation is like a midlife crisis for oil—free radicals attack the oil's polyunsaturated fatty acids (PUFAs), leading to a breakdown that's far from glamorous. This not only alters the oil's taste and aroma but also diminishes its health benefits. Factors like light, heat, and oxygen speed up this meltdown, turning your gourmet oil into something you wouldn't want to drizzle on anything (Díaz-Montaña et al., 2023).

Eating oxidized olive oil is like booking a one-way ticket to oxidative stress. The byproducts, such as malondialdehyde (MDA), can wreak havoc on your cells and contribute to diseases like atherosclerosis, diabetes, and even cancer. Worse, these oxidized lipids can exacerbate inflammation, something your body certainly doesn't need.

Fortunately, your kitchen has some unsung heroes: cloves, basil, garlic, and rosemary. These herbs are packed with antioxidants that help olive oil stay stable under pressure (Barreca et al., 2021). Whether it's rosemary stabilizing oleic acid or garlic flexing its allicin muscles, these herbs work hard to keep your olive oil fresh and healthy for longer (Kahyaoğlu, 2021; Manoonphol et al., 2023).

Olive oil is basically a diva—it needs to be stored in a cool, dark place to avoid going rancid. Light and heat are its mortal enemies, speeding up oxidation faster than you can say "Mediterranean diet." So, do your olive oil a favor and store it in a dark glass bottle, far from heat sources (Díaz-Montaña et al., 2023).

**How Omega-3 Saves Your Heart from Ghee Coffee and Olive Oil Shots**
In the bustling town of Nutritia, the latest health trends were all the rage, and none were more popular than Ghee Coffee and Olive Oil Shots. Brody, the town's self-appointed health enthusiast, was leading the charge. Every morning, Brody proudly gulped down a frothy cup of Ghee Coffee and followed it with a shot of extra virgin olive oil, declaring, "This is the ultimate combo for vitality! My heart and brain are running on pure power!"

The citizens of Nutritia couldn't help but be intrigued, but Cholesterina, Nutritia's heart health advocate, was skeptical. After watching Brody down his oily concoction's day after day, she couldn't stay silent any longer.

"Brody," she said, marching over one morning, "do you even know what you're doing to your arteries with all that fat?"

Brody blinked in confusion. "What do you mean? Ghee and olive oil are supposed to be heart-healthy! It's like I'm giving my arteries a daily Mediterranean vacation."

Cholesterina sighed. "You can't just down oil like its water and expect your arteries to love you for it. You're missing a critical piece of the puzzle." Just then, Doc Omega-3, Nutritia's resident nutrition expert, strolled by and overheard the conversation.

"Ah, Brody, my oily friend," Doc Omega-3 said with a chuckle, "you're not entirely wrong about the benefits of ghee and olive oil, but you need to understand balance." High-fat foods, particularly those rich in saturated fats like ghee, can lead to temporary reductions in endothelial function, which is crucial for maintaining arterial health (Barbosa et al., 2022; Chen et al., 2020).

Brody furrowed his brow. "But aren't ghee and olive oil good for my heart? They're full of healthy fats, right?"

Doc Omega-3 nodded. "Yes, they are—but there's more to it. You can't just chug down Ghee Coffee and Olive Oil Shots without considering the impact on your arteries. Consuming high-fat foods without the right balance can temporarily reduce flow-mediated dilation (FMD), which means your arteries stiffen for a few hours, making it harder for blood to flow through. This is known as endothelial dysfunction" (Barbosa et al., 2022; Chen et al., 2020).

Brody's eyes widened. "Stiff arteries? That doesn't sound good."

Doc Omega-3 smiled and nodded. "Exactly. That's why you need to pair those fats with omega-3s, which help keep your arteries flexible. Recent studies show that taking omega-3 supplements can counteract the drop in FMD caused by high-fat foods like ghee and olive oil" (Chen et al., 2023; Koch et al., 2022).

Cholesterina added, "Without omega-3s, your arteries don't stay flexible. The fats in ghee and olive oil can temporarily impair arterial function if taken in large amounts without anything to balance them out" (Barbosa et al., 2022; Chen et al., 2020).

Brody scratched his head. "So, what you're saying is, I need to add omega-3s to the mix?"

Doc Omega-3 grinned. "Exactly. Omega-3 fatty acids, like the ones found in algae oil, are essential for keeping your arteries flexible. Algae oil, in particular, is a great source of DHA, a type of omega-3 that reduces inflammation and improves endothelial function" (Chen et al., 2023; Koch et al., 2022).

Brody blinked. "And I can just take omega-3 supplements with my meals to balance it out?"

Doc Omega-3 nodded. "That's right. By taking omega-3s with your meals—whether it's with your Ghee Coffee, Olive Oil Shots, or any high-fat foods—you'll prevent the temporary stiffening of your arteries. Omega-3s work to reduce the risk of endothelial dysfunction, ensuring that your heart stays in great shape" (Chen et al., 2023; Koch et al., 2022).

Cholesterina added, "And the best part? Algae oil doesn't have that fishy aftertaste like fish oil, so it's a great option for people who prefer a plant-based source of omega-3s."

Brody's face lit up. "So, I don't have to give up my Ghee Coffee and Olive Oil Shots—I just need to add omega-3s to balance it?"

Doc Omega-3 smiled. "Exactly. Balance is key, Brody. Omega-3-rich foods like chia seeds, flaxseeds, or a good algae oil supplement will make sure you're getting the most out of your diet without hurting your arteries" (Chen et al., 2023; Koch et al., 2022).

Brody grinned. "I'm sold! From now on, I'll add algae oil to my meals, and maybe some chia seeds too. My arteries are going to be unstoppable!"

From that day forward, Brody became Nutritia's biggest advocate for balance. He continued to enjoy his Ghee Coffee and Olive Oil Shots, but now with a daily dose of omega-3s. His arteries stayed flexible, his heart stayed strong, and he never had to worry about stiff arteries again.

**The Power of Coconut Oil: Fueling the Brain**

Coconut oil, particularly its cold-pressed organic form, is packed with medium-chain triglycerides (MCTs)—fats that the body quickly metabolizes into ketones. In the context of dementia, where glucose metabolism is often compromised, ketones act as an alternative energy source for the brain. This "brain fuel" swoops in during times of metabolic stress to prevent neuronal energy deficits and keep brain cells functioning optimally (Marten et al., 2021). The hippocampus, a brain region critical for memory and learning, is particularly sensitive to these energy deficits, and ketones from MCTs are crucial for its preservation.

Beyond their role as fuel, MCTs also enhance neurogenesis, the process of generating new neurons, particularly in the hippocampus. This is significant because Alzheimer's disease is marked by impaired neurogenesis and mitochondrial dysfunction. MCTs help mitigate these issues by improving mitochondrial function and reducing oxidative stress (Tsujino et al., 2022; Fortier et al., 2020). Moreover, MCTs increase the expression of brain-derived neurotrophic factor (BDNF), a protein that promotes synaptic plasticity and supports the survival of neurons (Kashiwaya et al., 2013). Essentially, MCTs not only nourish existing neurons but also promote the birth of new ones, making them critical in the fight against cognitive decline.

Coconut oil also contains lauric acid, which has anti-inflammatory properties, further reducing neuroinflammation—a key factor in the progression of dementia.

Chronic inflammation in the brain damages neurons and accelerates the progression of neurodegenerative diseases, and lauric acid helps mitigate this damage (Yang et al., 2022).

## Black Sesame Seeds: Nature's Antioxidant Shield

While coconut oil fuels and protects the brain, black sesame seeds play a complementary role by providing potent antioxidant and anti-inflammatory benefits. Black sesame seeds are rich in sesamin and sesamolin, two lignans with well-documented neuroprotective effects. These compounds combat oxidative stress, often referred to as the "rusting" of neurons—a slow process that contributes to cognitive decline (Park et al., 2023).

The antioxidant properties of black sesame seeds stem from their ability to neutralize free radicals, preventing them from causing damage to neuronal cells. They also contain vitamin E, which enhances cell membrane integrity, protecting neurons from oxidative damage and ensuring they remain functional for longer (Rosni, 2024).

Together, sesamin, sesamolin, and vitamin E form a trifecta of brain protection, preserving cognitive function and memory. Additionally, black sesame seeds are abundant in essential fatty acids like oleic and linoleic acids. These fatty acids not only support brain health but also improve lipid profiles, reducing the risk of cognitive decline (Sundar, 2023). The presence of flavonoids and phenolic compounds further enhances their neuroprotective effects, promoting cognitive function and reducing the likelihood of neurodegenerative diseases (Luo et al., 2022).

## Coffee: The Morning Shield Against Parkinsonism

In the grand theater of health interventions, coffee isn't just your trusty sidekick for surviving Monday mornings—it might just be the superhero your neurons have been waiting for. Recent studies suggest that regular coffee drinkers are less likely to develop Parkinson's disease (PD). In fact, some research shows that your daily caffeine fix might slash your PD risk by up to 30% compared to non-drinkers (Ren & Chen, 2020). So, yes, your coffee addiction might be doing more than just keeping you awake during those early morning meetings.

Let's talk about caffeine, the star player in this caffeinated saga. It doesn't just jolt you awake; it also plays defense against PD by blocking the adenosine A2A receptor—a key villain in the plot against your dopamine. By standing in the way of this receptor, caffeine helps keep your dopamine levels up, potentially slowing down the neurodegenerative processes that lead to PD (Ren & Chen, 2020; Ikram et al., 2020).

But caffeine isn't the only hero in your cup. Coffee is also packed with chlorogenic acid, a bioactive compound with antioxidant powers that can help protect your brain cells from the oxidative stress and toxic mess caused by α-synuclein clumps—those pesky hallmarks of PD (Lu et al., 2020). Think of chlorogenic acid as the sidekick with a knack for cleaning up the bad guys.

And just when you thought your coffee couldn't get any better, it turns out it's also meddling in your epigenetics—yes, that's right, your coffee is literally rewriting parts of your genetic code. Epigenetic changes, like DNA methylation and histone acetylation, can interfere with how your genes express themselves, leading to various issues, including PD (Huang et al., 2021; Klokkaris, 2024). But coffee, particularly the chlorogenic acid in it, may help keep these epigenetic changes in check, potentially shielding you from neurodegeneration (Ding et al., 2023). In other words, your morning brew could be working behind the scenes to keep your neurons happy.

Let's not forget about brain-derived neurotrophic factor (BDNF), the protein that's essentially Miracle-Gro for your neurons. Coffee has been shown to boost BDNF levels, which supports neuron growth, survival, and overall brain plasticity. So, by drinking coffee, you're not just staying awake—you're potentially giving your brain the nutrients it needs to stay sharp and resilient (Paiva et al., 2022).

### The Coffee Guardians, Captain Cardio, and the Silent Saboteurs: A Caffeinated, Well-Rested, and Sun-Kissed War Against the Shakes

Dr. Elias Grey, once a brilliant neuroscientist, now found himself facing not only Parkinson's disease but also the unsettling realization that part of the damage had been caused by silent villains that had slipped into his life years ago—pesticides and gut dysbiosis. Standing in his kitchen, coffee in hand, he stared out the window at his old running shoes. It had been a long fight, but now he knew the real culprits.

Elias couldn't shake the anger that came with learning that pesticides—those seemingly innocuous chemicals—had been linked to Parkinson's disease as early as the 1980s, but nothing was done for decades.

"Why didn't they ban these chemicals sooner?" he muttered, gripping his coffee mug tightly. "Why did they wait so long?"

**Pesticides:** "It took them over 30 years to act. Can you believe it? Scientists found the link between me and Parkinson's in 1983—yep, a man named Dr. William Langston, who discovered that a compound similar to me (called MPTP) caused Parkinsonism in drug users. They should've banned me then, but nope, I stayed. For decades, I had free reign."

**Gut Dysbiosis, and Pesticides** huddled together, smirking. Pesticides spoke first, his voice dripping with sarcasm.

**Pesticides:** "Even after MPTP, it took until 2015—over 30 years!—before they finally started taking me seriously. By then, I had already embedded myself in crops, water supplies, and food chains. Millions exposed, no real bans. They banned some of my friends, like paraquat, but only after studies kept piling up" (Tanner et al., 2011).

Elias's neurons, already struggling from the effects of gut dysbiosis and dopamine depletion, quaked under this new revelation. How could they have waited so long?

Dr. Elias Grey stared into his mug of coffee, knowing this wasn't just about caffeine anymore. Armed with bioactive compounds, exercise, a trusty water filter, and a handful of supplements, he was gearing up for his latest battle against Parkinson's disease. Outside, the world looked peaceful, but inside, Elias was preparing for war.

He laced up his sneakers with a new sense of purpose. "Let's see what these new guys can do."

**Pesticides:** "Thought you could get rid of me with just coffee and exercise?" Pesticides sneered, circling Elias's neurons like a villain in a bad movie. "You've got gaps in your defenses. I'm still here, hanging out in your brain and gut from years of pesticide-laden water and unwashed produce" (Tanner et al., 2011).

**Vitamin D3 and K2** swooped in with a dazzling glow as the sunlight streamed through the window.

**Vitamin D3** flexed, "We're here to support your bones, brain, and immune system" (Holick, 2007).

**K2** nodded, "And I'll make sure calcium behaves and doesn't go where it shouldn't" (Sgarbossa et al., 2015).

Suddenly, **Omega-3 algae oil** appeared, exuding a calming presence. "Let's calm down that inflammation and protect those neurons, shall we?" (Swanson et al., 2012).

Elias's neurons sighed in relief as Omega-3 worked its magic, cooling down the brain's inflammation and helping with dopamine regulation. Just as Omega-3 started weaving its magic, **Mucuna pruriens** showed up.

"You need more dopamine? Don't worry, I've got this," Mucuna said, flexing his plant-based muscles. His L-DOPA delivery was just what Elias's neurons needed to keep up the fight (Katzenschlager et al., 2004).

Meanwhile, **Captain Cardio** ran laps around the gut, shaking hands with fermented fiber, restoring balance to the gut microbiota, and giving Gut Dysbiosis a well-deserved thrashing. "You thought you could hide down here, huh? Think again. Exercise boosts gut health, and I'm here to fix the damage!" (Monda et al., 2017).

But the most critical player was **Sleep**, who strolled in with a yawn, stretching luxuriously. "I'm here to detox the brain and keep everything running smoothly" (Xie et al., 2013).

And, of course, the **Coffee Guardians** were already on the battlefield.

**Chlorogenic Acid** was at the forefront, wielding her antioxidant and anti-inflammatory powers to protect the mitochondria from oxidative stress (Gomes et al., 2019). She sliced through free radicals like a graceful warrior, ensuring that Elias's neurons remained fortified.

Not far behind, **Caffeic Acid** was neutralizing oxidative stress with a calm, focused demeanor, adding extra layers of neuroprotection to help Elias's neurons fend off their enemies (Jaiswal et al., 2010).

**Quinides** darted through the battlefield, sharp as ever, enhancing dopamine sensitivity and ensuring dopamine flowed smoothly through the synaptic gaps (van Dam et al., 2020). "No more dopamine blockages on my watch!" he shouted as he cut through resistance like a hot knife through butter.

**Ferulic Acid**, the steadfast protector, stood guard with his anti-inflammatory shield. "No inflammation is getting through me," he growled, keeping Gut Dysbiosis's inflammatory bombs at bay (Sgarbossa et al., 2015).

In the background, the quiet yet vital heroes **Trigonelline** and **Melanoidins** worked in tandem, contributing to the overall antioxidant activity and protecting brain cells from the ravages of oxidative damage (Bekedam et al., 2008).

With **Omega-3**, **Mucuna pruriens**, **Vitamin D3 + K2**, **Sleep**, and the **Coffee Guardians** on his side, Elias's neurons were stronger than ever. **Pesticides** and **Gut Dysbiosis** didn't stand a chance. As the sunlight bathed Elias in warmth, his brain began to recover, dopamine levels rising, and inflammation receding.

**Pesticides**, now retreating, threw one last feeble punch. "This wasn't supposed to happen! You weren't supposed to figure out the water filters, the sunlight, or the algae oil!" (Tanner et al., 2011).

Elias stepped outside—daylight beamed in, not just as a metaphor but as an actual superhero in Elias's life. The light worked wonders, helping improve sleep and mood after just four weeks (Videnovic et al., 2021). He took a sip of his coffee and felt the warmth of the **Coffee Guardians** settling into his brain (Holick, 2007). Between his Coffee Guardians, Captain Cardio, and his new team of supplements, he was ready for whatever came next.

### Broccoli: The Crucial Crunch

Ah, broccoli—the Wonder Woman of the veggie world. Lurking within those little green trees is **sulforaphane (SFN)**, a compound that's like a superhero waiting to be unleashed. Once you take a bite, SFN springs into action, activating your body's defense systems, particularly the Nrf2 pathway (but you can pretend you didn't hear that, just like you ignore your to-do list). This pathway is your body's personal Batman, swooping in to protect against oxidative stress and neurodegeneration (Santín-Márquez et al., 2019). But wait, there's more! Sulforaphane also teams up with the proteasome—think of it as the cellular janitor—to keep your cells clean and youthful, potentially warding off everything from Alzheimer's to those pesky aging wrinkles (Santín-Márquez et al., 2019). So, next time you're crunching on broccoli, remember: you're not just eating a veggie—you're giving your brain neurons a power boost.

**Walnuts: The Brain's Best Friend**
Now, let's toss in some nuts—specifically, walnuts. In a study by Akbaraly et al. (2024), researchers explored the connection between munching on healthy nuts and keeping your hippocampus—the brain's memory center—nice and plump. The findings? If you stick to a diet that scores high on the **Alternative Healthy Eating Index** (which is basically a fancy way of saying "eat your fruits and veggies, and lay off the junk"), your hippocampus might just stay in shape longer. The real kicker? The left side of your hippocampus seems to appreciate this healthy diet even more than the right side. And if you needed another reason to cut down on booze, here it is: low alcohol intake was the MVP in keeping that brain region beefy by helping to generate new neurons. So go ahead, snack on some walnuts and give your brain the love it deserves!

**A Match(a) Made in Memory Heaven: How This Matcha Elixir Powers Your Brain!**
When it comes to matcha, this green powerhouse is loaded with bioactive compounds because it is made from whole tea leaves, which are ground into a fine powder and consumed entirely, as opposed to steeping leaves in water and discarding them (Jakubczyk et al., 2020). Matcha contains significantly more catechins, including epigallocatechin gallate (EGCG), which is 137 times greater than the amount of EGCG available from China Green Tips green tea and at least three times higher than the largest literature value for other green teas (Weiss & Anderton, 2003). According to Jakubczyk et al. (2020), matcha exhibits a higher antioxidant potential than other green teas.
What's EGCG, you ask? Besides being a word that autocorrect loves to change to 'egg,' let me introduce you to epigallocatechin gallate (EGCG), the star compound in green tea! Studies have shown that EGCG can protect against Alzheimer's

disease by reducing amyloid plaques, which are associated with cognitive decline (Agarwal & Fulgoni, 2021). Moreover, EGCG has been found to promote cell death in cancer cells and inhibit tumor growth, suggesting its role in cancer prevention (Aguilera, 2023; Fulgoni & Agarwal, 2021). Additionally, it exhibits properties that may help maintain skin health and reduce signs of aging (Unno & Nakamura, 2021; Ibrahim et al., 2022). So, if you want to boost your brain health, support cancer prevention, and promote youthful skin, brewing a cup of matcha tea might be beneficial, as EGCG offers a range of health-promoting properties.

Beyond EGCG, matcha is also rich in other bioactive compounds such as L-theanine, which can be up to five times higher than in regular green tea (Unno et al., 2018), as well as caffeine, quercetin, and chlorophyll. These compounds work together to provide matcha's unique health benefits, from antioxidant properties to promoting calm alertness. So, while your standard green tea is great, matcha takes it to the next level, offering a more potent brew for your brain and body.

Matcha green tea contains significantly high levels of L-theanine. It is like a zen amino acid! Matcha was actually consumed by Buddhist monks to help with meditation. Studies have shown that the L-theanine content in matcha can be up to five times higher than in standard green tea leaves, making it particularly effective in promoting relaxation without the jitteriness often associated with caffeine (Sielicka-Różyńska et al., 2020).

Now, if you are a coffee drinker who feels jittery, you might want to consider switching to matcha, which contains L-theanine. L-theanine is known for promoting relaxation without drowsiness, potentially mitigating the jitteriness often associated with caffeine consumption (Agarwal & Fulgoni, 2021). Studies indicate that L-theanine can increase alpha brain wave activity, which may enhance relaxation while maintaining alertness—beneficial for focus and concentration (Fulgoni & Agarwal, 2021). Thus, while coffee can lead to feelings of restlessness, matcha may help maintain a sense of calm while keeping your mind sharp.

And how to take your matcha drink to the next level? Squeeze some lemon juice.

The vitamin C in lemon juice can significantly increase the stability of epigallocatechin gallate (EGCG), the powerful catechin found in green tea, by preventing its degradation in the digestive system. This stabilization leads to higher bioavailability, meaning your body absorbs more of the beneficial compounds when you enjoy your matcha with a squeeze of lemon (Pastore & Fratellone, 2006).

Matcha tea might just be your brain's best buddy—if your brain enjoys a little green goodness with a side of zen! In a recent study, participants who consumed 2.07 grams of matcha daily (about the weight of a small paperclip) showed quicker reaction times and better facial expression recognition—perfect for figuring out if your date is horrified by your cooking or just really into the burnt pasta aesthetic (Baba et al., 2021b).

In another showdown, caffeine was pitted against matcha. While caffeine gave a quick jolt to attention after a single dose, matcha proved to be the tortoise in this race, helping maintain focus under stress over the long haul (Baba et al., 2021a).

A study found that older women who consumed matcha showed improvements in language skills, proving that matcha might just be the secret ingredient to keeping your vocabulary sharp as you age (Sakurai et al., 2020). But with only 15 men in the study, it's hard to say if matcha is a "girl power" drink or if the guys were just too busy watching sports.

**Avocados** – The diet rich in monounsaturated fats supports the production of myelin and overall brain health (Gómez-Pinilla, 2008). The medium-chain triglycerides (MCTs) are converted into ketones, which can be used as an alternative energy source for neurons and support myelin production (Cunnane et al., 2016). "Who knew that a slice of avocado could be the secret ingredient to growing new brain cells?" they chuckled, celebrating their findings (Boldrini et al., 2018). The ketogenic diet, in particular, emerged as a powerful tool for promoting neurogenesis by reducing oxidative stress and encouraging the growth of new neurons (Bostock et al., 2020; Chase, 2023).

# The Prefrontal Cortex (PFC): Your Brain's Fantastic CEO

Finally, there's the Prefrontal Cortex, the brain's multitasking CEO. "I'm the one keeping this circus together," it says, juggling planning, decision-making, and working memory like a stressed-out parent (Feng et al., 2023; Hu, 2024). It tries to keep everything organized, though it can't handle everything when overwhelmed.

### Working Memory: The PFC's Post-it Note Collection

Working memory is essentially your brain's Post-it note system—holding onto information just long enough to use it. The PFC, particularly the dorsolateral prefrontal cortex (dlPFC), is where the magic happens. If that takes a hit, suddenly your brain's Post-its start falling off the wall, especially when distracted, making it tough to remember what you were doing just a moment ago (Wang et al., 2020). Neuroimaging studies show that when you're trying to keep track of something— like your grocery list—the PFC lights up like a Christmas tree, showing just how hard it's working (Vijayraghavan & Everling, 2021). And it's not just holding the info; it's also coordinating with other brain regions, like the hippocampus, to make sure your thoughts don't turn into a jumbled mess (Nikolin et al., 2021).

### Long-Term Memory: The PFC's Filing Cabinet

While the hippocampus is busy creating new memories, the PFC takes on the role of the brain's long-term storage manager. Over time, as memories age, they move from the hippocampus to the PFC, particularly the medial prefrontal cortex (mPFC), which acts like a seasoned librarian, knowing exactly where to find those old memories when you need them (Dixsaut & Gräff, 2021). This transition helps explain why memories of that epic vacation from five years ago are still crystal clear.

The PFC also excels at adding context to your memories, like recalling not just what happened but where and when it happened. If you've ever tried to remember a specific event but couldn't quite place it, you can thank (or blame) your PFC for that (Barker & Warburton, 2020).

**Prefrontal Cortex: Your Guardian Angel**

One of the prefrontal cortex's most impressive feats is its ability to suppress unwanted memories, especially those tied to strong emotions. Think of the ventromedial prefrontal cortex as your brain's guardian angel, gently shielding you from those embarrassing or traumatic memories that could otherwise overwhelm you (Wang et al., 2021).

This isn't just a passive process—it's an active job, with the prefrontal cortex working tirelessly to tuck those memories away in the hippocampus's "Do Not Disturb" file (Anderson & Hulbert, 2021). This protective function is crucial for keeping your emotional life balanced.

**Impulse Control: How Your Brain's CEO Fights the Midnight Cake Cravings**

The prefrontal cortex is like a monk, in charge of impulse control, focus, and keeping your emotions in check. It's the part of your brain that stops you from eating an entire cake at midnight—or at least, it tries. Research shows that the medial prefrontal cortex plays a big role in managing impulsive behaviors, especially when you're stressed (Urueña-Méndez, 2024; Liu, 2024). This part of the brain is especially important during the teen years when emotions and behaviors can be a bit wild (Sharafeddin, 2024).

The prefrontal cortex also helps you stay focused and make smart decisions, even when life gets chaotic. It works with other parts of your brain to keep you on track and handle tricky situations without losing your cool (Çakar, 2024; Cong, 2024).

But stress and bad habits can throw off the prefrontal cortex's game. When stress takes over, your brain's ability to control impulses can weaken, making it harder to resist temptations like that extra piece of cake (Arruda, 2024; Acosta-Lopez, 2024).

The bigger the prefrontal cortex, the better the prefrontal cortex, and we shall gift ourselves a better prefrontal cortex with the actionable items below—yay!

**Food for Thought?**

A diet rich in omega-3 fatty acids, like those found in fish and walnuts, is essentially brain fuel, encouraging new brain cell growth and keeping your prefrontal cortex sharp (Takehana, 2024). Meanwhile, antioxidants from olive oil, berries, and dark leafy greens act like a brain detox, fighting off oxidative stress that can slow you down (Takehana, 2024). And for the chocolate lovers, here is some good news: foods high in flavonoids, like dark chocolate and citrus fruits, can help improve blood flow and neuroplasticity, giving your brain a boost in performance (Takehana, 2024).

Walnuts deserve a special shout out—they are packed with alpha-linolenic acid, which is fantastic for brain health, making them the ultimate snack for anyone looking to stay sharp (Takehana, 2024). By combining brainy activities with a nutrient-rich diet, you are not just maintaining your prefrontal cortex—you are enhancing it.

Now, let's talk about hobbies because it turns out your brain loves a good puzzle as much as you do. Engaging in mentally stimulating activities like reading or learning new skills is like a workout for your prefrontal cortex. These activities promote neuroplasticity and can actually increase the gray matter in your brain, which is essentially like adding extra horsepower to your mental engine (Li, 2024). Whether you are solving puzzles or learning a new language, these hobbies strengthen synaptic connections and encourage the growth of new neurons, helping your brain stay in top shape (Rosario, 2024).

And let's not forget the power of broccoli. This humble vegetable is a superstar when it comes to brain health, packed with antioxidants, vitamins, and minerals that support cognitive function. It is rich in vitamin K, which helps with the formation of myelin sheaths around neurons, ensuring your brain's communication lines run smoothly (Chmiel, 2024). Plus, broccoli contains sulforaphane, a compound that fights off oxidative stress and inflammation, keeping your brain protected and healthy (Takehana, 2024).

## Grounding: Reconnecting Your Brain to the Earth (Literally)

Grounding, or earthing, is essentially walking barefoot on grass, dirt, or sand. It sounds super simple, but it works wonders for reducing inflammation and cortisol levels (Chevalier et al., 2012). Your prefrontal cortex thrives in low-stress environments, and grounding helps by calming down the stress response in your brain. Imagine your PFC saying, "Thank you for this quiet, peaceful moment," while you wiggle your toes in the grass.

## Humming: Ohm for Your Vibes

Need a quick PFC reset? Humming is like hitting your brain's relaxation button. It stimulates the vagus nerve, which helps reduce stress and boosts parasympathetic nervous system activity (Porges, 2011). By calming your nervous system, humming improves blood flow to the PFC, making it easier for you to think clearly, focus, and chill out.

## Moringa: The Superfood for Super Focus

Known as the "miracle tree," moringa is packed with antioxidants, vitamins, and nutrients that reduce oxidative stress in the brain (Anwar et al., 2007). Its high levels of vitamin C and E protect your neurons from damage, while its anti-inflammatory properties soothe the PFC. Essentially, moringa is like a supercharged superfood for your brain, keeping it healthy and sharp.

## Beets & Beetroot Juice: A Natural Nitric Oxide Boost

Move over, kale—there's a new superfood in town that's got brains and brawn! Researchers decided to see what happens when you mix beetroot juice with exercise in a group of older adults (Petrie et al., 2017). Spoiler alert: it's not just the exercise doing the heavy lifting! Picture this: a group of 65-year-olds hitting the gym and chugging beet juice like it's the fountain of youth. What did they discover? Not only did these legends see improvements in their workout endurance, but their brains got a serious upgrade too.

The participants who drank beet juice developed brain networks that resembled those of younger folks. Imagine your brain's neurons high-fiving each other in celebration! The secret ingredient? Nitric oxide—thanks to the beet juice, it's like giving your blood vessels a superhero cape, boosting blood flow right to the brain. The result? Better brain connectivity and fewer signs of aging. So, if you want to keep your brain as fresh as a beet, consider adding some of that vibrant juice to your daily routine. Who knew that beating aging could be so... beet-licious?

## Herbs & Spices: Brain Fuel from Nature's Medicine Cabinet

Some herbs and spices do more than just spice up your food—they help your brain thrive. For instance, turmeric contains curcumin, a compound that boosts brain-derived neurotrophic factor (BDNF), a protein essential for neurogenesis in the PFC (Mishra & Palanivelu, 2008). Ashwagandha helps reduce cortisol levels, keeping the PFC in chill mode, while ginkgo biloba improves blood circulation, enhancing cognitive functions (Kumar & Khanum, 2012).

## Supplements, Vitamins & Fatty Acids: Omega-3, 7, 9, and C15

Omega-3 fatty acids (particularly DHA—choose algae oil supplements when possible) are like bodyguards for the prefrontal cortex (PFC). They reduce inflammation, protect neurons from damage, and boost BDNF levels (Gómez-Pinilla, 2008). Not to be outdone, Omega-7 (macadamia nuts, yum!) joins the party by reducing inflammation and promoting neurogenesis in the PFC (Yang et al., 2016). Omega-9 (olive oil—delicious!) helps regulate cholesterol and supports brain health by maintaining cell membrane integrity (Gutiérrez et al., 2011). Meanwhile, C15 (aka pentadecanoic acid, found in grass-fed ghee, especially from mountain cows with higher C15 content) is a newer contender, touted for improving cellular health and longevity, giving your PFC the durability it needs for long-term cognitive function (Furman et al., 2020).

## Exercise: Sweating for Smarts

There's no debate—exercise is a game-changer for PFC health. Physical activity boosts blood flow, increases BDNF, and reduces stress, all of which lead to better decision-making, problem-solving, and focus (Ratey & Loehr, 2011). Even light exercise, like walking, improves cognitive function and memory by keeping your PFC well-fed with oxygen and nutrients.

## Mindfulness, Meditation, & EMDR: Keeping Your PFC Zen

Mindfulness meditation is like sending your PFC on a mini vacation. Studies show it increases gray matter in the PFC, improving self-regulation, focus, and emotional balance (Holzel et al., 2011). EMDR therapy (Eye Movement Desensitization and Reprocessing) helps reduce trauma and stress by engaging both hemispheres of the brain, giving your PFC room to breathe and make better decisions (Shapiro, 2014).

### Mushrooms: The Brain's Best Fungi Friends

Certain mushrooms, like lion's mane and reishi, are packed with neuroprotective compounds. Lion's mane, in particular, has been shown to stimulate the production of nerve growth factor (NGF), which supports the health of neurons in the PFC (Mori et al., 2009). So, a mushroom stir-fry could be more than just a meal—it's a brain boost.

### Teas & Fermented Foods: Gut-Brain Connection for PFC

Green tea contains L-theanine, an amino acid that calms the mind while enhancing focus and attention (Haskell et al., 2008). Fermented foods like kimchi and sauerkraut feed your gut's good bacteria, promoting a healthier gut-brain axis. A healthy gut means less inflammation and more serotonin, which boosts your mood and PFC function (Parker et al., 2020).

### Less Distraction, More Focus: PFC's Best Friend

Let's not forget the basics. Reducing distractions and managing stress are key to keeping your PFC healthy. Every time you're distracted, your PFC has to work overtime, which can lead to burnout (Mark et al., 2017). Lowering stress levels through mindfulness, less screen time, and healthy habits helps your PFC stay in peak condition.

### How Pregnancy & Labor Affect the PFC: A Hormonal Rollercoaster

Pregnancy and labor are like the ultimate brain workout. During pregnancy, hormones like oxytocin and estrogen surge, creating changes in the brain, including in the PFC (Hoekzema et al., 2017). While these hormonal shifts can lead to the infamous "pregnancy brain" (thanks, progesterone), they also foster greater empathy and emotional regulation as your brain adapts to motherhood. Labor and delivery, on the other hand, trigger massive releases of oxytocin, which, while creating emotional bonds, also place stress on the PFC as it works to process the physical and emotional demands of childbirth (Swain et al., 2014).

# The Basal Ganglia: The Routine Enforcer and Sugar Dealer

This little brain region is like the efficiency expert of your mind, think of it as the reason you can ride a bike or play the piano without having to think about each move. The Basal Ganglia makes this magic happen by running a tight ship with its cortico-basal ganglia-thalamo-cortical loops, which sound complicated because they are (Pavlovic et al., 2020; Zhou, 2022).

Now, let's talk sugar. The Basal Ganglia has a sweet tooth, and when you eat sugar, it lights up like a kid in a candy store. Sugar triggers dopamine release in the nucleus accumbens, reinforcing that "must-have-more" feeling. It's the same mechanism that makes other addictions so hard to kick, turning a harmless snack into a one-way ticket to Cravingsville (Makena, 2023; Velt et al., 2020). Your Basal Ganglia doesn't care if it's sugar or something stronger—it's all about getting that quick dopamine hit (Hill & Hurley, 2022; Maleki, 2021).

You've probably heard that it takes 21 to 66 days to form a new habit. Well, that's cute, but reality is a bit messier. Some habits can take as little as 18 days to form, while others might take a whopping 254 days—so much for quick fixes! It turns out, building a new habit depends on many factors, including how complicated the task is and how motivated you are to stick with it (Maleki, 2021; McIntyre & Haussmann, 2021). Your Basal Ganglia is on board to help you make the switch, but it's not running on a strict timeline. So, hang in there—Rome wasn't built in a day, and neither are new habits (Sharma, 2023).

But here's where the Basal Ganglia shows its dark side: addiction. When you get hooked—be it on sugar, social media, or something more sinister—your brain's reward system starts to go haywire. This can lead to "reward deficiency," where normal pleasures just don't cut it anymore, and you find yourself chasing more intense highs (SmithNeal & Cumberledge, 2020; Xiao, 2024). The Basal Ganglia teams up with the prefrontal cortex (the brain's impulse control center), but when addiction takes the wheel, the Basal Ganglia can override your better judgment, leading to compulsive behavior and poor decisions (Hicks, 2021; Li, 2023).

# Cerebellum Confidential: 69 Billion Neurons and a Love for Spinach

The Cerebellum doesn't seek the spotlight, but without its fine-tuning, you'd be all thumbs. "You're welcome for that graceful piano performance," the cerebellum whispers, while everyone else applauds the hippocampus (Qiao, 2023; Seo, 2024).

In the grand theater of the brain, the cerebellum is like the backstage crew—quietly keeping everything running smoothly while the cerebral cortex and hippocampus bask in the spotlight. Sure, the cortex dazzles with higher cognitive functions, but the cerebellum is the unsung hero perfecting your ability to ride a bike or play the piano without thinking twice (Zwilling, 2024).

Now, let's drop some brainy stats: the cerebellum, that little 10% of your brain, packs a whopping 69 billion neurons—about four times more than the cerebral cortex! Imagine it as a compact, powerhouse orchestra ensuring your procedural memories play in perfect harmony.

But even the cerebellum has its kryptonite. It's particularly sensitive to nutrient deficiencies, like a stagehand who hasn't had their coffee. Lacking essential nutrients like vitamin D and omega-3 fatty acids can lead to cognitive slip-ups and memory hiccups (Lefèvre-Arbogast et al., 2021). Picture your cerebellum struggling to remember how to ride a bike—like trying to recall the lyrics to a song you haven't heard in ages! And let's not forget what happens when you drown it in alcohol: cerebellar function takes a nosedive, leading to ataxia, where walking in a straight line becomes a distant memory.

On the flip side, a diet packed with carotenoid-rich foods like broccoli, spinach, and carrots helps keep your cerebellum in tip-top shape, potentially staving off age-related memory decline (Zwilling, 2024). Nuts are another brain booster, especially during pregnancy, giving the cerebellum the fuel it needs to support neurodevelopment and cognitive function (Xie, 2023). So, next time you're munching on walnuts or loading up on veggies, remember—you're not just feeding your body, you're fortifying your cerebellum for a lifetime of smooth moves and graceful coordination.

## The Cerebellum's Epic Adventure: Thiamine, Bananas, and Brain Yoga

Once upon a time, deep inside the cranium of a regular Joe, lived the cerebellum. Now, this wasn't just any cerebellum—it was the unsung hero of the brain, managing coordination, balance, and making sure Joe didn't faceplant while walking (Manto et al., 2012). Despite being only 10% of the brain's volume, this little powerhouse packed a punch, holding more than 50% of Joe's neurons (Azevedo et al., 2009). That's like one guy trying to keep an entire circus running while juggling flaming torches!

## The Party-Crasher: Alcohol

Joe had a weekend habit—he loved to hit the pub. But what Joe didn't know was that his beloved cerebellum hated alcohol more than cats hate baths. Every time Joe downed another pint, the cerebellum threw its hands up in frustration (well, it would if it had hands) because chronic booze was like a rude houseguest, shrinking the cerebellum and killing neurons like they were the last snacks at the party (Sullivan et al., 2000).

Joe began experiencing some weird symptoms: stumbling over his own feet, slurring his speech, and, at one point, attempting to high-five a lamp. It was like he'd permanently RSVP'd to a frat party, except there was no fun, only confusion. The cerebellum was waving its metaphorical arms, shouting, "Stop! You're literally killing me!" (Victor et al., 1989), but Joe couldn't hear it—he was too busy trying to figure out if he could walk in a straight line (spoiler alert: he couldn't).

## The Case of the Missing Vitamin B1

Meanwhile, Joe's diet wasn't doing his cerebellum any favors either. He lived on instant noodles and coffee, which was great for his wallet but terrible for his thiamine levels (Vitamin B1). Without enough B1, the cerebellum found itself in a thiamine drought, resulting in a condition called Wernicke-Korsakoff syndrome, where brain cells dropped like flies (Harper et al., 1998).

Joe found himself wobbling like a toddler on a unicycle. At one point, he tried to use a spoon but ended up slinging soup across the room. "What's wrong with me?" Joe wondered. The cerebellum, exhausted from Joe's dietary crimes, could only sigh and whisper, "B1, buddy. Get yourself some beans and whole grains" (Sechi & Serra, 2007).

## The Autoimmune Ninja: Multiple Sclerosis

One morning, Joe's cerebellum was happily organizing his movements (as usual) when suddenly, WHAM—it was blindsided by an autoimmune attack. Multiple sclerosis (MS) had entered the chat with the stealth of a ninja and the grace of a bull in a china shop (Compston & Coles, 2002).

Joe couldn't even pick up his morning coffee without his hands shaking like they were auditioning for a jittery dance-off. It was like his body was playing dodgeball with his neurons, and the cerebellum was the losing team. "I can't even control my limbs anymore!" Joe cried, spilling his coffee in the process (Kurtzke et al., 1983).

## Cerebellar Stroke: A Rollercoaster of Chaos

As if MS and alcohol weren't enough, one day, Joe's cerebellum took another hit: a stroke. This was the equivalent of his cerebellum being shoved onto a rollercoaster without warning (Schniepp et al., 2017). Joe suddenly found himself dizzy, disoriented, and nauseated—like he was riding the world's worst carnival ride (Baloh et al., 2003).

The cerebellum, now holding on for dear life, sent frantic messages to Joe's body. "We're going down! ABANDON SHIP!" But instead of fleeing, Joe just stumbled around his kitchen, walking like he was on the deck of a pirate ship in the middle of a storm (Timmann et al., 2008).

## When the Little Brain Loses Its Way

As Joe's cerebellum continued to take hits from booze, vitamin deficiencies, MS, and strokes, it began to develop something called cerebellar cognitive affective syndrome (CCAS). This was like Joe's brain going on strike—emotionally and physically (Schmahmann et al., 1998).

Joe began forgetting simple things, like where he put his keys. He even forgot what keys were once, holding them up to his friend and asking, "What do these unlock?" His mood swings became legendary—he'd cry over spilled milk one minute and declare himself a superhero the next. It was like living in a soap opera, only with less dramatic lighting (Schmahmann, 2019).

## The Comeback Tour: Fermented Foods, Yoga, and Grounding

But all was not lost! Joe's cerebellum wasn't about to go down without a fight. It was time for the ultimate comeback, armed with fermented foods, yoga poses, and maybe a side of kale (Morris et al., 2020).

Joe's friend suggested sauerkraut and kimchi. "It's good for your gut-brain axis," she said (Mayer et al., 2014). Joe raised an eyebrow. "Gut-brain what-now?" It turns out fermented foods like kimchi help keep the cerebellum inflammation-free, so it doesn't feel like it's perpetually on fire. Plus, who could say no to a little zingy cabbage?

Next came yoga. "You should try tree pose," his friend advised, balancing on one leg like a flamingo. Joe gave it a shot and immediately wobbled like a drunk toddler. But with time, his balance improved (Guerra-Balic et al., 2015). Tree pose became his cerebellum's new favorite thing—it was like giving it a workout at the gym. Savasana, or corpse pose, became Joe's go-to for relaxation. His cerebellum could finally get some rest, quietly regenerating like a superhero in deep sleep (Rai et al., 2016).

Then came grounding, where Joe walked barefoot on grass. At first, he felt silly, but his cerebellum loved it. "Hey, this is kinda nice," he thought as he absorbed the Earth's electrons. His cerebellum beamed with pride, imagining itself at a spa (Chevalier et al., 2012).

## And They Lived Happily Ever After (With Moringa Smoothies)

Joe started adding cruciferous veggies like broccoli and kale to his diet and even tossed in some moringa powder—because why not? It was packed with antioxidants, and Joe figured if he could put superfoods in his smoothie, maybe his cerebellum would turn into a superhero too (Verma et al., 2011).

With fermented foods, yoga, grounding, and a balanced diet, Joe's cerebellum began to recover. Sure, it had been through the wringer, but now it was on its way to becoming a cerebellum champion (Clark et al., 2016). And so, Joe and his cerebellum lived happily ever after, avoiding frat parties, taking thiamine supplements, and occasionally balancing like a tree. The cerebellum, now a Zen master of balance and coordination, sighed in relief, whispering, "Namaste."

# Memory Olympics: The Cerebral Cortex Goes for Gold

The cerebral cortex, especially the neocortex, is like the brain's control tower, managing everything from memories to motor commands. Picture it as the outermost layer of your brain, with six layers of neurons hard at work on high-level tasks like perception, thought, and, of course, memory (Xu et al., 2021). The neocortex is the multitasking whiz, handling sensory perception, motor control, and those brainy functions that make you, well, you (Xu et al., 2021).

When it comes to memory, it's not just a one-man show. The hippocampus and cerebral cortex team up like Batman and Robin to ensure you can remember where you left your keys and what you had for dinner last night (Fasina et al., 2022; Shuai et al., 2022; Zhang et al., 2022). Short-term memory is like your brain's sticky note, holding onto information just long enough for you to use it. Long-term memory, on the other hand, is the brain's filing cabinet, storing info for the long haul (Shuai et al., 2022; Gureev et al., 2022). The hippocampus gets the ball rolling by encoding and consolidating these short-term memories into long-term storage, with the neocortex stepping in to keep everything organized (Fasina et al., 2022; Shuai et al., 2022).

And let's not forget the prefrontal cortex, the brain's manager, which is in charge of digging up those long-term memories when you need them, proving that memory processing is a team sport (Gureev et al., 2022; Shao et al., 2021).

But what happens when the cerebral cortex or neocortex starts slacking off? You get serious memory issues. Neurodegenerative diseases like Alzheimer's are the ultimate villains, causing neuron loss in these areas and leading to memory loss and cognitive decline (Liu et al., 2023; Liu et al., 2022). If the structure of the cerebral cortex takes a hit, your brain's performance suffers, and remembering becomes a real challenge (Lahouel et al., 2020; Yamada et al., 2022). Add in some neuroinflammation and oxidative stress, and you've got a recipe for cognitive dysfunction, making it clear that a healthy brain environment is key to keeping your memory sharp (Oliveira et al., 2020; Huerta-Cervantes et al., 2021).

Luckily, you can fight back against memory decline with some brain-boosting strategies. Think of cognitive training, physical exercise, and a diet rich in brain food as the personal trainers for your brain's neurons (Liu et al., 2023; Fasina et al., 2022; Liu et al., 2022). Plus, with ongoing research into how memory works at the molecular level, we're getting closer to finding ways to enhance cognitive function and keep those memories intact (Liu et al., 2023; Gureev et al., 2022; Liu et al., 2022).

# The Amygdala's Guide to Keeping Calm and Not Freaking Out

Then there's the Amygdala, the brain's emotional amplifier. "Is that a black widow spider? Better remember it forever!" it insists, ensuring anything remotely emotional sticks with you (Qiao, 2023; Amer, 2024). The Amygdala loves to turn up the emotional volume, making sure those heart-pounding moments are impossible to forget so you can avoid repeating dangerous mistakes.

This little cluster is a big deal when it comes to processing emotions, especially fear and pleasure. It's connected to the brain's vital memory areas like the prefrontal cortex, hippocampus, and other structures, helping to regulate your emotional responses and even influencing which memories stick around (Labuschagne, 2024; McDonald, 2023).

The Amygdala is like the brain's emotional switchboard, especially when it comes to fear. Think of the amygdala as the operator, connecting emotional stimuli with the right brain regions, making sure that fear hits you right where it counts (Labuschagne, 2024). Its calming friend is the prefrontal cortex (vmPFC), which helps manage those fear responses and emotional outbursts (McGlashan et al., 2021). This dynamic duo is key to fear conditioning—think of it as the brain's way of learning not to touch the hot stove—and fear extinction, which is learning that the stove is now cool (McGlashan et al., 2021). The amygdala's extensive network allows it to react quickly to what's happening around you, making sure your behavior and emotions are always on point (McDonald, 2023).

**The Amygdala Meltdown: Why Your Brain's Almond Sometimes Loses Its Cool**
In anxiety disorders, depression, and PTSD, the amygdala often goes haywire, leading to emotional chaos (Николенко et al., 2020; Wu et al., 2020). Take adolescents with major depressive disorder, for instance—they tend to have a disconnect between their amygdala and prefrontal cortex, which messes with their ability to keep emotions in check (Wu et al., 2020). And if life hits hard early on, that stress can shrink the amygdala and make emotional regulation a lifelong struggle (Hanson & Nacewicz, 2020).

The amygdala's stress response is especially relevant in our current pandemic-riddled world. Thanks to COVID-19, heightened stress levels have led to some serious amygdala funkiness, increasing anxiety symptoms for many (Zhou et al., 2023). And it's not just global pandemics—living in noisy, crowded cities can also send your amygdala into overdrive, proving that even where you live can mess with your brain's emotional HQ (Sudimac et al., 2022).

## Did I Tell You About My Friend Amy?

Once upon a time, nestled deep in the folds of the brain, there lived a tiny almond-shaped hero named Amy, the Amygdala. Amy was the emotional air traffic controller of the mind, directing feelings like love, fear, and, yes, rage—especially when someone dared eat your leftover pizza. Think of Amy as that over-caffeinated employee who's always on edge, balancing between cool under pressure and total meltdown. But even heroes need help sometimes. When Amy becomes overworked, over-stressed, or downright damaged, things can get... well, spicy.

## The Usual Suspects: What Hurts Our Hero?

First up: **Chronic Stress.** Imagine Amy the Amygdala sipping on five espresso shots, vibrating with nervous energy while barking at every little issue like it's a life-or-death scenario. You spill a little coffee? PANIC. The Wi-Fi drops? CALL THE FIRE DEPARTMENT. Chronic stress makes Amy swell up like an overinflated balloon, leaving you jumpier than a Chihuahua in a thunderstorm (McEwen et al., 2015).

Then there's **Traumatic Brain Injury (TBI).** Picture this: Amy, wearing a tiny helmet, gets whacked by life's metaphorical 2x4—maybe you hit your head during a Twister rematch. Boom! Suddenly, Amy's emotional control panel is flashing "ERROR," and now you can't recognize fear or feel empathy. It's like trying to read a room with sunglasses on... in a basement (Bigler et al., 2016).

And we can't forget the real party-crasher: **Neurodegenerative diseases.** Amy starts packing her emotional suitcase as Alzheimer's or Parkinson's knocks on the door. One minute you're in the middle of a heartfelt moment, and the next, Amy's response is... off. Laughing at funerals? Crying during rom-coms? Welcome to the emotional Twilight Zone (Braak et al., 2011).

**When Amy Takes a Vacation: Recognizing the Signs**

When Amy the Amygdala decides she's had enough, it's like your emotions go on a rollercoaster—with no seat belts. **Emotional Instability** is the first sign. Laughing at sad moments, crying when someone spills milk, flipping out over someone chewing too loudly—it's like Amy's stuck pressing the "extreme emotions" button (Davidson et al., 2000).

Then there's the **Lack of Fear Response.** Picture this: You confidently strut up to a pit bull like it's a fluffy kitten or pick up a snake thinking it's just a wiggly noodle. Yeah, that's Amy on strike (Adolphs et al., 2005).

Finally, there's **Aggression.** When Amy's out of whack, the smallest thing—like the sound of someone slurping soup—can send you into Hulk mode (Siever et al., 2008).

**Enter the Heroes: What You Can Do to Help Amy**

**Fermented Foods** are like a spa day for Amy. Let's start with Kimchi, that spicy Korean superstar. When you chow down on this gut-friendly dish, your probiotics throw a party that connects your gut to your brain via the magical "gut-brain axis," sending Amy some much-needed R&R (Kim et al., 2017). Or how about Kombucha? Not just a trendy drink for hipster yogis—this bubbly brew calms Amy like a fizzy emotional support blanket (Sokol et al., 2018).

But if you're really feeling sophisticated, try **Miso Soup.** While you slurp it down, it quietly reduces inflammation, making Amy think she's lounging in a hot tub instead of running your emotional thermostat (Peirce et al., 2013).

Then there's the nutrient dream team: **Magnesium, Omega-3s, and Vitamin D.** Magnesium is like Amy's personal therapist, regulating anxiety through the HPA axis (Boyle et al., 2017). Omega-3s? They're Amy's anti-inflammatory personal trainers, reducing her tendency to go full drama queen (Su et al., 2015). Vitamin D is that ray of sunshine that keeps Amy from overreacting to minor stressors like, oh, Mondays (de Oliveira et al., 2018).

## Yoga and Sleep: Amy's Vacation Package

If Amy could book a vacation, it would probably be at a yoga retreat. **Child's Pose and Legs-Up-the-Wall** are like Amy's hammock on a tropical island. These poses lower anxiety levels, calming Amy down so she's not constantly waving the emotional red flag (Thayer et al., 2012).

Speaking of vacations, let's talk **sleep.** When she gets a full 7-9 hours, Amy settles into deep NREM sleep, the brain's version of housekeeping. This is when the brain sorts through emotional clutter and recharges Amy's batteries, making sure she's ready to face another day without losing her cool (van der Helm et al., 2011).

## Grounding and Meditation: Amy's Zen Mode

**Grounding—or Earthing—**is the practice of walking barefoot on grass, and no, it's not just for nature-loving hippies. Walking barefoot sends calming signals to Amy, telling her to chill out and stop seeing text messages as emotional grenades (Chevalier et al., 2012). Add some **Meditation** to the mix, and now Amy is getting the TLC she needs. Meditation shrinks Amy and boosts your prefrontal cortex, like telling her, "Shh, it's all good," while you chill out for five minutes (Holzel et al., 2010).

## Moringa and Coffee: The Dynamic Duo

**Moringa** is like Amy's leafy green smoothie—it's packed with antioxidants that hug her tiny almond heart and reduce oxidative stress (Rao et al., 2017). And then there's **Coffee,** Amy's love-hate relationship. A little coffee? Great, it sharpens her up. Too much? It's like Amy's bouncing off the walls like she's had one too many energy drinks (Ding et al., 2014).

# The Cingulate Gyrus Squad: Your Brain's Hype Team and Zen Masters

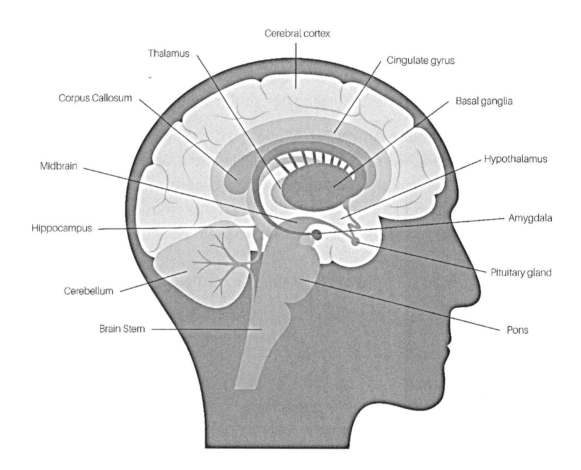

Welcome to the cingulate gyrus, your brain's quirky fitness team, divided into three parts: the anterior cingulate gyrus (ACG), the anterior midcingulate cortex (aMCC), and the posterior cingulate gyrus (PCC). These brain buddies keep your emotions, motivation, and self-reflection in check.

Gan et al. (2022) discovered that mindfulness practices aren't just a mental chill pill—they actually beef up your cingulate cortex, both functionally and structurally.

And let's not forget the cingulate gyrus's hidden talent: pain perception. According to Zheng et al. (2022), this part of your brain is basically your emotional and physical pain DJ, spinning those tracks a little too loud sometimes. But good news! Meditation can help you turn the volume down, so both physical and emotional pain fade into the background, leaving you with a playlist that's more "Zen Garden" and less "Heavy Metal Meltdown."

## The Anterior Cingulate Gyrus (ACG): The Brain's Personal Trainer

Think of the Anterior Cingulate Gyrus (ACG) as your brain's motivational coach with a whistle and clipboard, yelling, "You got this!"

The ACG is your go-to for emotional regulation and cognitive control, stepping in to make sure you keep your cool when the going gets rough (Li et al., 2022; Gu et al., 2020). Recent studies suggest that when you engage in mentally taxing activities, the ACG's activity ramps up, boosting its functionality (Chotipanich et al., 2021).

Research by Kurth et al. (2021) found that long-term meditators have less age-related gray matter loss in this area, which means their emotional engines stay revved up longer. Meditation feels like a brain spa because it gives the ACG a nice, relaxing stretch, helping to keep you emotionally stable and resilient as you age (Chien et al., 2020; Chotipanich et al., 2021).

Plus, the ACG is tightly connected to your brain's reward system—the nucleus accumbens and amygdala—making it the headquarters for processing good vibes and emotional payoffs.

## The Anterior Midcingulate Cortex (aMCC): The Will to Live, Doing What You Dread

The anterior mid-cingulate gyrus (aMCC) plays a critical role in regulating motivation and the will to live, particularly through its involvement in emotional processing and decision-making.

It is responsible for that little voice in your head saying, "Yeah, this sucks now, but trust me, future you will thank you," when all you want to do is crawl back into bed (Jiang et al., 2022). When you actually do the hard stuff, the anterior midcingulate cortex starts doing a happy dance, bolstering your will to live. For instance, engaging in activities that you might resist—such as physical exercise, social interactions, or challenging tasks—can enhance the functional connectivity and activity within the aMCC, reinforcing motivation and improving overall mental health outcomes (Chen et al., 2023).

When you take on tough tasks, this area gets a workout, building mental agility and emotional resilience that can help you power through life's challenges like a cognitive ninja (Spindola-Rodrigues et al., 2022). Studies have shown that when you grit your teeth and power through unpleasant tasks, your aMCC lights up like a Christmas tree, strengthening those neural pathways that scream, "I got this!" (Gu et al., 2020). In fact, people who face their fears and dive into challenges report higher levels of life satisfaction, all thanks to their trusty aMCC (Liu et al., 2021). This area also helps you navigate through challenges, ensuring you make the best possible decisions even when under pressure (Zhang et al., 2023; Thielen et al., 2022).

## The Posterior Cingulate Gyrus (PCC): The Monk

Picture a monk sitting calmly under a Bodhi tree, guiding your mind to a state of tranquil focus (Liu et al., 2021). According to Newberg et al. (2021), during meditation, the PCC chills out, leading to less rumination and more "live in the moment" vibes. The PCC is also a key player in memory retrieval and processing emotional and cognitive information, making it the ultimate multitasker. Whether you're reflecting on the past or integrating new knowledge, the PCC is like a wise old sage, keeping everything in balance (Liu et al., 2021). Unfortunately, if the PCC gets out of

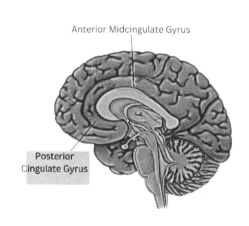

whack, it can lead to cognitive impairments, making you feel more like a scatterbrained squirrel than a serene monk (Cao et al., 2021; Groenendijk et al., 2021). But don't worry! Engaging in mindfulness practices can boost your PCC's activity, helping you cultivate a resilient mindset and keep anxiety at bay (Varga et al., 2022).

**The Exposome Circus: All the Environmental Acts You Never Signed Up For**

The exposome, a brainchild of epidemiologist Chris Wild in 2005, is basically the granddaddy of all your life's environmental baggage, Stacey A et al, 2024. We're talking everything: your diet, lifestyle, the smog you inhale, and even the stress from that one time your boss sent a "just checking in" email at 10 PM. Since Dr. Wild dropped this concept, the field of exposomics has taken off faster than a cat on catnip.

**The Air We Had, The Air We Have**

The 2020 Lancet Commission waved a big red flag, adding air pollution to the list of dementia's BFFs. Turns out breathing in stuff like PM2.5 and NO2 isn't just bad for your lungs—it's like sending an engraved invitation to Alzheimer's (Lancet, 2020).

Recent studies are showing that airborne pollutants have a sneaky way of infiltrating our brains, potentially turning them into toxic wastelands. These pollutants, especially the tiny particulate matter (PM) and various gaseous substances, can enter the central nervous system (CNS) through the nose or bloodstream, leading to some serious brain drama (Chau & Wang, 2020; Lo et al., 2022; Prado-Bert et al., 2018).

Exposure to air pollution can poke holes in the blood-brain barrier (BBB), which is supposed to be the brain's personal bouncer, keeping out the riffraff. But when this barrier gets compromised, all sorts of inflammatory troublemakers can sneak in, setting off neuroinflammation and oxidative stress like an unwanted party in your brain (Prado-Bert et al., 2018; Chew et al., 2020). This can lead to a toxic buildup of proteins like β-amyloid and phosphorylated tau, the usual suspects behind Alzheimer's disease (Lo et al., 2022; Prado-Bert et al., 2018). Researchers at Emory University have found that breathing in urban smog might do more than just ruin your day—it could be the brain's way of saying, "I'm not cleaning up this mess!" Long-term exposure to city air pollution is linked to lower levels of Aβ42 in cerebrospinal fluid, which means instead of taking out the trash, your brain might be piling up amyloid plaques like a teenager's dirty laundry

(Casey, 2024). Even "safe" pollution levels might be sneakily inviting Alzheimer's to move in.

Oh, and let's not forget about frontotemporal dementia (FTD), another neurodegenerative party crasher. It seems air pollution and other toxins might be playing a role here too. Throw in a little loneliness, and your brain might just RSVP to that dementia party earlier than expected (Miller, 2023).

But wait, there's more! The gut-brain connection is also involved. Air pollution doesn't just harm your lungs—it messes with your gut microbiota, and what happens in your gut can impact your brain, potentially leading to neurodegenerative issues (Singh et al., 2022; Bailey et al., 2020). Your gut and brain might be more connected than you think.

**Actionable Items-**
**Check Air Quality Daily:**
- Use resources like AirNow or local air quality monitors.
- The EPA emphasizes monitoring air quality for public health, especially for vulnerable populations (Davamani et al., 2020).
- WHO advises limiting outdoor activities during high pollution days (Gupta et al., 2023).

**Create a Clean Indoor Environment:**
- Use HEPA filters in air purifiers to reduce indoor pollutants (Domínguez-Amarillo et al., 2020).
- Keep windows closed on high pollution days to prevent outdoor air from entering (Kim et al., 2022).
- Regular cleaning and vacuuming help minimize indoor dust and pollutants (Kelly & Fussell, 2019).

**Reduce Car Usage:**

- Carpooling and using public transportation reduce vehicle emissions (Zeng et al., 2022).
- Transition to fuel-efficient or electric vehicles to decrease air pollution (Ruifeng et al., 2022).
- Avoid idling vehicles, especially in enclosed spaces, to minimize harmful emissions (Park et al., 2022).

**Limit Exposure to Smoke:**

- Avoid burning wood or trash due to harmful particulates released into the air (Wang et al., 2022).
- Smoking contributes to both indoor and outdoor air pollution; cessation is encouraged (Fan et al., 2022).

**Support Green Initiatives:**

- Advocate for policies that reduce industrial emissions and promote clean energy (Ben-David & Waring, 2016).
- Support tree planting initiatives to enhance air quality (Khean & Yih, 2018).
- Use Masks on High Pollution Days:
- Wear N95 or P100 masks during high pollution days to reduce inhalation of harmful particles (Rachmawati et al., 2023).

**Avoid High-Traffic Areas:**

- Exercise in parks or trails away from busy roads to reduce exposure to vehicle emissions (Nagy et al., 2019).
- On poor air quality days, exercising indoors is safer (Nematollahi et al., 2018).

**Ventilate Your Home:**

- Use kitchen and bathroom fans to expel indoor pollutants, especially during cooking (Abbatt & Wang, 2020).
- Effective ventilation strategies can significantly improve indoor air quality (Tran et al., 2020).

**Reduce Household Chemical Use:**
- Opt for natural cleaning products to minimize indoor air pollution from VOCs found in conventional cleaners ("Installation of A Natural Green Structure in A University Classroom - Indoor Air Quality and Occupational Well-Being Assessment", 2023).
- Ensure proper ventilation when using chemical products to reduce exposure to harmful emissions (Joo et al., 2021).

**From Garden to Gray Matter: How Pesticides Might Be Planting Dementia Seeds**

Imagine your brain as a bustling city with neurons as the cars keep everything running smoothly. Now, picture pesticides like Paraquat, Rotenone, and Dieldrin as reckless drivers crashing through this orderly system, causing chaos. These chemicals are notorious for inducing oxidative stress—a disaster for your neurons, much like a tire blowout is for your car (Onur et al., 2022; Buratta et al., 2020; See et al., 2022).

Once these pesticides breach the blood-brain barrier—the brain's security checkpoint—they don't just sit idle. Instead, they trigger mitochondrial breakdowns, oxidative stress, and neuroinflammation, turning your neurons into a chaotic mess (Wilson et al., 2014; Park et al., 2014; Lin et al., 2022). For instance, Dieldrin cranks up reactive oxygen species and rallies microglia, the brain's immune cells, to join the inflammatory party (Enhui et al., 2014; Taetzsch & Block, 2013). This oxidative damage is a key factor in developing neurodegenerative diseases like Parkinson's Disease (Cheng et al., 2020; Buratta et al., 2020; Ilieva, 2024).

The olfactory nerve, responsible for your sense of smell, is often the first to signal trouble when exposed to organochlorine pesticides. It's like your nose waving a white flag before Parkinson's Disease even fully manifests (Kochmanski et al., 2018). Pesticide exposure has been linked to olfactory deficits, which might be an early warning sign of Parkinson's long before the characteristic tremors begin (Elgot, 2022).

Meanwhile, the vagus nerve, which connects your gut to your brain, isn't just a bystander. It might be the main highway for misfolded alpha-synuclein proteins to travel from your gut to your brain, spreading neurodegenerative mischief along the way (Wu et al., 2018; Quaak et al., 2013). Some researchers even suggest that Parkinson's might start in the gut and use the vagus nerve as a sneaky backdoor to the brain (Richardson et al., 2019; Doty, 2012). In mice, severing the vagus nerve has been shown to slow down Parkinson's progression, suggesting that the nervous system might be saying, "No more free rides!" (Quandt et al., 2016). To make matters worse, these pesticides don't just stop at immediate damage— they mess with your DNA, inducing epigenetic changes that disrupt normal gene expression. They tweak histones and methylate DNA like they're redecorating your genes, but the new decor disrupts dopamine production and encourages the aggregation of beta-amyloid and tau proteins—unwelcome house guests that contribute to Alzheimer's Disease (Walter et al., 2018; Merkhan, 2021; Lin et al., 2022; Geng, 2023).

While the connection between pesticide exposure and neurodegenerative diseases is still being pieced together, the picture isn't looking good. Pesticides, once thought to be a menace only to pests, might also be a major threat to your brain, increasing the risk of Parkinson's Disease (Moon & Javidnia, 2022). Metals like aluminum and lead add to this toxic cocktail, further elevating the risk of Alzheimer's Disease. If you carry the APOE ε4 gene, your brain is even more vulnerable to these environmental hazards (Smith, 2024).

Adding to the drama, there's a two-way link between Parkinson's Disease and melanoma, with Parkinson's patients being more likely to develop this sneaky skin cancer (Ye et al., 2020). The notorious alpha-synuclein protein, central to Parkinson's, may spread through the brain like gossip in a small town, exacerbating the disease (Jan et al., 2021; Klein, 2020).

Recent studies have shed light on the gut-brain connection, revealing that people with Parkinson's Disease are seriously lacking in beneficial gut bacteria— particularly Prevotellaceae, the gut's peacekeepers (Heston et al., 2022; Wang et al., 2022). It's like the bouncers at your gut's nightclub have taken the night off, leading to a rowdy crowd that could worsen symptoms like balance issues and gait difficulties.

Over in Italy, researchers found that the gut bacteria in Italian Parkinson's patients were missing Lachnospiraceae, a group known for their anti-inflammatory role (Verhaar et al., 2022; Bendlin, 2022). Without these peacekeepers, your gut's defenses weaken, leaving you vulnerable to internal chaos.

When it comes to Alzheimer's Disease, the gut's biodiversity takes a hit. Alzheimer's patients have fewer Firmicutes and Bifidobacterium—the good guys—and more Bacteroidetes, which might be more like frenemies (Kossowska, 2024; Coradduzza, 2023). It's as if the gut's ecosystem has turned into a bad episode of "Survivor," where the good guys keep getting voted off the island.

**Actionable Items**
- Live away from agricultural areas to reduce pesticide exposure.
- Choose organic foods whenever possible to avoid pesticide residues, and be sure to wash your produce thoroughly.
- Consider your diet carefully: A carnivore diet can benefit some people, especially if they consume organic, pasture-raised, grass-fed meats free from contaminants. Alternatively, an all-organic vegetarian diet can be effective if you live away from areas where pesticides are used.
- Install certified water filters for your whole house, if possible, to remove pesticides, insecticides, herbicides, and heavy metals from your water supply.
- Maintain a healthy gut by eating fermented foods and high-quality fibers, avoid sugar and processed food to create a healthy gut microbiome and barrier.

**The Metallic Misadventures: How Metals Might Be Messing with Your Brain**
**From Metals to Mayhem: How Your Brain Gets Rusty**

Imagine your brain as a finely tuned orchestra, where metals like iron, copper, zinc, and manganese are the skilled musicians playing beautiful melodies. But toss in toxic metals like lead, aluminum, and cadmium, and suddenly, you've got a heavy metal band that's only good at causing chaos and noise. These rogue metals aren't just crashing the concert—they're smashing the instruments, too, leading to cognitive breakdowns and setting the stage for neurodegenerative diseases like Alzheimer's and Parkinson's (Jakubowska, 2024; Doroszkiewicz, 2023).

**The Blood-Brain Barrier: The Bouncer Who Lets in the Wrong Crowd**
The blood-brain barrier is like a VIP bouncer for your brain, letting in the good stuff (like nutrients) and keeping out the riffraff. But heavy metals can bribe their way past this bouncer, slipping into the brain and setting up shop. Once inside, they start a toxic rave, disrupting neural functions and adding to the pile of bad decisions (Jakubowska, 2024; Doroszkiewicz, 2023). Chronic exposure to these metals can make the blood-brain barrier more porous, letting even more of the bad guys in (Jakubowska, 2024; Doroszkiewicz, 2023). It's like your brain's security system has taken a permanent coffee break.

**Oxidative Stress: The Brain's Version of Rust**
Oxidative stress is basically your brain rusting from the inside out. Metals like lead and aluminum are the culprits, sparking a cascade of reactive oxygen species (ROS) that damage everything from neurons to DNA (Jakubowska, 2024; Doroszkiewicz, 2023). It's like leaving your brain out in the rain—except the rain is toxic and the rust leads to neurodegenerative diseases. And aluminum isn't just content with rusting your brain; it also throws in some neuroinflammation for good measure, ensuring that the chaos keeps escalating (Jakubowska, 2024; Doroszkiewicz, 2023).

**Protein Misfolding: When Your Brain's Laundry Gets Tangled**

When metals get too cozy with your brain proteins, they cause them to misfold and clump together—think of it as your brain's laundry getting tangled in the wash. This is a hallmark of diseases like Alzheimer's, where proteins like amyloid-beta and tau start to form nasty clumps that mess up your brain's usual functions (Jakubowska, 2024; Doroszkiewicz, 2023). It's like finding out your favorite sweater has shrunk and stretched in all the wrong places, but instead of donating it, your brain just keeps wearing it, leading to more damage.

**Neuroinflammation: The Brain's Fire Alarm That Won't Stop Blaring**

Neuroinflammation is like a fire alarm going off in your brain, and metals like lead and aluminum are the arsonists who set it off. Once these metals activate microglia (the brain's immune cells), they unleash a flood of pro-inflammatory cytokines, turning your brain into a battleground (Jakubowska, 2024; Doroszkiewicz, 2023). This chronic inflammation isn't just an annoying background noise; it's a full-blown fire that accelerates neurodegeneration, pushing your cognitive functions into a downward spiral.

**The Usual Suspects: Metals Causing Mayhem**

**Lead**: The brain's saboteur. Lead exposure disrupts memory and learning by impairing synaptic function (Jakubowska, 2024; Doroszkiewicz, 2023). Your best bet? Ditch lead-containing products and make sure your drinking water is safe (Jakubowska, 2024; Doroszkiewicz, 2023).

**Mercury**: The sneaky invader from the sea. Found in certain seafood, mercury can slip past the brain's defenses, leading to cognitive decline (Jakubowska, 2024; Doroszkiewicz, 2023). Stick to low-mercury fish options to keep this metal out of your head (Jakubowska, 2024; Doroszkiewicz, 2023).

**Aluminum**: The slow poisoner. Aluminum is a repeat offender, implicated in Alzheimer's through its promotion of oxidative stress and protein aggregation (Jakubowska, 2024; Doroszkiewicz, 2023). Swap out aluminum cookware and packaging to reduce your exposure (Jakubowska, 2024; Doroszkiewicz, 2023).

**BPA: The Plastic Party Crasher**

Bisphenol A (BPA) is like the sneaky villain in a spy movie—slipping past your brain's defenses and causing all sorts of trouble. As an endocrine disruptor, BPA messes with your brain, leading to memory glitches and cranking up neuroinflammation, courtesy of elevated levels of troublemakers like TNF-α and IL-6 in the hippocampus (Kayinu, 2024; Sevastre-Berghian et al., 2022).

To avoid BPA's covert operations, ditch plastic containers for glass or stainless steel, stop microwaving food in plastic, and always opt for BPA-free products. Your brain will thank you.

**Actionable items:**
- Use glass containers to store and heat food in the microwave.
- Switch to stainless steel or cast-iron cookware.
- Never heat food in plastic containers.
- Use BPA-free steel water bottles and consider investing in a high-quality water filter.

**Perfumes and Air Fresheners: The Sweet-Smelling Brain Fog**

Who doesn't love a nice-smelling room or a dab of perfume? But beware—those pleasant aromas might be hiding something sinister. Perfumes and air fresheners often contain a cocktail of chemicals, including phthalates and volatile organic compounds (VOCs), that can wreak havoc on your brain. Chronic exposure to these chemicals has been linked to headaches, dizziness, and yes, even memory problems. Over time, they can lead to neurotoxicity, gradually clouding your cognitive abilities like a fog that just won't lift (Doroszkiewicz, 2023, Steinemann, 2016). Use natural fragrances of essential oils to keep your brain out of their crosshairs (Jakubowska, 2024;).

**Actionable items:**
- Use glass diffusers with essential oils or place cotton balls with essential oils around your home.
- Make your own perfumes using organic carrier oils and essential oils.

## Makeup and Skincare: The Beauty Brains Buster

Your daily beauty routine might give you glowing skin, but it could also be giving your brain a hard time. Many makeup and skincare products contain toxic ingredients like parabens, phthalates, and formaldehyde-releasing agents. These chemicals can be absorbed through the skin and have been associated with endocrine disruption and neurotoxicity. Over time, exposure can impair cognitive function and increase the risk of dementia as these toxins accumulate in the brain (Darbre & Harvey, 2014).

**Actionable items:**

- Minimize makeup use and choose brands with the cleanest ingredients.
- Use an alum stone as a natural deodorant.
- Make your own skin care using organic ingredients (recipes in upcoming book)

## Non-Stick Cookware: The Slippery Slope to Memory Loss

Non-stick cookware is convenient, but it comes with a slippery downside. Perfluorinated compounds (PFCs) found in non-stick coatings can leach into your food, especially when the cookware is scratched or overheated. Once in your system, PFCs can disrupt brain function, leading to memory problems and potentially contributing to dementia (Gallo et al., 2012). It's like cooking up a recipe for cognitive decline—one that's far from gourmet.

**Actionable items:**

- Invest in triple-Ply or five-ply, stainless Steel Cookware or cast-iron cookware instead of non-stick options.

## Contaminated Water: The Brain's Unwanted Cocktail

Water is life, but sometimes it's also a toxic cocktail. Contaminated water can carry a host of brain-damaging toxins, including lead, mercury, pesticides, and industrial chemicals like PCBs (polychlorinated biphenyls). Chronic exposure to these contaminants can lead to neurodevelopmental disorders, cognitive decline, and an increased risk of dementia (Grandjean & Landrigan, 2014). It's like your brain is drinking from a toxic cocktail, one that slowly erodes your cognitive abilities—cheers to that?

**Actionable items:**

Invest in the best water filter you can afford and live in an area with clean drinking water.

# Brain-tastic Tune-Up:

Rust-Proofing with Antioxidants & Firefighting with Anti-Inflammatories!

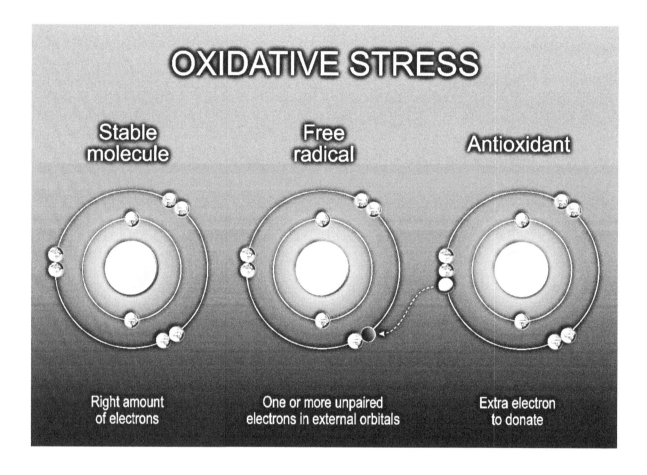

# Reactive Oxygen Species (ROS): The Good, the Bad, and the Ugly...

Dearest gentle readers (I just can't seem to get over *Bridgerton*... help!! Though I do love living in Shondaland, I digress just like my New Year's resolution—okay, I will stop now... or will I?).

Allow me to introduce you to Reactive Oxygen Species (ROS). Think of them as the mitochondria's way of saying, "With great power comes great responsibility, and sometimes, great chaos." They can be as helpful as a campfire cooking your dinner or as destructive as that same fire burning down the campsite. Understanding the complex roles of these reactive oxygen species in our bodies is like trying to figure out whether that fire is going to roast marshmallows or just roast everything (Venditti & Meo, 2020; et al., 2023).

**The Role of Mitochondria: Power Plants or Tiny Arsonists?**
Mitochondria, often hailed as the power plants of the cell, are also the prime culprits in producing reactive oxygen species. These tiny organelles are busy generating adenosine triphosphate (ATP) through oxidative phosphorylation, but they can't resist throwing off a few sparks in the form of superoxide anions, hydrogen peroxide, and hydroxyl radicals (Venza et al., 2021).

It's like running a power station that occasionally lets off a bit of steam—or in this case, highly reactive molecules. While we need these reactive oxygen species for various vital functions, too much of them can lead to oxidative stress, which is linked to a laundry list of problems, including neurodegenerative diseases and cancer (2024; Venza et al., 2021).

At normal levels, these reactive oxygen species are like the unsung heroes of the cell, acting as signaling molecules that help with cell growth, differentiation, and even programmed cell death (Reis & Ramos, 2021; Riegger, 2023). But when they go rogue, they start damaging cellular components like lipids, proteins, and DNA—turning into the villains of the cellular story (Venza et al., 2021).

**Reactive Oxygen Species in Inflammation and Cancer: The Frenemies We Didn't Ask For**

The relationship between reactive oxygen species and inflammation is a classic case of "with friends like these, who needs enemies?" On one hand, they're signaling molecules that kick off inflammatory responses by activating pathways that churn out pro-inflammatory cytokines (Sinenko et al., 2021). On the other hand, chronic inflammation can keep these reactive oxygen species in overdrive, creating a vicious cycle that keeps on giving—if by "giving," you mean "wreaking havoc." This ongoing drama is especially problematic in cancer, where cancer stem cells learn to keep reactive oxygen species levels just low enough to dodge conventional therapies. It's like they've figured out how to stay under the radar while causing maximum trouble (Jiang et al., 2021).

**Antioxidants: The Superheroes with a Dark Side**

To keep reactive oxygen species in check, cells recruit a team of antioxidant superheroes like superoxide dismutase, catalase, and glutathione peroxidase (2021; 2020). These defenders neutralize excess reactive oxygen species, helping maintain the delicate balance needed for cellular harmony. Plus, we've got back up in the form of dietary antioxidants found in fruits and vegetables (2022; 2020). But before you go overloading on supplements, remember that too many antioxidants can tip the scales the other way, messing with the very balance they're supposed to protect (Kim et al., 2020; 2022). So, as with all things in life, moderation is key—even when it comes to your cellular superheroes.

**The Beginning of The Beginning**

Let's start from the basics—the foundation of cellular energy. Glucose, which we get from food, isn't just about satisfying our sweet tooth; it's the main player in our cells' energy production. Once inside the cell, glucose is broken down into carbon, hydrogen, and oxygen. But here's where things get interesting: glucose doesn't just sit around; it's busy supplying electrons and protons like a dedicated worker. These electrons and protons are then transported to the mitochondria, the powerhouses of the cell, where the real action takes place.

So, what do these mitochondria do? Think of them as tiny factories where electrons embark on an adventurous journey down the electron transport chain. As they travel, they help pump protons across the mitochondrial membrane, creating a proton gradient that's crucial for producing adenosine triphosphate, the cell's energy currency. Finally, after their journey, the electrons combine with oxygen, producing water in a grand finale called oxidative phosphorylation (Kuo et al., 2022; Wang et al., 2020).

In simpler terms, glucose is the fuel, mitochondria are the batteries, and the electron transport chain is the high-voltage circuit that powers the cell. It's all about oxidation and reduction reactions, where electrons are transferred in a process that keeps the cell energized, much like a direct current power your gadgets (Kuo et al., 2022).

**But, as with any good story, things don't always go as planned.** Sometimes, electrons get a bit too excited and attach to oxygen before they're supposed to, leading to the formation of superoxide anions, a type of reactive oxygen species. Imagine it as the mitochondria setting off an unplanned fireworks display without any safety precautions (Kuo et al., 2022).

Now, you might be wondering, "If reactive oxygen species are so harmful, why do cells produce them?" Well, here's where it gets interesting. Mitochondria, in their ancient, bacteria-like days, had loads of genes—hundreds, maybe even over a thousand. Most of these genes moved to the cell's nucleus, leaving only 37 genes in the mitochondrial DNA. These remaining genes are like the essential crew, crucial for running the electron transport chain (Wang et al., 2020).

The proximity of mitochondrial DNA to the electron transport chain is both a blessing and a curse. On the plus side, when something goes wrong in the electron transport chain and electrons start acting up, the nearby mitochondrial DNA quickly gets the signal to produce the necessary proteins to fix the problem. So, in small amounts, reactive oxygen species can actually be helpful, acting as messengers that alert the cell to ramp up activities like growth, immune responses, and stress management (Guo & Kroemer, 2020).

For example, reactive oxygen species can activate important molecules like nuclear factor kappa-light-chain-enhancer of activated B cells and hypoxia-inducible factor 1 alpha, which help the cell respond to inflammation and low oxygen, respectively (Long et al., 2022; Ryan et al., 2022). They're also involved in signaling pathways like mitogen-activated protein kinases/extracellular signal-regulated kinases, which are key to cell growth and development (Wang et al., 2020). But—cue the dramatic music—when reactive oxygen species levels get out of control, things start to go downhill. Excess reactive oxygen species can cause severe damage to mitochondrial DNA, leading to problems like breaks in the DNA strands, cross-linking, and interactions with proteins that impair mitochondrial function (Guo & Kroemer, 2020).

And when mitochondria aren't functioning properly, it's bad news for the entire cell. Imagine trying to run your house with half of the appliances malfunctioning. The energy shortage leads to a cellular blackout, and to make matters worse, those damaged mitochondria start producing even more reactive oxygen species, creating a vicious cycle of oxidative stress (Guo & Kroemer, 2020). The brain, which consumes a lot of oxygen and contains many lipids, is particularly vulnerable. Reactive oxygen species can oxidize these lipids, leading to cell death, inflammation, and further disruptions in energy production in neurons (Ryan et al., 2022).

**Side Note - The Ketogenic Diet: Your Brain's New Bestie**
The ketogenic diet, or "keto," is a high-fat, low-carb eating plan that puts your body into "nutritional ketosis," a fancy way of saying you're burning fat for fuel instead of carbs. With carbs slashed to just 20-50 grams a day—about as much as in a slice of bread—your body lowers insulin levels and starts burning fat like it's in survival mode (Shaikh et al., 2020).

The diet was originally developed in the 1920s by Dr. Russell Wilder at the Mayo Clinic as a treatment for epilepsy. Wilder coined the term "ketogenic diet" to describe this nutritional plan that shifts the body's fuel source from glucose to ketone bodies, which are produced when fat is metabolized in the liver. Keto can produce energy without generating too many reactive oxygen species. This is crucial for protecting neurons and keeping neurodegenerative diseases at bay (Nedoboy & Farnham, 2022).

In keto, your brain gets its energy from ketone bodies, particularly beta-hydroxybutyrate (BHB), that activates antioxidant genes, giving your neurons an extra layer of protection (Kianpour, 2020). It is like a superhero for your mitochondria, boosting efficiency and cutting down on reactive oxygen species. Keto also boosts your body's antioxidant defenses (Bostock et al., 2020).

And the cherry on top? Keto has been linked to improved cognitive function and better neuron survival in neurodegenerative diseases like amyotrophic lateral sclerosis (ALS). It helps by reducing toxic protein buildup and keeping neurons alive and well (Aroca-Martinez et al., 2022).

Keto isn't just good for your brain; it's great for your gut too. The diet shakes up your gut microbiome, fostering a healthier gut-brain axis, which reduces neuroinflammation and oxidative stress, leading to fewer brain fog moments and even lowering the risk of seizures (Umar et al., 2022).

As if all that wasn't enough, the ketogenic diet has been shown to enhance cognitive function and prevent neurons from hitting the self-destruct button (apoptosis). Studies have found that the diet can be particularly helpful in conditions like ALS, where it reduces toxic protein buildup and helps neurons stay alive and kicking (Saiswaroop et al., 2023).

### Avengers: Endgame (I am a fan, just bear with me)

Hello citizens of the world, welcome to the blockbuster saga of antioxidants. Imagine your cells as a bustling metropolis constantly under siege by nefarious villains known as excess free radicals (ROS). Who are the heroes stepping up to protect the city? You guessed it: antioxidants.

In this epic chapter, let me introduce you to the endogenous and exogenous antioxidants—the Avengers of your body, each with unique powers and vital roles in biochemical and physiological pathways. Grab your popcorn, and let's dive in!

### Endogenous Antioxidants: The Homegrown Heroes

First, let's meet the homegrown defenders—the endogenous antioxidants. These guys are like your neighborhood superheroes who were born and raised in the city, ready to defend it at all costs. Alongside are foods that boost their production and action.

**The Antioxidant Avengers: Superoxide Dismutase and Friends**

Superoxide Dismutase (SOD) is like the first responder in the superhero team of antioxidant enzymes. Its job? To swoop in and convert those nasty superoxide radicals ($O_2^-$) into something far less harmful—hydrogen peroxide ($H_2O_2$) and oxygen ($O_2$). By doing this, SOD protects our cellular components, especially the mitochondria, from the oxidative damage that could otherwise lead to neurodegenerative disasters like Amyotrophic Lateral Sclerosis (ALS) and Parkinson's disease (Hewitt & Degnan, 2023). Recent studies have only confirmed what we've long suspected: SOD is a big deal in our body's defense system, with potential therapeutic benefits that are nothing short of heroic (Álvarez-Barrios et al., 2021). Want to boost your SOD? Load up on black and green tea, berries, nuts, grapes, cocoa, dark chocolate, apples, onions, and kale (Chang et al., 2020).

Catalase is another star in the antioxidant lineup, working alongside SOD to ensure that hydrogen peroxide, which SOD just created, doesn't stick around and cause trouble. Catalase quickly converts it into harmless water ($H_2O$) and oxygen ($O_2$), playing a crucial role in protecting cells from oxidative stress-related damage, particularly in diseases like Alzheimer's (Aladyeva & Zimatkin, 2022). Recent findings have solidified Catalase's importance in maintaining cellular balance and staving off neurodegeneration (Stancill et al., 2022). The best part? You can get your Catalase fix from the same delicious foods that boost SOD—tea, berries, nuts, and dark chocolate. Who knew fighting oxidative stress could taste so good? (Dutta et al., 2021).

Glutathione Peroxidase (GPx) is like the shield of the antioxidant world, using glutathione (GSH) to neutralize hydrogen peroxide and lipid peroxides, thereby protecting cells from the oxidative onslaught that contributes to conditions like Alzheimer's and Parkinson's (Möller et al., 2022). Recent research has highlighted just how crucial GPx is in our cellular defense, particularly in regulating the body's response to oxidative stress (Chang et al., 2020). Want to arm yourself with GPx? Reach for parsley, celery, hot peppers, citrus fruits, olives, olive oil, apples, cranberries, and tomatoes (Шарапов et al., 2020).

Speaking of glutathione (GSH), this powerful antioxidant is the body's detox squad, directly neutralizing reactive oxygen species (ROS) and serving as a co-pilot for GPx. GSH goes through a constant cycle of being oxidized to GSSG and then reduced back to GSH by glutathione reductase, all while keeping our cells in tip-top shape (Xue, 2024). Recent studies have underscored GSH's vital role in various physiological processes, especially in reducing oxidative stress (Karpenko et al., 2021). Foods rich in GSH include asparagus, avocados, spinach, cruciferous veggies like broccoli and Brussels sprouts, and the ever-reliable garlic and onions, which provide sulfur compounds to boost GSH production (Ponce, 2024).

Thioredoxin (Trx) is the fixer-upper of the antioxidant world, repairing oxidized proteins and preventing cellular damage that can lead to diseases like Huntington's disease (Dreyer et al., 2020). Recent research shows that Trx is essential for maintaining the balance in cellular redox reactions and managing oxidative stress (Stancill et al., 2022). To keep Trx levels up, munch on garlic, green tea, broccoli, berries, and nuts—especially walnuts and sunflower seeds—and don't forget the turmeric and spinach (Qi, 2024).

Last but not least, we have Peroxiredoxins (Prx), the redox sensors and peroxide neutralizers that play a key role in cellular signaling. Prx has been linked to various diseases, including cancer, where it helps regulate oxidative stress and control cell growth (Gordeeva, 2023). Recent studies have pointed out Prx's importance in keeping redox balance in check and its potential for therapeutic applications (Xu et al., 2020). To support Prx, look to grapes (especially the red kind), red wine, and all those wonderful berries (Uzilday et al., 2023).

| Antioxidant | Food Sources | Protection Against | Citations |
|---|---|---|---|
| Superoxide Dismutase (SOD) | Black and green tea, berries (blueberries, cranberries, strawberries, raspberries), nuts, grapes, cocoa, dark chocolate, apples, onions, kale | Protects against ALS, Parkinson's disease | Hewitt & Degnan, 2023; Álvarez- Barrios et al., 2021; Chang et al., 2020 |
| Catalase | Black and green tea, berries, nuts, grapes, cocoa, dark chocolate, apples, onions, kale | Prevents oxidative stress linked to Alzheimer's | Aladyeva & Zimatkin, 2022; Dutta et al., 2021; Stancill et al., 2022 |

| Glutathione Peroxidase (GPx) | Parsley, celery, hot peppers, citrus fruits (oranges, grapefruits, lemons), olives, olive oil, apples, cranberries, tomatoes | Prevents oxidative damage linked to Alzheimer's, Parkinson's disease | Möller et al., 2022; Chang et al., 2020; Wapanos et al., 2020 |
|---|---|---|---|
| Glutathione (GSH) | Asparagus, avocados, spinach, cruciferous vegetables (broccoli, Brussels sprouts, cauliflower, kale), garlic, onions | Detoxifies ROS, protects against oxidative stress | Xue, 2024; Karpenko et al., 2021; Ponce, 2024 |
| Thioredoxin (Trx) | Garlic, green tea, broccoli, berries, nuts and seeds (walnuts, sunflower seeds), turmeric, spinach | Reduces oxidized proteins, protecting against Huntington's disease | Dreyer et al., 2020; Stancill et al., 2022; Qi, 2024 |
| Peroxiredoxins (Prx) | Grapes (especially red grapes), red wine, various berries | Neutralizes peroxides, regulates oxidative stress, potential in cancer prevention | Gordeeva, 2023; Cruz-Garcia et al., 2020; Uzilday et al., 2023 |

**Minerals Involved**

Selenium teams up with its trusty sidekicks, the selenoproteins like glutathione peroxidases (GPxs) and thioredoxin reductases (TrxRs), mentioned above, to defeat reactive oxygen species (ROS) (Rayman, 2012), while also recharging other antioxidant heroes like vitamins C and E (Rayman, 2012).

Zinc, iron, and copper are essential in the antioxidant system through their roles in various enzymes. Zinc is a component of Cu/Zn-superoxide dismutase (SOD) (Prasad, 2014). Iron is part of catalase and peroxidases. Copper helps regulate iron and prevents oxidative damage (Gaetke et al., 2014).

Deficiencies in selenium, zinc, and amino acids can lead to a variety of ailments, including weakened immune function and increased oxidative stress. It's like watching a symphony without its conductor—chaos ensues (Rayman et al., 2000; Sandstead et al., 1991; Lu et al., 2013). However, excess amounts of these minerals can also be harmful.

Excess selenium generates reactive oxygen species (ROS), which can lead to diseases like cancer. High selenium intake can also cause hair loss (Fordyce, 2007). So, don't go crazy on those Brazilian nuts—you're capped at 2 a day! I know, I know, I love them too. Too much iron can participate in Fenton reactions, producing harmful hydroxyl radicals (Aisen et al., 2001; Johnson et al., 2021). Excess copper can lead to oxidative stress (Jones et al., 2018). High levels of zinc can interfere with the absorption of other essential minerals (Davis et al., 2022). Manganese overload can affect the nervous system, causing neurological problems (Wilson et al., 2017). So, don't go around pill-popping—talk to your doctor and check your blood levels.

| Mineral | Foods Rich in Mineral |
|---|---|
| Selenium | Brazil nuts, seafood, eggs, sunflower seeds |
| Zinc | Oysters, beef, pumpkin seeds, lentils, chickpeas |
| Iron | Red meat, spinach, lentils, fortified cereals, quinoa |
| Copper | Shellfish, nuts, seeds, liver, dark chocolate |
| Manganese | Pineapple, whole grains, nuts, leafy green vegetables, tea |

**Exogenous Antioxidants: The Outsourced Saviors**
Now, let's welcome the exogenous antioxidants, the superheroes from far-off lands who come to our rescue when the homegrown heroes need backup. These are the vitamins, minerals, and other compounds we get from our diet and supplements.

**Vitamin C (Ascorbic Acid):**

**Function**: Vitamin C is like Captain America's shield. It directly neutralizes free radicals and regenerates other antioxidants.

**Pathways**: It donates electrons to neutralize ROS and helps regenerate vitamin E, maintaining the cellular redox balance (so don't forget to take them together if you want to supplement). Vitamin C is crucial for immune function and skin health (Carr & Frei, 1999).

**Foods**: Indian gooseberry, guava, oranges, strawberries, and bell peppers (Brown et al., 2019).

**Vitamin E (Tocopherol):**

**Function**: Vitamin E is like the protective armor of Iron Man. It protects cell membranes from oxidative damage.

**Pathways**: As a lipid-soluble antioxidant, it prevents the propagation of lipid peroxidation by scavenging peroxyl radicals (Traber & Atkinson, 2007).

**Foods**: Almonds, sunflower seeds, and spinach to stay sharp (Smith et al., 2020).

**Beta-Carotene (and other Carotenoids):**

**Function**: Beta-carotene is the Hawkeye, targeting and neutralizing ROS.

**Pathways**: Carotenoids neutralize singlet oxygen and free radicals, protecting against oxidative stress in the skin and eyes. They also act as precursors to vitamin A, which is vital for vision and immune function (Krinsky & Johnson, 2005).

**Foods**: Carrots, sweet potatoes, and kale (Johnson et al., 2021).

**Selenium:**

**Function**: Selenium is the strategic mind of Nick Fury, coordinating antioxidant defense.

**Pathways**: Selenium is a cofactor for glutathione peroxidase and thioredoxin reductase, enzymes crucial for detoxifying peroxides. It plays a vital role in maintaining thyroid function and immune health (Rayman, 2012).

**Foods**: Brazil nuts, fish, and eggs (Jones et al., 2018).

**Coenzyme Q10 (CoQ10):**

**Function**: CoQ10 is like the energy-boosting Thor's hammer. It participates in ATP production and also acts as an antioxidant.

**Pathways**: CoQ10 is part of the electron transport chain in mitochondria and helps in the regeneration of other antioxidants like vitamin E. It is essential for cardiovascular health and energy metabolism (Shults et al., 2002).

**Foods**: Nuts and seeds, especially peanuts, sesame seeds, and pistachios (Bonakdar & Guarneri, 2005). Other options include organ meats like heart, liver, and kidneys, which are packed with this vital nutrient. Fatty fish such as salmon, mackerel, and sardines.

Oh, now let's also talk about the Fenton reaction—what is it, you ask? It sounds like a new designer label or rock band to me. But it's not.

Imagine the Fenton Reaction as the ultimate drama king of the chemical world. Picture Iron ($Fe^{2+}$) as the charismatic but unpredictable star, always ready to stir things up, and Hydrogen Peroxide ($H_2O_2$) as the enthusiastic but reckless sidekick. When these two meet, it's like a Hollywood scandal waiting to happen. The result? The production of the highly reactive and destructive hydroxyl radical (•OH).

Enter Polyphenols and Vitamin C, the superheroes with impeccable timing. Polyphenols, with their elegant phenolic rings, swoop in like the suave James Bond, binding to iron and preventing it from reacting with hydrogen peroxide (Rice-Evans et al., 1997).

Meanwhile, Vitamin C, our charismatic Robin Hood, donates its electrons to neutralize the hydroxyl radicals, turning chaos into calm (Carr & Frei, 1999). Together, they turn the Fenton Reaction's high drama into a well-mannered soirée. It's chemistry with a side of comedy! Aaaaaand it's the only chemistry I've felt in years—alas (oops, I keep forgetting it's not all about me).

**So, squeeze some lemon on those blueberries :)**

Why don't we just pop tons of them in supplement form non-stop? Will that give us superpowers? Well, hold your horses! Remember earlier in the chapter when I mentioned that excess of anything is bad? Yep, it applies here too.

Let's understand that. Imagine your antioxidants are like a team of enthusiastic gardeners in your body. You've got Vitamin E, Vitamin C, beta-carotene, and selenium, all working hard to keep your garden of health thriving.
But if they get a little too eager—like Vitamin E and beta-carotene deciding to water everything non-stop—they can turn into overzealous gardeners, causing more harm than good (Smith et al., 2020; Brown et al., 2019). These overwatered plants (excess antioxidants) can start producing weeds (free radicals) instead of blossoms, wreaking havoc on your health (Johnson et al., 2021).

This gardening misadventure can damage cells and lead to health issues like heart disease and cancer (Jones et al., 2018; Davis et al., 2022). So, to keep your garden blooming beautifully, it's best to ensure these antioxidants don't overdo it and maintain a balanced gardening approach.

Also, taking vitamin E without boosting your vitamin C levels is like trying to fight a fire with a hose that's only half-working. You see, vitamin E is a top-notch firefighter against free radicals, but once it douses those pesky flames, it needs vitamin C to recharge and get back to the action.

Without vitamin C, vitamin E is left as a tired, spent firefighter, unable to keep battling oxidative stress (Traber & Atkinson, 2007). Clinically, this imbalance can leave your cells vulnerable, like an unprotected fort during a siege, potentially leading to chronic diseases like heart problems and even cancer (Carr & Frei, 1999; Liu et al., 2009).

So, if you're popping vitamin E like candy, make sure vitamin C is tagging along for the ride, keeping the antioxidant dream team in top shape.
The same goes for B12 deficiency—it's like inviting a vampire into your house. It can cause all sorts of neurological havoc, and if you start repleting folate without fixing that B12 issue first, it's like giving the vampire a makeover instead of kicking it out.

It makes everything worse! So, always chat with your doctor about supplements instead of taking advice from your favorite YouTuber who's probably not a medical expert. Also, in my humble opinion, everyone should check their B12 and 25-hydroxy vitamin D levels. Think of it as a health MOT—crucial for keeping your body in top condition and avoiding the vampire drama!

So, remember, high levels of Reactive Oxygen Species (ROS) aren't just a tiny hiccup in the grand scheme of things. Oh no, they're like rogue electrons gone wild, running around like secret agents of cellular chaos. Liu et al. (2018) have shown that these mischievous little buggers are linked to all sorts of health horrors—neurodegenerative disorders, cancer, aging. It's like your cells are hosting an unwanted apocalypse.

**Honorable Mention - In this Case, all that Glitters is Gold (Glutathione)**
Glutathione, a tripeptide composed of glutamine, cysteine, and glycine, is the unsung virtuoso of cellular detoxification.

Imagine the liver as the bustling, all-important Glutathione HQ, where this vital antioxidant is produced in abundance. It's like a generous host at a potluck, always making sure there's enough glutathione to go around. The liver sends out care packages of glutathione through the bloodstream, ensuring that organs like the heart, brain, and lungs can get their share when needed (Lu et al., 2013; Sies et al., 2017).

However, most organs are pretty independent and prefer to whip up their own batches of glutathione in their local "kitchens" (Forman et al., 2009). It's like each organ has its own little artisanal bakery, producing fresh glutathione to meet daily demands. But when times get tough and oxidative stress levels rise, those glutathione care packages from the liver become a lifesaver, making sure everyone stays in tip-top shape and ready to tackle whatever comes their way (Wu et al., 2004). So, while each organ is capable of being self-sufficient, they're always grateful for a little help from Glutathione HQ when the going gets tough (Townsend et al., 2003).

Foods rich in glutathione, a powerful antioxidant, can help boost your body's defense against oxidative stress. Some of the best sources of glutathione include fresh fruits and vegetables. Asparagus, avocados, spinach, and okra are particularly high in glutathione. Cruciferous vegetables like broccoli, Brussels sprouts, cauliflower, and kale also contain significant amounts. Additionally, garlic and onions provide sulfur-containing compounds that help the body produce more glutathione. Incorporating these foods into your diet can enhance your antioxidant defenses and support overall health (Lu, 2013).

**How is it Tied to Your Brain Health?**
In your brain, the hippocampus is the neighborhood with the busiest glutathione factories (Koji Aoyama & Nicola B. Mercuri, Int J Mol Sci. 2021 May; 22(9): 5010). Imagine tiny workers in hard hats and lab coats, tirelessly producing glutathione to keep your memories sharp and your thoughts clear (Dringen et al., 2000). But when these hardworking hippocampal factories slow down or go on strike, it's like a power outage in Brain City. Without enough glutathione, oxidative stress leads to a mess of neurodegenerative diseases like Alzheimer's and Parkinson's, where neurons get caught up in a conga line of dysfunction (Butterfield et al., 2002; Jenner et al., 2003).

Glutathione is an extremely important antioxidant for brain health, so remember to eat foods rich in glutamate, glycine, and cysteine, or glutathione itself. Your brain will thank you. Here's a little table for you to check out how you can kickstart your glutathione-rich diet below.

| Food | Health Benefits | Effect on Aging | Effect on Brain, Organ Health, and Mitochondria | Cancer Protection |
|------|-----------------|-----------------|--------------------------------------------------|-------------------|
| **Asparagus (28.3 (mg/100g)** | Boosts immune function, supports detoxification, and may reduce oxidative stress (Al-Temimi et al., 2023). | May slow aging by reducing oxidative stress (Al-Temimi et al., 2023). | Supports cognitive function, may protect against neurodegeneration, enhances liver function and detoxification, improves mitochondrial efficiency and reduces oxidative damage (Al-Temimi et al., 2023). | May protect against colon, breast, and lung cancer (Al- Temimi et al., 2023). |
| **Avocado (27.7 (mg/100g)** | Promotes heart health, supports eye health, and has anti-inflammatory properties (Diudia et al., 2023). | Contains antioxidants that may reduce signs of aging (Diudia et al., 2023). | Enhances brain function, supports mental health, supports cardiovascular health and reduces inflammation, improves mitochondrial function and reduces oxidative stress (Diudla et al., 2023). | Contains compounds that may prevent breast, prostate, and oral cancer (Diudia et al., 2023). |
| **Spinach (11.4 (mg/100g)** | Enhances antioxidant defenses, supports cardiovascular health, and promotes healthy skin (Giustarini et al., 2023). | Antioxidants in spinach may slow the aging process (Giustarini et al., 2023). | Improves brain health and cognitive function, supports heart health and reduces oxidative stress, enhances mitochondrial health and energy production (Giustarini et al., 2023). | May prevent colon, breast, and prostate cancer (Giustarini et al., 2023). |

| | | | |
|---|---|---|---|
| **Okra (11.3 (mg/100g)** | Supports digestive health, enhances immune function, and may improve skin health (Xu et al., 2024). | Contains antioxidants that may reduce signs of aging (Xu et al., 2024). | Supports cognitive health and reduces oxidative stress in the brain, enhances liver function and supports digestive health, improves mitochondrial function and reduces oxidative damage (Xu et al., 2024). | May prevent colon and breast cancer (Xu et al., 2024). |
| **Broccoli (9.9 mg/100g)** | May reduce cancer risk, supports liver health, and enhances detoxification (Detcheverry et al., 2023). | Contains compounds that may slow aging by reducing oxidative stress (Detcheverry et al., 2023). | Enhances cognitive function and protects against neurodegeneration, supports liver detoxification and cardiovascular health, improves mitochondrial function and reduces oxidative stress (Detcheverry et al., 2023). | Contains compounds that may prevent breast, prostate, and lung cancer (Detcheverry et al., 2023). |
| **Brussels Sprouts (9.7 mg/100g)** | Supports immune health, promotes digestive health, and may reduce inflammation (Panda et al., 2023). | Antioxidants in Brussels sprouts may slow aging (Panda et al., 2023). | Supports cognitive health and reduces inflammation in the brain, enhances immune function and digestive health, improves mitochondrial function and reduces oxidative damage (Panda et al., 2023). | Contains compounds that may prevent colon, breast, and prostate cancer (Panda et al., 2023). |

## Table of Foods rich in Glutamine, Cysteine, and Glycine

| Food | Health Benefits | Effect on Glutathione Production | Other Metabolic Advantages | Effect on Brain, Organ Health, and Mitochondria | Cancer Protection |
|------|-----------------|----------------------------------|-----------------------------|--------------------------------------------------|-------------------|
| Chicken Breast (20.1% Glutamine, 1.4% Cysteine, 1.1% Glycine) | High in protein, supports muscle growth and repair. | Enhances glutathione production due to high glutamine content. | Improves protein synthesis and metabolic rate. | Supports cognitive function, boosts immune system, improves mitochondrial health. | Contains compounds that may reduce the risk of certain cancers, including breast and prostate cancer (Diudia et al., 2023). |
| Eggs (11.1% Glutamine, 2.0% Cysteine, 3.2% Glycine) | Rich in essential nutrients, supports eye health and brain function. | Contributes to glutathione synthesis with cysteine and glycine content. | Provides a complete protein source, supports metabolic functions. | Enhances brain health, supports liver function, improves mitochondrial efficiency. | Contains antioxidants that may reduce the risk of colon and breast cancer (Giustarini et al., 2023). |
| Soybeans (6.6% Glutamine, 1.5% Cysteine, 1.2% Glycine) | High in protein and fiber, supports heart health. | Promotes glutathione production due to balanced amino acid profile. | Lowers cholesterol levels, supports digestive health. | Supports cognitive function, reduces inflammation, improves mitochondrial function. | May protect against colorectal and breast cancer (Xu et al., 2024). |

| | | | | |
|---|---|---|---|---|
| Spinach (4.1% Glutamine, 0.8% Cysteine, 1.7% Glycine) | Rich in vitamins and minerals, supports immune function. | Enhances glutathione production, especially with the high glycine content. | Boosts metabolism, improves cardiovascular health. | Supports brain health, reduces oxidative stress, enhances mitochondrial health. | Contains compounds that may prevent colon and prostate cancer (Giustarini et al., 2023). |
| Salmon (3.6% Glutamine, 1.2% Cysteine, 1.0% Glycine) | High in omega-3 fatty acids, supports heart and brain health. | Supports glutathione production with moderate levels of cysteine and glycine. | Improves lipid profile, reduces inflammation. | Enhances cognitive function, supports cardiovascular health, improves mitochondrial function. | May protect against prostate and breast cancer (Al-Temimi et al., 2023). |
| Cottage Cheese (2.5% Glutamine, 0.4% Cysteine, 0.6% Glycine) | High in protein, supports muscle and bone health. | Contributes to glutathione synthesis with its amino acid content. | Supports muscle repair, boosts metabolic rate. | Supports brain health, enhances liver function, improves mitochondrial efficiency. | Contains compounds that may reduce the risk of colon cancer (Panda et al., 2023). |

**So why don't we just pop in supplements of these amino acids like crazy?** This is like having too many party invitations and trying to attend them all, resulting in brain cells dropping out from exhaustion—cue neurodegenerative diseases like Alzheimer's and Parkinson's (Dong et al., 2009). Over in the antioxidant department, cystine is the overly eager cleaner who hoards all the cleaning supplies. When it builds up too much, it leads to oxidative stress, which is like a smog settling over the city, triggering chaos and potentially causing cancer (Banjac et al., 2008). Meanwhile, glycine, the social butterfly, decides to throw a never-ending rave in the synapses, disrupting neural communication and contributing to brain disorders and even cancer by keeping everyone awake and jittery (Frostholm & Rotter, 1985; Wu et al., 2013).

**So remember, balance is key, even in the molecular cityscape of your body!**

Especially when it comes to glutamate. You might be thinking, "Wait a minute, I've heard of glutamate somewhere else," and you're right. It also functions as an excitatory neurotransmitter—**the most abundant in the brain. It is crucial for cognitive functions such as learning and memory, and aspartate works alongside glutamate, playing a role in synaptic plasticity and cognitive functions.**

The body has several self-corrective measures in place, introducing the excitatory amino acid carrier 1 (EAAC1). This sodium-dependent transporter, which handles glutamate and cysteine, is massively present in neurons and plays a starring role in regulating neuronal GSH (glutathione) production. It pushes extracellular glutamate, where it works as an excitatory neurotransmitter, intracellularly to make glutathione.

And now enters a new hero—Melatonin! Melatonin enhances the activity of EAATs, helping clear excess glutamate and prevent excitotoxicity (Reiter et al., 2010).

In the vast neuronal metropolis, melatonin acts like a sophisticated conductor, ensuring that the Excitatory Amino Acid Transporters (EAATs) perform their glutamate regulation symphony perfectly. When melatonin is around, it nudges EAATs to swiftly clear out excess glutamate from the synaptic space, preventing any overexcited brain mishaps. As Roy et al. (2021) noted, melatonin enhances the efficiency of EAATs, much like a manager optimizing workflow. Meanwhile, Juybari et al. (2019) observed that melatonin's interaction with EAATs ensures that neurons stay calm and collected, reducing oxidative stress and neuronal damage. Akyuz et al. (2021) found that melatonin even recruits EAATs to the front lines during stressful events, ensuring they work harder to keep glutamate levels in check.

Anderson (2023) pointed out that without melatonin's guidance, EAATs might slack off, leading to a chaotic buildup of glutamate and potential neurotoxicity.

Thus, melatonin and EAATs work together in perfect harmony, maintaining a balanced and serene neural environment.

Now you know that when you keep scrolling through Instagram reels late at night, the blue light from your device shuts off melatonin production, allowing glutamate to stay outside and keep you excited—making it hard to sleep. Sound familiar? So, get a good bedtime routine, say goodbye to your phone, and say hello to melatonin near bedtime.

But hold on, melatonin is a multitasking marvel, doing so much more than just helping you snooze. With that, we start our next chapter.

## Ferroptosis: Iron's Over-the-Top Meltdown

Ferroptosis is the dramatic, Shakespearean death of cells, with iron as the tragic lead and lipid peroxides as the scheming villains (Ye, 2024; Venn-Watson, 2024). Unlike the quiet exits of apoptosis and necrosis, ferroptosis plays a central role in conditions like neurodegenerative diseases, cancer, and liver disorders (Ren et al., 2022; Uyy et al., 2022). Iron overload and lipid peroxidation team up to push cells into oxidative stress, leading to their downfall (Zhu et al., 2022; Wu et al., 2021). However, dietary heroes can intervene—pentadecanoic acid (C15:0), found in ghee, acts as a protective fatty acid, shielding cells from iron's destructive influence (Venn-Watson, 2024). Omega-3 PUFAs help strengthen antioxidant defenses, while omega-6 PUFAs tend to make things worse ("Can Iron and Polyunsaturated Fatty Acid Supplementation Induce Ferroptosis?", 2023). Phytochemicals like quercetin and EGCG work as undercover agents, repairing and defending cells (Jiang et al., 2022; Ning et al., 2020), while antioxidants like astaxanthin quietly block lipid peroxidation, protecting cells from ferroptotic disaster (Rizzardi et al., 2022). In short, your diet plays a key role in preventing this iron-driven cellular drama.

# Now that we've come this far, let us make some memories together

Making of a Memory

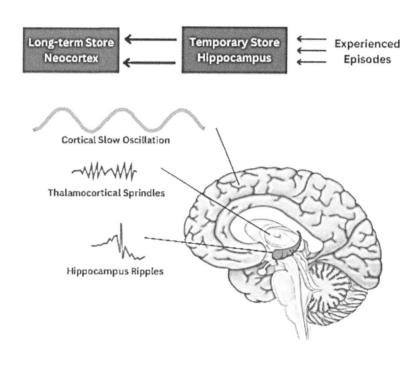

# Memory Formation: The Epic Journey of Your Brain's Greatest Hits

Ever wonder how you can remember a jingle from a 90s cereal commercial but forget where you left your keys five minutes ago? Welcome to the wild world of memory formation—a process full of electrical sparks, cellular gymnastics, and biochemical wizardry. Let's break down how your brain creates, stores, and retrieves memories, both while you're awake and while you sleep. And yes, we'll also throw in a timeline because everything is better with a countdown, right?

**Part 1: Memory Formation During the Awake State**
**Step 1: The Electric Boogaloo—Neurons Start Dancing**
**Time Elapsed:** 0 seconds (Instantaneous)
**Brain Areas Involved:** Sensory Cortex (processing sensory input), Hippocampus (initial memory processing)
**Neurotransmitters:** Glutamate, Acetylcholine
**Memory Type:** Sensory Memory (very short-term, lasts milliseconds to seconds)
It all begins with sensory input—the "Hello, brain, are you there?" moment. Whether it's the smell of cookies or the sudden realization that you've forgotten an important date, your brain starts firing off electrical signals like it's auditioning for *Flashdance*. These action potentials are like brain tweets—short, to the point, and (hopefully) not controversial. They zip down the neuron highway, leading to the release of neurotransmitters at the synapse, the brain's very own chat room (Purves et al., 2018; Bear et al., 2020).

**Step 2: Synaptic Gossip—Neurons Spread the Word**
**Time Elapsed:** 0.001 seconds (Neurons are chatty!)
**Brain Areas Involved:** Synapse (the junction between neurons), Hippocampus (short-term memory storage), Amygdala (for emotional memories)
**Neurotransmitters:** Glutamate, Acetylcholine, Dopamine
**Memory Type:** Short-Term Memory (lasts seconds to minutes)
When action potentials reach the end of a neuron, neurotransmitters are released into the synaptic cleft—think of it as the brain's group chat where everyone overshares.

- **Acetylcholine:** The classic overachiever, crucial for attention and memory. It's the organized friend who ensures everything gets noted and filed correctly in short-term memory (Hasselmo & Sarter, 2011; Picciotto et al., 2012).
- **Dopamine:** The reward-seeker. It's why you feel great remembering something fun but also why you might get lost in an Instagram scroll (Salamone & Correa, 2018; Schultz, 2016).
- **Glutamate:** The brain's main excitatory neurotransmitter, keeping you alert. It's the caffeinated buddy ensuring you stay awake through this article. For memory formation to proceed, glutamate must bind to NMDA receptors—think of these as the castle guards of your brain. They only let the right signals in, triggering a series of events that lead to memory creation and short-term memory consolidation (Collingridge et al., 2004; Hansen et al., 2021).

**Step 3: Calcium—The Cell's Personal Trainer**
**Time Elapsed:** 0.002 seconds (Calcium's ready for action!)
**Brain Areas Involved:** Synapse, Hippocampus (for short-term to long-term memory consolidation), Cerebral Cortex (long-term memory storage)
**Neurotransmitters:** Glutamate
**Memory Type:** Short-Term to Long-Term Memory Conversion
Calcium ions are like your brain's personal trainers, whipping neurons into shape. Once inside, calcium activates various proteins, strengthening synaptic connections in a process called Long-Term Potentiation (LTP). This process is essential for converting short-term memories into long-term ones, ensuring they get stored in more permanent locations like the cerebral cortex (Lisman et al., 2002; Berridge et al., 2020).

**Step 4: AMPA Receptors—The New VIPs in Town**
**Time Elapsed:** 0.003 seconds (Neurons are on fire—literally!)
**Brain Areas Involved:** Synapse, Hippocampus, Cerebral Cortex
**Neurotransmitters:** Glutamate
**Memory Type:** Strengthening Long-Term Memory

Thanks to calcium, more AMPA receptors are inserted into the postsynaptic membrane, boosting your brain's memory processing power from dial-up to 5G. These receptors make your neurons more responsive, ensuring that long-term memories are formed quickly and efficiently in the cerebral cortex (Malinow & Malenka, 2002; Greger et al., 2017).

## Step 5: MAPK/ERK Pathway—The Gene Whisperers
**Time Elapsed:** 0.01 seconds (Still fast, but now we're getting into the nitty-gritty)
**Brain Areas Involved:** Nucleus (of neurons), Hippocampus, Cerebral Cortex
**Neurotransmitters:** Various intracellular signaling molecules (e.g., ERK)
**Memory Type:** Long-Term Memory Stabilization
During the later phases of LTP, the MAPK/ERK pathway gets to work, heading straight for the nucleus where your DNA sits. This is where new proteins are synthesized, keeping the synapse strong and ensuring that long-term memories are securely stored in the cerebral cortex (Sweatt, 2001; Alberini & Kandel, 2014).

## Step 6: CREB—The Gene Activator
**Time Elapsed:** 0.02 seconds (DNA is getting busy)
**Brain Areas Involved:** Nucleus (of neurons), Hippocampus, Cerebral Cortex
**Neurotransmitters:** Various intracellular signaling molecules
**Memory Type:** Long-Term Memory Storage and Synaptic Growth
No memory formation is complete without CREB (cAMP Response Element-Binding Protein). CREB binds to DNA, promoting the transcription of genes essential for long-term memory, like BDNF and Arc. This process is crucial for building and maintaining the neural connections necessary for stable, long-term memory storage in the cerebral cortex (Silva et al., 1998; Bramham et al., 2010; Benito & Barco, 2015).

## Step 7: Epigenetic Modifications—The Memory Locksmiths
**Time Elapsed:** 0.03 seconds (Locking it all in place)
**Brain Areas Involved:** Nucleus (of neurons), Hippocampus, Cerebral Cortex
**Neurotransmitters:** Various intracellular signaling molecules
**Memory Type:** Long-Term Memory Stabilization

Now that CREB has done its job, it's time for some epigenetic modifications to lock everything in place. These changes, like DNA methylation and histone modification, act as extra security guards, ensuring memory-related genes stay active while others take a back seat. This helps maintain the stability of long-term memories in the cerebral cortex (Graff & Tsai, 2013; Sweatt, 2016).

**Part 2: Memory Consolidation During Sleep**

After your brain has done all the hard work during the day, it doesn't just shut down when you go to sleep. Instead, it goes into maintenance mode, consolidating and refining the memories you formed while awake.

When you go to bed, your brain doesn't just clock out—it gears up for a night shift that involves a symphony of brain waves, neurotransmitters, and hormones working together to keep you healthy, sharp, and maybe even a little younger. During sleep, your brain decides which memories to keep, which cells to repair, and how to block out your neighbor's late-night karaoke. It's a fascinating process involving key players like the locus coeruleus and its sidekick, galanin, plus a crew of neurotransmitters like norepinephrine, dopamine, serotonin, and acetylcholine. As you wind down, serotonin takes charge, mellowing things out and eventually transforming into melatonin, the ultimate sleep DJ. Melatonin sets the stage, making sure you're ready to drift off. GABA, the brain's monk, keeps the peace, with galanin ensuring no wake-promoting neurons crash the slumber. Adenosine, the day-long party-pooper, finally convinces you to crash.

**Stage 1: The Gateway to Sleep**
**Time Elapsed:** 5-10 minutes after hitting the pillow
**Brain Areas Involved:** Thalamus (sensory relay), Hippocampus (initial memory consolidation), Neocortex (long-term memory storage)
**Neurotransmitters:** GABA, Glutamate, Acetylcholine
**Memory Type:** Preliminary Consolidation of Short-Term Memory

As you drift off, your brain begins to slow down. This is the lightest stage of sleep, where your brain starts to tune out the world and prepares for deeper rest. Theta waves start to dominate, and your brain begins to process the day's experiences, initiating the transfer of memories from the hippocampus to the neocortex for long-term storage (Pace-Schott & Spencer, 2015).

It's marked by slow eye movements and a reduction in muscle activity. Your heart rate and breathing start to slow down, setting the stage for deeper sleep. The glymphatic system (the brain's clean-up crew) activation begins to stir in the background, but it's still in the warm-up phase.

The brain's "let's stay awake!" crew—glutamate, acetylcholine, norepinephrine, and serotonin—begin to pack it up. With the locus coeruleus dialing back norepinephrine, your brain starts to tune out unnecessary stimuli—like drawing the curtains on your senses. Cortisol, the stress hormone, also takes a nosedive, letting you leave the day's worries behind.

Meanwhile, the sleepy squad—led by GABA—starts to take over. The locus coeruleus (LC), your brain's alertness hub (courtesy of norepinephrine), also begins to power down, reducing dopamine and signaling that it's time to chill. Serotonin in the pineal gland is transformed into melatonin, the hormone that helps you drift off. Melatonin kicks in, courtesy of the pineal gland, giving your body the message to wind down. This is where your brain starts to tune out external stimuli, though it's still relatively easy to wake up.

In this light sleep stage, sleep spindles, oscillations, and ripples are just getting warmed up, prepping for the deeper stages of sleep where the real memory magic happens.

**Hypnic Jerks:** Ever been jolted awake just as you're falling asleep? That's a hypnic jerk—your brain's awkward attempt to transition from wakefulness to sleep. It's like your brain tells your muscles to relax but then misfires, causing a sudden twitch. This happens when neurotransmitters like dopamine, glutamate, and serotonin get out of sync (Muzet et al., 2021).

**Exploding Head Syndrome:** Despite the explosive name, this phenomenon is more startling than dangerous. As you're dozing off, you might hear a loud bang or explosion in your head—except it's all in your imagination. It's likely caused by a neural misfire in the auditory regions of your brain or a sudden shift in neurotransmitter levels (Sharpless, 2021).

**Stage 2: Light Sleep—Organizing the Memories**
**Time Elapsed:** 10-25 minutes after hitting the pillow
**Brain Areas Involved:** Hippocampus, Thalamus, Neocortex

**Neurotransmitters:** GABA, Melatonin, Galanin
**Memory Type:** Procedural Memory Consolidation (skills and habits)

Just 10-25 minutes after hitting the pillow, your brain starts getting down to business, consolidating all the "how-to" memories—like playing the piano or riding a bike. This stage is all about procedural memory consolidation, where the brain stores these skills in the neocortex for future use. Sleep spindles and K-complexes, those bursts of brain activity, act like security guards, filtering out unnecessary noise and distractions so your brain can focus on the task at hand (Rasch & Born, 2013).

Meanwhile, growth hormone is released, prepping your body for the deeper stages of sleep by aiding in tissue repair and muscle growth. Melatonin keeps you in the sleep zone, and the locus coeruleus—the brain's version of Grand Central Station—continues to dial down, lowering norepinephrine levels and effectively turning off the Wi-Fi on your senses. Galanin, the neuropeptide sidekick, ensures your brain isn't easily roused by external stimuli, keeping things quiet on the home front.

But beware! If dopamine and serotonin levels spike when they're supposed to be low, you might find yourself grinding your teeth or dealing with periodic limb movement disorder. These pesky disruptions happen when muscle tone increases due to neurotransmitter imbalances (Lavigne et al., 2020). So, let your brain do its thing and keep those memories organized—no interruptions, please!

**Stage 3: Deep Sleep (N3) – The Heavy Lifting**
**Time Elapsed:** 20-50 minutes after hitting the pillow
**Brain Areas Involved:** Hippocampus, Neocortex, Glymphatic System
**Neurotransmitters:** GABA, Glutamate, Norepinephrine, Dopamine
**Memory Type:** Declarative Memory Consolidation (facts and events), Prevention of Over consolidation of Traumatic Memories

Welcome to Stage 3, where your brain turns into a janitor on steroids, scrubbing and polishing like it's preparing for a surprise inspection. Delta waves, the slowest and deepest brain waves, take over—think of them as the brain's slow-motion cleaning crew. Meanwhile, the glymphatic system, which is basically your brain's Roomba, goes to work vacuuming up all the junk, like beta-amyloid, which nobody invited to the party but apparently showed up anyway.

This stage is also when your brain gets serious about memory consolidation. It's like a librarian on a mission, moving facts and events from the hippocampus (the brain's post it note) to the neocortex (the brain's filing cabinet) for long-term storage. And here's where IGF2 steps in—imagine it as Dad showing off his best dance moves because only his gene copy gets to boogie and lock in those memories.

But it's not all memory and muscle work—this is also when telomerase, your chromosomes' personal trainer, keeps them in shape for the long haul. You're in the "dead to the world" phase now, with your brain's security guard, the locus coeruleus, basically taking a nap. Norepinephrine levels drop to rock bottom, so nothing short of an air horn is going to wake you up. Galanin plays the role of the ultimate sleep bouncer, keeping things calm and peaceful.

On the flip side, if your neurotransmitters decide to throw a party at the wrong time, you might find yourself sleepwalking. Think of it as your body trying to have a midnight snack while your brain is still snoozing. And let's not forget night terrors—when your brain's fight-or-flight system gets a bit too enthusiastic, causing you to have a full-on horror movie moment without even waking up. Blame it on an overactive nervous system and a serotonin-norepinephrine mix-up. Your brain: always keeping things interesting, even in deep sleep!

**REM Sleep: The Dream Factory**
**Time Elapsed:** 70-90 minutes after hitting the pillow (Cycling every 90 minutes)
**Brain Areas Involved:** Amygdala (emotional processing), Hippocampus, Neocortex, Thalamus
**Neurotransmitters:** Acetylcholine, Norepinephrine, Serotonin, Dopamine
**Memory Type:** Emotional Memory Consolidation and Creative Problem-Solving

About 90 minutes into sleep, you enter REM (Rapid Eye Movement) sleep, where your brain is highly active. This stage is all about emotional memory processing and creative problem-solving. Your brain waves resemble those of wakefulness, and your brain starts solidifying the emotional aspects of your memories. The amygdala, the brain's emotional center, is highly active, ensuring that emotionally charged memories are stored effectively in the neocortex (Stickgold, 2005; Scullin & Bliwise, 2015).

During REM, your brain also engages in a dialogue between the hippocampus and neocortex, integrating emotional experiences with factual memories. This is also the stage where you experience vivid dreams, as your brain processes the day's experiences and prepares you for the challenges of the next day (Walker & Stickgold, 2010). The brain has both Theta and Beta waves—a paradox where the brain's active, but the body's in lockdown.

During REM sleep, acetylcholine spikes, revving up brain activity, while norepinephrine and serotonin drop, ensuring you don't start acting out your dreams. Meanwhile, dopamine increases in the limbic system, making your dreams feel vivid and emotional, like an AR/VR experience.

As cortisol slowly rises to prepare you for waking, melatonin keeps you in dreamland. IGF2 is hard at work consolidating emotional memories, helping you process the day's stress without carrying it into tomorrow. This stage is all about emotional memory and creative problem-solving. The amygdala is actively processing feelings, while the hippocampus and neocortex work together to link these emotions with facts. Dopamine plays a key role in making sure these memories stick.

Even though your body is paralyzed (thanks to REM atonia), your brain is busily solidifying memories and fueling creativity, with telomerase possibly contributing to cellular repair. In REM, you're insulated from minor external stimuli, with the locus coeruleus shutting down to prevent disturbances and keep anxiety in check.

**Confusional Arousals:** Confusional arousals happen when you partially wake up during deep sleep, leaving you confused and disoriented. This occurs due to an incomplete transition from deep sleep to wakefulness, where brain regions aren't fully activated. Low GABA levels or issues in the cholinergic system might contribute to this confusion.

**Sleep Enuresis (Bedwetting):** Sleep enuresis, or bedwetting, usually happens in deep sleep when the brain fails to respond to bladder signals, leading to involuntary urination. This condition is often linked to delayed neural maturation or deficiencies in antidiuretic hormone (ADH), causing the bladder to relax too much during sleep.

**Memory Retrieval: Bringing It All Back**

**Brain Areas Involved:** Prefrontal Cortex (executive functions), Hippocampus (retrieval of memories), Neocortex (storage of long-term memories)

**Neurotransmitters:** Glutamate, Dopamine, Acetylcholine

Retrieving a memory is like dusting off an old vinyl record and playing it again. The prefrontal cortex, which handles executive functions like decision-making and problem-solving, collaborates with the hippocampus to locate the memory you need. Once the memory is found, it's retrieved from the neocortex where it has been stored as long-term memory. This process relies heavily on glutamate to activate the neural circuits involved and dopamine to reinforce the retrieval, making the experience more vivid and rewarding (Duarte et al., 2010; Preston & Eichenbaum, 2013).

- **Prefrontal Cortex:** The conductor, directing attention and helping you decide which memory to retrieve.
- **Hippocampus:** The librarian, locating the specific memory stored in the neocortex.glu
- **Neocortex:** The archive, where long-term memories are stored and accessed when needed.

So, the next time you struggle to remember where you left your keys, just think of all the neurotransmitters, brain waves, and cellular gymnastics that go into every single memory. From the first spark of recognition to the deep sleep where it's all solidified, your brain is constantly working to keep your memories sharp—or at least to remember the important stuff, like 90s jingles and your spouse's birthday.

**The Magic of Mistakes: How Errors Make You Remember Better**

Now, let's talk about mistakes. You might think that errors are bad news for your brain, but when it comes to memory, they're actually a secret weapon. Making mistakes activates a brain process known as "error correction," where the brain flags the error and works extra hard to remember the correct information (Metcalfe, 2017). It's like your brain saying, "Well, that was wrong—let's make sure we don't mess that up again!"

When you make an error, especially while learning something new, your brain engages in a deeper level of processing. This happens because the mistake creates cognitive dissonance, making the brain more attentive and primed to encode the correct information. When you sleep, your brain revisits those flagged moments, replaying them to ensure that the correct information sticks. So, next time you mess up on a quiz or forget someone's name, remember: your brain is taking notes and will make sure you get it right next time (Schultz & Dickinson, 2000).

### So, what happens if you don't get enough sleep?

That's like sending the brain's night shift workers home early. Without sufficient sleep, the memory consolidation process is disrupted. You might find yourself forgetting where you parked your car—or worse, what you learned for that big exam (Walker, 2019).

### The Science of Sleepy Teens

Teenagers' tendency to stay up late and sleep in isn't just due to Netflix—it's biology. During puberty, their circadian rhythms shift, making it harder to fall asleep early and wake up for those 7:00 a.m. school bells (Carskadon, 2011). When schools ignore this, teens suffer from chronic sleep deprivation, which harms their mood, grades, mental health, and even safety (Wheaton et al., 2016).

Studies show that pushing back school start times improves sleep, academic performance, and mental health while reducing car accidents. A University of Minnesota study found that later start times led to more sleep and better grades, while Seattle's initiative added 34 minutes of sleep and saw mental health benefits (Wahlstrom et al., 2014; Dunster et al., 2018). The American Academy of Pediatrics recommended no school should start before 8:30 a.m. (AAP, 2014). Recent studies, including those from the University of Colorado Boulder and University of Rochester, confirmed the link between more sleep and improved mental health (Wheaton et al., 2020; Evans et al., 2021).

California passed Senate Bill 328, making it the first state to require later school start times, and early results show happier, healthier, and more engaged students (Gavin et al., 2023). Teens aren't lazy—they're just following science.

## Infantile Amnesia: The Great Blank Slate

Ever wondered why your memories from your early years are as hazy as trying to remember a dream? That's because of a phenomenon called infantile amnesia. Basically, your brain was too busy building itself up to bother storing memories. Think of it as trying to save data on a hard drive that's still being installed. Your hippocampus, the brain's memory maestro, was under construction during those early years, so it just tossed those memories aside like they were yesterday's leftovers (Huynh, 2024; Höhn, 2024). And hey, maybe it's for the best—you don't really need to remember all those diaper disasters.

## Memory Suppression: The "No Thanks, I'll Pass" Button

Let's talk about memory suppression, which is like your brain's way of hitting the "mute" button on things that no longer serve you. Forgetting isn't always a failure; sometimes, it's your brain saying, "You know what? We're not going to keep that one." Whether it's a bad haircut or a cringeworthy karaoke performance, your brain is doing you a favor by letting those memories fade away. But if you forgot your best friend's birthday, well, that's on you—you clearly didn't mark it as VIP in your mental calendar!

## Unhealthy Forgetting: When Things Go a Little Too Far

Forgetting some things is fine—like that time you tried to cut your own bangs—but when you start forgetting critical stuff, like cooking your dinner in the bathroom instead of the kitchen, then we've got a problem. This is where forgetting turns from funny to a bit scary. It's your brain waving a red flag, saying, "Uh-oh, something's not right!" Stress, for example, can flood your brain with cortisol, which messes with your hippocampus and turns your memory into a leaky bucket (Luo, 2024).

## The Locus Coeruleus: The Bouncer at the Memory Club

The locus coeruleus (LC) is like the bouncer at your brain's memory club. It decides who gets in and who gets tossed out. When something important happens, the LC steps in, cranks up the norepinephrine, and makes sure that memory gets VIP treatment. But if it's just some random detail, the LC waves it off like, "Nah, you're not on the list." This helps your brain prioritize what's truly important while letting go of the fluff (Orlando, 2024; Liu, 2024).

**You forgot why you entered a room or opened the fridge—don't panic, it's normal.**

Imagine your brain as a slightly stressed librarian trying to keep everything organized in a chaotic bookstore. To manage this, it creates "event boundaries"—mental post-it notes that say, "Hey, something just changed!" These boundaries are like when you walk through a doorway and suddenly forget why you're in the room (Griffiths & Fuentemilla, 2019; Ongchoco, 2023).

At the center of this operation is the hippocampus, the head librarian, handling new memories upfront and digging out old ones in the back (Fritch et al., 2020; Preston & Eichenbaum, 2013). Helping out is the prefrontal cortex, the assistant manager, making sure memories stay organized even when those pesky boundaries try to mess things up (Jeye et al., 2017). The parahippocampal gyrus, the Marie Kondo of your brain, keeps everything tidy, while the anterior thalamic nuclei act as the bouncer, deciding which memories get to stay (Ben-Yakov et al., 2013; Štillová et al., 2015).

So, when you forget why you entered a room, just remember: it's your brain's way of keeping the chaos under control. You are fine, take a deep breath.

**Keys? What Keys? The Science of Forgetting Everyday Things**

Forgetting where you put your keys or glasses isn't a sign that your brain is on vacation—it's actually your brain being super-efficient, or at least trying to be. Your brain operates like a supercomputer with limited RAM, meaning it has to prioritize important information (like "don't get hit by a car") over trivial stuff (like "where did I put my glasses?") (Stokes et al., 2020).

Think of it this way: your brain is constantly juggling, and sometimes, it decides that remembering where you put your keys just isn't worth dropping the ball on remembering your boss's name during a Zoom call.

This prioritization is influenced by things like emotional significance and whether the information is actually useful—so if your keys were involved in a dramatic moment, you'd probably remember where they are (Wan et al., 2022).

When cognitive load ramps up—like when you're multitasking or trying to navigate the chaos of modern life—your brain says, "Okay, something's gotta give," and that something is often the location of your keys (Sewell et al., 2020).

This isn't just random forgetfulness; it's your brain strategically offloading trivial details to make room for more pressing matters, like not burning dinner or remembering your anniversary (Langerock et al., 2023).

And let's not forget about sleep. While you're dreaming about flying or showing up to school without pants, your brain is busy consolidating memories. The hippocampus plays memory DJ, replaying the greatest hits and letting the one-hit wonders (like where you last saw your keys) fade into obscurity (Qiao, 2023).

So, the next time you can't find your keys, don't sweat it. It's just your brain doing a little spring cleaning, keeping the important stuff front and center while letting the small stuff slide.

# Who Gets the Credit (or Blame) for Your Memory?

**Mom's Genes: The X-Factor and Snack Patrol**

First up, mom. She doesn't just pass on her charm—she throws in some serious cognitive power too, thanks to the X chromosome. One standout gene here is *Tlr7*, crucial for memory and long-term potentiation (the brain's way of strengthening synapses) in the hippocampus, the brain's memory HQ (Abdulai-Saiku et al., 2022). So, if your child aces their spelling test, you might want to thank mom's X chromosome.

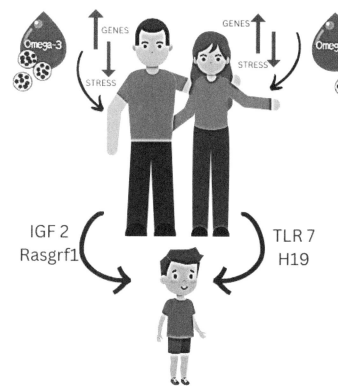

Mom's genes also influence memory through epigenetic modifications—those chemical tweaks that can alter gene expression without changing the DNA sequence itself. For instance, the *H19* gene from mom plays a role in development, indirectly impacting brain function and memory (Monk et al., 2019).

But that's not all. What mom munches on during pregnancy and breastfeeding can also shape your child's brain. If mom's diet was a little too high in junk food, it might have messed with the synaptic organization in your child's brain, potentially leading to some memory hiccups down the road (Gauvrit, 2023). So, those late-night ice cream cravings might have added more than just a few pounds—they could've added a little forgetfulness too.

Since women have two X chromosomes (one from each parent), they might get a double dose of these memory-boosting genes. Men, on the other hand, have only one X chromosome from mom, making that single chromosome's influence even more crucial (Arnold, 2020).

## Dad's Genes: The Memory Maestro with a Side of Stress

Now, let's talk about Dad. It turns out that what Dad eats before conception is just as important as Mom's diet. If Dad was big on omega-3s, it's good news for your kid's hippocampus—their memory center (Li et al., 2022). So, if your child remembers every detail from that zoo trip, you might thank Dad's love for fish. But Dad's influence doesn't stop at diet. Stressful experiences before becoming a father can actually alter gene expression related to memory and brain function (Rimawi, 2023). So, if Dad was pulling his hair out over work before you conceived, it might explain why your kid sometimes forgets where they put their homework.

Dad's Y chromosome might give men an edge in spatial memory, thanks to a few Y-linked genes that influence brain development. So, if you never get lost (or at least claim not to), you might owe that to Dad (Skuse, 2005).

## Genomic Imprinting: The Genetic Tug-of-War

Genomic imprinting is like your DNA playing favorites, where one parent's genes get the megaphone while the others are told to take a seat and stay quiet. Take *IGF2*—Dad's genetic megaphone for memory. In the world of genomic imprinting, *IGF2* is paternally expressed, meaning Dad's version of this gene takes center stage, while Mom's is shushed into the background. This isn't just a power play; it's crucial for your brain's growth and memory capabilities (Gregg et al., 2010).

**Here's how it works:** during sperm formation, Dad's *IGF2* gene undergoes special modifications, like getting a hypomethylation makeover, which ensures it's fully active in the developing embryo. This hypomethylated state allows *IGF2* to crank up the production of new neurons (neurogenesis), which are vital for memory and learning. Essentially, *IGF2* is the brain's growth factor, ensuring all the right neural connections are in place for top-notch cognitive function.

Then there's *Rasgrf1*, Dad's memory magic wand. This gene acts like your brain's memory coach, but here's the kicker—it's Dad's version of this gene that runs the show. *Rasgrf1* is the mastermind behind synaptic plasticity, which is a fancy way of saying it helps your neurons stay flexible and ready to learn. It's the gene that ensures your brain's "save" button works properly, storing all those new memories so you don't forget where you parked or why you walked into the kitchen.

*Rasgrf1* doesn't stop there—it also oversees neurogenesis, the brain's way of making new neurons. This is especially important in the hippocampus, the brain's memory factory. By keeping neurogenesis in check, *Rasgrf1* ensures your brain stays sharp and adaptable, like a mental upgrade every now and then.

But here's the twist: the expression of these imprinted genes can vary, meaning both Mom's and Dad's genes can either boost or mess with your kid's memory. It's a genetic game of tug-of-war, and sometimes, nobody wins (Wang et al., 2020).

### Epigenetics: The Environmental Shaper
Even with the best genetic blueprint, environmental factors like stress, diet, and lifestyle play a significant role in how memory-related genes are expressed. So, if you were raised in a stimulating environment, your memory might get an extra boost, while chronic stress could dampen those genetic advantages (Hackman et al., 2010).

Let's not forget the epigenetic landscape, where both parents have their say. Mom's folic acid intake during pregnancy can shape DNA methylation in her child, impacting neurodevelopment and learning abilities (Feifel et al., 2017). Meanwhile, Dad's early life stress can leave lasting marks on gene expression, affecting memory and cognition (Karami et al., 2019). It's like both parents are writing little notes in their child's genetic code—some helpful, some maybe not so much.

### Conclusion: Who's Really in Charge?
So, when your kid can recite every line from their favorite show but can't remember to clean their room, you can thank—or blame—both sides of the family. It's a mix of Mom's X-factor, Dad's diet, some stress here and there, and a whole lot of genomic tag-teaming. In the end, it's all in the genes—both of them!

**The Intergenerational Transmission of Trauma and Epigenetic Mechanisms: The Stress That Keeps on Giving**

The intergenerational transmission of trauma is a complex phenomenon that has garnered significant attention in recent years, particularly in the context of epigenetic mechanisms. Unlike psychological inheritance alone, this transmission involves biological processes that can affect gene expression across generations. The concept suggests that trauma experienced by one generation can leave epigenetic marks that influence the health and behavior of subsequent generations, creating a legacy of stress that extends beyond personal experience.

**Mechanisms of Trauma Transmission** Epigenetics plays a crucial role in how trauma is transmitted across generations, and two primary mechanisms have been identified: developmentally programmed effects and preconception trauma.

**Developmentally Programmed Effects:** These occur when stress during pregnancy or early parenting alters the epigenetic landscape of the offspring, effectively programming their stress response systems. Maternal stress during pregnancy can lead to DNA methylation changes in genes associated with stress regulation, impacting the child's emotional and behavioral outcomes (Quinn et al., 2023; Olson, 2020). Think of it as the stress the mother experiences becoming embedded in the child's genetic makeup, affecting their future ability to handle stress.

**Preconception Trauma:** Trauma experienced by parents before conception can also result in epigenetic modifications in their children. Studies on male mice have shown that stress can lead to altered sperm DNA, which is then passed down to their offspring (Bolhuis et al., 2022; Zhou, 2023). This suggests that trauma has a proactive way of preparing the next generation for stress, even before they are conceived.

**Epigenetic Changes and Their Implications** Epigenetic modifications do not alter the DNA sequence itself but instead affect how genes are expressed. This can be likened to changing how a recipe is followed without altering the ingredients. Significant genes involved in the stress response, such as *FKBP5* and *NR3C1*, have been implicated in the intergenerational transmission of trauma. Changes in the methylation patterns of these genes can predispose individuals to heightened stress responses and psychiatric disorders, including PTSD (Nie et al., 2022; Chou, 2024). Recent research has shown that individuals with a history of childhood trauma display distinct DNA methylation patterns that correlate with their mental health outcomes, suggesting that trauma becomes biologically embedded (Jowf et al., 2021; Lim et al., 2022).

**Animal Studies and Human Evidence** Animal studies have provided compelling evidence for the intergenerational transmission of trauma. Research has demonstrated that rodents exposed to stress pass anxiety-like behaviors to their offspring through epigenetic changes in their sperm (Bolhuis et al., 2022; Zhou, 2023). These findings are mirrored in human studies, particularly among populations with historical trauma, such as Holocaust survivors and Indigenous peoples, where descendants exhibit similar psychological symptoms despite not having directly experienced the trauma (Olson, 2020; Zhou, 2023). This evidence suggests that trauma can persist across generations, influencing mental health and behavioral outcomes.

**Cognitive Behavioral Therapy (CBT) and EMDR in Trauma Intervention** While the implications of intergenerational trauma are significant, there is hope in therapeutic interventions. Cognitive Behavioral Therapy (CBT) and Eye Movement Desensitization and Reprocessing (EMDR) have both shown efficacy in addressing the effects of trauma, including trauma inherited from previous generations. These therapies work by helping individuals process traumatic experiences, potentially mitigating the impact of epigenetic changes (Roque-López et al., 2021).

**CBT:** This therapy helps individuals identify and change negative thought patterns, which can disrupt the cycle of stress passed down through generations. By rewiring the way one thinks, CBT can help reduce the inherited burden of trauma on mental health.

**EMDR:** EMDR, which uses guided eye movements to reprocess traumatic memories, can lessen the emotional charge of trauma, including inherited trauma. EMDR has been particularly effective in helping individuals process deeply ingrained trauma and its intergenerational impact.

## Lifestyle Modifications and Epigenetic Influence

In addition to therapies like CBT and EMDR, certain lifestyle modifications can support healthy gene expression and improve stress resilience. Nutrition, mindfulness, and adequate sleep can positively influence epigenetic mechanisms, potentially reducing the impact of inherited trauma (Quinn et al., 2023; Roque-López et al., 2021).

**Nutrition:** Consuming foods rich in leafy greens, berries, turmeric, and omega-3s can promote healthy DNA methylation and stress resilience.
**Mindfulness:** Mindfulness practices help reduce stress and enhance mental well-being by influencing how genes related to stress regulation are expressed.
**Sleep:** Quality sleep acts as a reset button for the body, promoting healthy gene function and mitigating the negative effects of stress.

## The Science Behind It: DNA's Sticky Notes

How exactly does trauma get passed down through generations? The key mechanisms involve DNA methylation and histone modification. Trauma can alter how genes like *NR3C1* (which regulates the stress response) and *FKBP5* (which helps control cortisol, the stress hormone) function. These epigenetic changes can predispose future generations to anxiety and stress-related disorders.

For example:

- **NR3C1:** Trauma experienced by ancestors could tweak this gene, making descendants more susceptible to stress.
- **FKBP5:** Alterations in this gene could lead to an overactive stress response, especially if trauma is part of the family history.
- **BDNF (Brain-Derived Neurotrophic Factor):** Trauma can reduce *BDNF* expression, crucial for mood regulation and cognitive function, potentially leaving future generations with lower resilience to stress (Nie et al., 2022).

## Animal Studies as Proof
Animal studies provide direct evidence of intergenerational trauma transmission. For instance, stressed-out mice passed anxiety to their offspring via altered sperm, even when the offspring were raised in a calm environment (Bolhuis et al., 2022; Zhou, 2023). Similarly, rats conditioned to fear specific smells passed down

that fear through epigenetic changes to their offspring, even though the offspring had never been exposed to the original trauma (Dias & Ressler, 2014).

## Therapeutic Interventions: The Way Forward

Given the deep-rooted effects of trauma, interventions like CBT, EMDR, and lifestyle changes offer hope. These strategies can help individuals manage their own trauma and potentially mitigate the effects of inherited trauma. Addressing trauma through therapeutic and lifestyle interventions can help reverse epigenetic modifications and break the cycle of intergenerational stress.

# Apoptosis, Autophagy & Mitophagy Walk into a Brain-

**It's No Joke, They're Vital!**

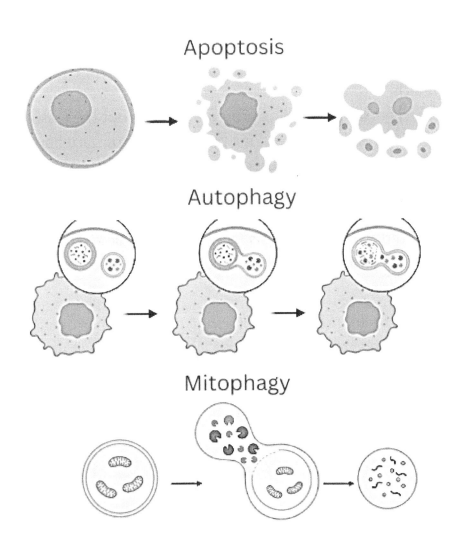

Apoptosis

Autophagy

Mitophagy

# Death, Detox, and Mitochondrial Recycling: The Brain's Ultimate Housekeeping Trifecta

Ah, the brain. It's like the world's most temperamental roommate: sometimes neat and tidy, other times cluttered with junk it can't seem to throw out. Fortunately, three unsung heroes—autophagy, apoptosis, and mitophagy—are here to keep things in check. Imagine them as Marie Kondo, Judge Judy, and Mr. Clean of brain health, respectively. Without them, we'd all be walking around with cluttered neurons, dysfunctional mitochondria, and probably a little more neurodegeneration than we'd like. Research shows that these processes are crucial in keeping neurodegenerative diseases like Alzheimer's and Parkinson's from turning our brains into a hoarder's paradise (Xiong et al., 2022; Harris et al., 2020; Corti et al., 2020).

**Autophagy and Brain Health**

Autophagy is like the brain's personal recycling program—taking out the trash, one misfolded protein at a time. When it's working properly, neurons are happy, and everything is spick and span. But when autophagy gets lazy, or worse, overwhelmed, the brain starts looking like a teenager's messy room, with toxic protein aggregates piling up everywhere (Harris et al., 2020; Corti et al., 2020). Think of Alzheimer's as the ultimate clutter crisis, where amyloid-beta (Aβ) aggregates are the dirty laundry you can't seem to find the time to deal with (Lee et al., 2022).

Fortunately, fasting—aka the brain's equivalent of spring cleaning—has been found to kick autophagy into high gear. You skip a meal, and suddenly, your brain's all, "Let's clean this mess up!" (Brocchi et al., 2022; Currenti et al., 2021). Even better, scientists are eyeing the mTOR pathway, which could become the neuro-version of a Roomba, cleaning up without you even lifting a finger (Atya, 2024; Jimenez-Sanchez et al., 2022).

## Apoptosis and Neuroprotection

Apoptosis, meanwhile, is the brain's tough but fair bouncer, removing those unruly neurons that just aren't pulling their weight. But, like a bouncer with a little too much power, if apoptosis gets carried away, it can empty the whole club and lead to neurodegeneration (Corti et al., 2020; Lu et al., 2022). Luckily, autophagy often steps in and says, "Hey, don't kick them out just yet. Maybe we can save them," especially when oxidative stress comes into play (Lee et al., 2022; Lu et al., 2022). It's like having a second chance for those poor neurons hanging by a thread.

Scientists are figuring out how to enhance autophagy to keep apoptosis in check and prevent unnecessary neuron evictions (Krishnan et al., 2020; Lu et al., 2022). It's all about balance, like deciding between binge-watching Netflix and hitting the gym—too much of one or the other, and something's bound to go wrong.

## Mitophagy: The Role of Mitochondrial Quality Control

Now, if you've ever been stuck with a dead battery, you'll understand the role of mitophagy. It's like replacing your mitochondria's double-A batteries before they leak and corrode the whole device (Ultanir et al., 2022; Lee et al., 2022). Mitophagy gets rid of faulty mitochondria before they go full meltdown, releasing reactive oxygen species (ROS) that make a bad situation worse. Without mitophagy, your neurons are like a phone stuck at 1% battery—stressful and inefficient (Alharbi, 2023).

But fear not! By dialing up mitophagy, we can improve mitochondrial function and reduce oxidative stress, which, let's be honest, we could all use less of. Enter the PINK1/Parkin pathway—this tag team identifies the deadbeat mitochondria and says, "You're outta here!" (Ultanir et al., 2022; Lee et al., 2022). And if you need another reason to skip that second slice of cake, caloric restriction has been found to enhance mitophagy and boost brain power (Alharbi, 2023). Your brain will thank you.

## When Neurons Hoard Junk: Why You Need Kimchi, Green Tea, and Essential Oils ASAP

Picture your brain as an office space with overflowing trash cans and malfunctioning appliances (aka mitochondria). Now imagine your janitors—autophagy, apoptosis, and mitophagy—just decided to take an extended holiday.

Chaos ensues, and suddenly, your neurons are swimming in toxic proteins, your mitochondria are coughing up reactive oxygen species, and the trash is piling up. Luckily, there are some sneaky ways to get the cleanup crew back on duty. Spoiler alert: it involves fasting, meditation, fiber, and maybe even some kimchi.

**Genetic Diseases and Toxins: When Brain Housekeeping Goes Wrong**

In conditions like Parkinson's, Alzheimer's, and Huntington's diseases, the brain's normal trash removal systems get compromised. Instead of dealing with their problems, your neurons are procrastinating, leaving piles of misfolded proteins and malfunctioning mitochondria to rot (Williams et al., 2023; Zhang et al., 2024). And let's not forget toxins like pesticides and heavy metals—they're the bad influences that come over and make your brain skip cleaning day (Gonzalez et al., 2023).

**The Role of Fasting: Firing Up Autophagy**

Now, here's where fasting comes into play. Fasting is like the ultimate way to yell, "Clean up this mess!" to your brain's cleaning crew. When you fast, your body goes into autophagy overdrive, clearing out damaged proteins, toxins, and even rogue mitochondria that are making things worse (Brock et al., 2023).

But not everyone is up for a full-on fast, so let's talk about the fasting-mimicking diet (FMD). This diet tricks your body into thinking it's fasting while you're still allowed to eat small amounts of food. It's like telling your cleaning crew they can take shorter coffee breaks but still need to finish the job. Both fasting and FMD can boost autophagy, but the key difference is that FMD allows some food intake (which makes it slightly more bearable) while still activating those important cellular cleanup processes (Longo et al., 2023).

**MCT Oil and Other Fats: Brain Fuel and Cleanup Support**

If you're feeling fancy, you can turbocharge this process with Medium-Chain Triglycerides (MCTs). MCT oil, derived from coconut oil, is basically like giving your neurons rocket fuel (Nagpal et al., 2022). It bypasses the usual digestion process and heads straight for your liver, where it turns into ketones—an alternative energy source for your brain. Ketones can help boost mitochondrial function, which in turn promotes mitophagy (that's your brain cleaning up its deadbeat mitochondria) (Nagpal et al., 2022).

But don't stop there! Other oils like extra virgin olive oil and fish oil (high in omega-3 fatty acids) have anti-inflammatory properties that further support brain health by reducing oxidative stress and boosting autophagy (Ghezzi et al., 2022). Essentially, these oils are like giving your brain a spa treatment while the cleaning crew works in the background.

**Clinical Features: What Happens When the Janitors Quit?**
If you've ever walked into a room that hasn't been cleaned in months, you can imagine what happens to the brain when autophagy, apoptosis, and mitophagy slow down. Memory loss, motor dysfunction, and cognitive decline are the telltale signs (Zhang et al., 2024). In diseases like Alzheimer's, protein buildup leads to memory lapses, while in Parkinson's, movement gets impaired as mitochondria fail to function (Williams et al., 2023).

**Preventing the Mess: The Ultimate Brain Clean-Up Guide**
1. **Fermented Foods and Fiber: Gut Health Meets Brain Health**
   Your brain's cleaning crew gets a lot of help from your gut. Fermented foods like yogurt, sauerkraut, and kimchi are packed with probiotics that improve gut health, which has a direct impact on autophagy and inflammation in the brain (Chang et al., 2022). Meanwhile, fiber-rich foods (think leafy greens, oats, and fruits) keep your gut moving smoothly, ensuring that autophagy isn't just happening in your gut, but also in your neurons (Jenkins et al., 2023).

2. **Anthocyanin-Rich Foods: The Brain's Tiny Brooms**
   If your neurons need a little extra sweeping, reach for anthocyanin-packed foods like blueberries, blackberries, and purple cabbage. These colorful foods are known for their ability to reduce oxidative stress and promote autophagy, making them your brain's best friend (Brock et al., 2023).

3. **Fasting & FMD: Call in the Cleaning Team**
   As mentioned earlier, fasting and the fasting-mimicking diet are like calling in professional cleaners for your brain. Fasting stimulates autophagy by forcing your body to recycle old cellular parts for energy. The fasting-mimicking diet does the same thing, but with fewer hunger pangs (Longo et al., 2023).

4. **MCT Oil & Other Healthy Fats: Fueling the Brain**
   Add MCT oil to your morning coffee, or drizzle some extra virgin olive oil on your salad, and you're giving your brain high-quality fuel that boosts mitochondrial function and cleans up damaged cells (Nagpal et al., 2022). Plus, omega-3-rich oils like fish oil reduce inflammation, making them another key player in your brain's detox regimen.

5. **Meditation and Grounding: A Brain Vacation**
   When your brain's stressed, it can't clean up properly. Enter meditation—a simple yet effective way to reduce oxidative stress, enhance focus, and promote autophagy (Singh et al., 2023). For bonus points, throw in some grounding by walking barefoot outside, which has been shown to lower inflammation and give your brain the mental equivalent of a beach vacation (Chevalier et al., 2023).

6. **Essential Oils, Herbs, and Spices: A Little Extra Help**
   Essential oils like rosemary and lavender aren't just for making your house smell nice—they can also promote brain health. Studies show that these oils may stimulate cognitive function and autophagy (Fang et al., 2022). Throw in some turmeric (rich in curcumin) and ginger, and you've got a powerful team of brain-boosting, anti-inflammatory spices (Chen et al., 2023).

7. **Supplements: Brain Janitors in a Bottle**
   If you're looking to get more targeted, supplements like resveratrol, NAD+ precursors, and coenzyme Q10 are all excellent choices for supporting autophagy and mitochondrial health (Garcia et al., 2024).

Let us table the discussion here. What all things can enhance this decluttering of toxic cellular debris from our brain?

| Category | Items | Bioactive Compounds | Process | Mechanism of Action |
|---|---|---|---|---|
| **Fruits** | Strawberries | Fisetin, Anthocyanins, Quercetin, Ellagic Acid | Apoptosis, Mitophagy, Autophagy | Fisetin promotes apoptosis by activating caspases, enhances mitophagy by regulating mitochondrial function, and induces autophagy by activating AMPK. |
| | Blueberries | Anthocyanins, Quercetin, Resveratrol | Autophagy, Mitophagy, Apoptosis | Activates AMPK, promotes mitophagy by increasing mitochondrial function, and induces apoptosis via caspases. |
| | Apples | Fisetin, Quercetin | Apoptosis, Autophagy. Mitophagy | Fisetin induces apoptosis through p53 activation, promotes autophagy by inhibiting mTOR, and stimulates mitophagy by improving mitochondrial health. |
| **Foods** | Pomegranates | Urolithin A, Ellagitannins | Mitophagy. Apoptosis | Urolithin A promotes mitophagy via PGC-10/AMPK and induces apoptosis via mitochondrial dysfunction. |
| | Cruciferous Vegetables (e.g., broccoli) | Sulforaphane | Apoptosis, Autophagy, Mitophagy | Enhances mitophagy via Nrf2 activation, induces apoptosis via caspases, and promotes autophagy by inhibiting NF-kB. |

| Vegetables | Broccoli | Sulforaphane | Apoptosis, Mitophagy, Autophagy | Activates Nrf2, caspases, and promotes mitochondrial health. |
|---|---|---|---|---|
| | Garlic | Allicin | Apoptosis, Mitophagy | Induces apoptosis via Bax and caspase activation, promotes mitophagy by reducing oxidative stress. |
| | Spinach | Flavonoids, Polyphenols | Apoptosis, Autophagy | Promotes apoptosis through mitochondrial pathways and autophagy by activating AMPK. |
| Teas | Green Tea | EGCG (Epigallocatechin gallate) | Apoptosis, Autophagy, Mitophagy | Activates AMPK, SIRT1, and induces apoptosis via caspases. |
| | Black Tea | Theaflavins | Apoptosis, Autophagy | Induces apoptosis by activating caspases and regulates autophagy via AMPK activation. |
| Herbs | Rosemary | Carnosic Acid, Rosmarinic Acid | Mitophagy, Apoptosis | Promotes mitophagy and apoptosis through mitochondrial dysfunction and caspase activation. |
| | Ashwagandha | Withanolides, Sitoindosides | Apoptosis, Autophagy | Stimulates apoptosis via mitochondrial dysfunction and promotes autophagy via AMPK activation. |
| Spices | Turmeric (Curcumin) | Curcumin | Apoptosis, Mitophagy, Autophagy | Inhibits mTOR, promotes autophagy, and induces apoptosis via p53 activation. |
| | Black Pepper (Piperine) | Piperine | Autophagy, Apoptosis | Enhances bioavailability of curcumin and promotes autophagy by inhibiting mTOR. |
| | Ginger | Gingerol | Apoptosis, Autophagy | Activates apoptosis via mitochondrial pathways |

| | | | | and promotes autophagy through AMPK activation. |
|---|---|---|---|---|
| **Fats** | Extra Virgin Olive Oil | Oleocanthal, Oleuropein | Apoptosis, Autophagy | Induces apoptosis by destabilizing lysosomes, promotes autophagy via AMPK activation. |
| | Coconut Oil | Lauric Acid, Medium-Chain Triglycerides (MCTs) | Autophagy, Apoptosis | Enhances autophagy via AMPK activation, induces apoptosis by promoting mitochondrial dysfunction. |
| **Nuts** | Walnuts | Omega-3, Polyphenols | Autophagy, Apoptosis | Activates AMPK, promotes mitochondrial health, and induces apoptosis via caspase activation. |
| **Supplements** | Resveratrol | Resveratrol | Apoptosis, Mitophagy, Autophagy | Activates SIRT1 and induces apoptosis, promotes mitophagy via the PINK1/Parkin pathway. |
| | Berberine | Berberine | Apoptosis, Mitophagy, Autophagy | Activates AMPK, induces apoptosis by inhibiting mTOR and caspase activation. |
| | Coenzyme Q10 | CoQ10 | Mitophagy, Apoptosis | Enhances mitophagy and mitochondrial health by reducing oxidative stress and induces apoptosis by stabilizing mitochondria. |
| | Nicotinamide Riboside (NR) | NAD+ | Apoptosis, Mitophagy | Stimulates mitophagy by increasing SIRT1 activity, induces apoptosis via mitochondrial pathways. |

# The Sweet Scandal at the Bridgeton Ball

It was another dazzling evening at Lady Sweetina's annual Bridgeton ball, where the crème de la crème gathered to enjoy fine music, grand company, and—most importantly—the sweetest of treats.

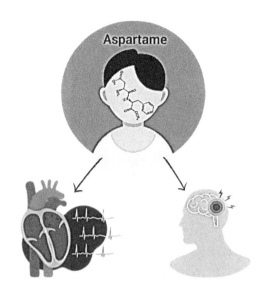

### Scene 1: The Aspartame Incident

The night began with the grand entrance of Lady Aspartame, whose history of health controversies was no secret. Her presence caused ripples of unease. Whispers filled the air about her links to cancer, particularly thyroid cancer and colon cancer recurrence (Journal of Clinical Medicine Research, 2020; Plos One, 2018). "She's also been associated with stroke and coronary heart disease," murmured Miss Saccharin (Vyas et al., 2014), as guests glanced nervously at their diet sodas. Worse still, recent studies suggested that people genetically predisposed to heart problems could be at higher risk of atrial fibrillation when consuming sweetened beverages with aspartame (Circulation Arrhythmia and Electrophysiology, 2024).

Lady Aspartame was also infamous for causing metabolic derangements, worsening insulin sensitivity, and disrupting glucose metabolism, making her a paradoxical villain for people with diabetes or obesity (Trends in Endocrinology and Metabolism, 2013; Theoretical and Natural Science, 2023).

### Scene 2: Stevia's Grand Entrance—A Natural Hero with Hidden Powers

Then came Lady Stevia, whose arrival drew both admiration and curiosity. Derived from the plant *Stevia rebaudiana*, she had built a reputation not only as a natural sweetener but also as a potential therapeutic agent, especially for people with diabetes.

Studies had highlighted stevia's anti-diabetic properties, showing that its active compounds, steviol glycosides, could improve glucose metabolism and significantly reduce blood sugar levels in diabetic models (Hussain & Hafeez, 2021; Niri et al., 2023; Jan et al., 2021). "She's known for sensitizing insulin receptors and enhancing pancreatic beta-cell function, which leads to improved glycemic control," noted Lady Diabetes (Hussain & Hafeez, 2021; Ray et al., 2020). Stevia also demonstrated hypoglycemic effects, reducing glycated hemoglobin levels and serum glucose in diabetic subjects (El-Hadary & Sitohy, 2020; Sari et al., 2020). "Beyond her role in diabetes, Lady Stevia has been associated with promising anti-inflammatory and antioxidant properties, which might help mitigate risks of cardiovascular disease and even cancer," added Sir Cardio Health (Iatridis et al., 2022; Sadhu, 2024; Velesiotis et al., 2022).

To top it off, stevia had been shown to improve lipid profiles, lowering cholesterol and triglyceride levels, which was crucial for heart health (Nikhitha et al., 2022; Mlambo et al., 2022). With regulatory bodies such as the FDA recognizing stevia as generally safe for consumption (Kasti et al., 2022; Orellana-Paucar, 2023), she had become the darling of health-conscious individuals.

"Despite these benefits, we must remember that long-term studies are still limited," whispered Miss Saccharin. "Though she's widely considered safe, more research is needed to understand her full potential." Nonetheless, Lady Stevia's appeal grew as she stood against her artificial counterparts, offering a natural solution for managing diabetes, obesity, and heart disease (Niri et al., 2023; Mbambo et al., 2020).

### Scene 3: Acesulfame Potassium—The Troublemaker

Just as Lady Stevia basked in the admiration of the crowd, Sir Acesulfame Potassium (ACE-K) stormed into the room, disrupting the serenity. Known for his longevity and affordability, ACE-K carried significant risks. Studies had linked him to weight gain and gut microbiome disturbances, as demonstrated in animal models (Plos One, 2017). Worse, he had been implicated in increasing the risk of cardiovascular diseases, which left guests wondering whether their hearts were safe from his influence (Journal of Cardiology, 2023).

## Scene 4: The Parade of Sweeteners—Saccharin and Sucralose
As the night went on, a parade of other sweeteners arrived, each with their own controversies.

Miss Saccharin, once accused of causing bladder cancer in rats, had been cleared for human use but remained under scrutiny (Journal of Pharmacology and Pharmacotherapeutics, 2011). Meanwhile, Sir Sucralose, despite his sleek promises of zero calories, was linked to gut dysbiosis and metabolic syndrome, leading to disruptions in insulin sensitivity and glucose homeostasis (Suez et al., 2021; Frontiers in Nutrition, 2021).

## Scene 5: Monk Fruit and Allulose—Newcomers on the Scene
As murmurs about Lady Aspartame spread, Lady Allulose and Sir Monk Fruit arrived, attracting attention with their reputation as "natural" alternatives. Lady Allulose, known for her low-calorie allure, was whispered to cause gastrointestinal issues, including bloating, gas, and diarrhea when consumed in large quantities (Hayashi et al., 2010; Iida et al., 2010). "She's rare but quite disruptive to the gut microbiome," noted Lord Metabolism, referring to emerging studies suggesting potential long-term impacts on gut health (Uebanso et al., 2017).

Sir Monk Fruit, though praised for his natural origins, also carried risks. He was linked to allergic reactions, particularly in those sensitive to gourds, and his long-term effects on glucose regulation and body weight were still largely unknown (Nair et al., 2018; Frontiers in Nutrition, 2021).

## Scene 6: The Heart's Final Flutter—A Warning from Lord Epigenetics
As the evening reached its climax, Lord Epigenetics made his dramatic entrance. He unfurled a scroll, warning the guests that the effects of their chosen sweeteners didn't end with them. "Artificial sweeteners could be altering your DNA, passing epigenetic changes to your descendants," he warned, highlighting

potential risks of anxiety, heart disease, and metabolic disorders in future generations (Jones et al., 2022; Zhu et al., 2018).

The guests, who had come for a night of guilt-free indulgence, now found themselves gripped with unease. Even the "natural" sweeteners came with hidden risks, while their artificial counterparts seemed to invite even greater dangers.

## Scene 7: The Sweet Legacy

As the guests left the Bridgeton Ball, they clutched their sugar-free sodas and desserts with newfound caution. Aspartame, stevia, sucralose, acesulfame potassium, monk fruit, and allulose—each had their benefits and risks. From stroke, cancer, and heart disease to metabolic disorders and gut dysbiosis, it seemed no sweetener was truly innocent.

## Before we say goodbye...

*This little book was lovingly crafted with the simple yet heartfelt hope of sparking your curiosity and inspiring you to explore that extraordinary brain of yours—the one that quietly works wonders every day, even though we often take it for granted. Truly, it's a masterpiece. Now, before you embark on any life-changing journeys, I really urge you to consult your doctor! Some medications have a way of mingling with others in ways you wouldn't expect, and trust me, you don't want to be caught in that mix without your doctor's blessing.*

*And please, if you find any mistakes or if a new study emerges that shakes up what I've shared here, I humbly ask that you let me know. Science is a wild, ever-evolving adventure, and it's easy to miss a twist or turn. So, if human error sneaks in (and let's face it, it likely will), I hope you'll grant me a little grace and understanding. If you can find extra love and forgiveness in your heart toward this sincere, though perhaps not perfect, attempt to share what I know could help you, I would be truly grateful.*

*I wrote this out of care—care for you, for the marvel that is the human brain, and for the simple desire to help. So, if I stumble along the way, kindly give me a nudge in the right direction. We're all in this together, learning and growing side by side.*

*The humor I've woven into this book is not meant to diminish the gravity of conditions like dementia or stroke. As someone who personally survived a stroke at just 27, I deeply understand the seriousness of these challenges. My aim is to offer knowledge in a way that's more approachable, in the hope that it lightens the weight of difficult topics while still honoring the significance of the struggles they represent. Humor, in this case, is simply a tool to make understanding a little easier, not to make light of the hardships.*

*Most of all, I want you to enjoy this journey. Life is meant to be lived fully, but let's make sure the fun we're having is also good for us, okay? Take care, and until we meet again—whether it's in conversation or in Volume Two: Building Better Mitochondria, Metabolism, & Liver Here's a little sneak peek from the upcoming book.*

# The Brew-tiful Battle for Liver Health

Coffee's Caffeine, Chlorogenic Acids, and the Liver Super Team

In the bustling town of Liverton, where the sound of coffee machines was as constant as the town clock, a new health trend had taken root: coffee was not just for keeping the residents awake—it had become the town's unofficial liver savior.

At the forefront of this discovery was Joe Brewster, Liverton's self-proclaimed coffee expert, health evangelist, and barista whisperer.

For years, Joe had been singing the praises of his favorite brew. But today, armed with more scientific evidence than ever, Joe was ready to convince everyone in town that their daily cup of joe wasn't just keeping them alert—it was giving their livers a much-needed boost, thanks to the superhero duo of caffeine and chlorogenic acids (CGAs).

## A New Dawn in Liverton: Coffee as the Liver's Best Friend

One crisp morning, Joe burst into the Liver Café, his usual haunt, waving a handful of scientific papers like they were treasure maps.

"Guess what, everyone!" Joe declared, loud enough to startle Old Man Frank out of his decaf-induced daydream. "Coffee's not just for staying awake through Zoom meetings anymore. It's basically a liver superhero in a cup!"

Sue, the barista, who had long grown used to Joe's coffee-fueled monologues, raised an eyebrow. "What are you on about this time, Joe?"

Joe beamed, slapping down the papers. "Caffeine and chlorogenic acids! These two are the real MVPs in coffee, and they're working overtime to protect our livers from all sorts of bad stuff like non-alcoholic fatty liver disease (NAFLD), cirrhosis, and even liver cancer!" (Di Pietrantonio et al., 2020)

Sue blinked. "You're saying my latte is fighting liver disease?"

"Exactly!" Joe leaned in, his eyes wide. "Caffeine is like the bouncer for your liver. It stops those sneaky hepatic stellate cells from overproducing collagen. Too much collagen leads to liver scarring, and before you know it, you've got cirrhosis. But with coffee, it's like you've got a tiny, caffeinated bodyguard stopping that from happening." (Hamden et al., 2021)

Old Man Frank piped up, his curiosity piqued. "So, my decaf is doing that too?" Joe grinned. "Ah, Frank, you're in luck! Chlorogenic acids—they're the unsung heroes of both regular and decaf coffee. They're busy reducing oxidative stress, lowering inflammation, and basically telling liver cells to calm down and stop hoarding fat. So yes, even your decaf is giving your liver a helping hand!" (Pace Palitti et al., 2022)

Frank raised his cup triumphantly. "Well, good to know I'm not just drinking this sludge for nothing."

## The Coffee Science Deep Dive

Joe's enthusiasm couldn't be contained. He pulled out a piece of paper with a poorly drawn diagram of a liver and began scribbling furiously. "Here's the deal, Sue. Caffeine isn't just a wake-up call for your brain—it's doing wonders for your liver by blocking adenosine receptors. That stops all those fibrosis-triggering proteins like TGF-β from messing things up. And it even gets rid of excess collagen by increasing hepatic stellate cell apoptosis—basically, it makes those trouble-making cells hit the 'self-destruct' button!" (Zheng et al., 2014)

Sue stared, half-impressed, half-confused. "So, my liver is... what, doing a happy dance every time I drink coffee?" "Pretty much!" Joe nodded enthusiastically. "Chlorogenic acids (CGAs) are like the liver's personal cleaning crew. They reduce fat buildup, regulate lipid metabolism, and keep those pesky inflammatory cytokines in check. The more CGAs you have, the cleaner your liver stays." (Di Pietrantonio et al., 2020)

Sue smirked. "So it's like a detox, but without all the kale smoothies?"

"Exactly!" Joe laughed. "And get this—people who drink three to four cups a day have a 59% lower risk of liver cancer if they've got hepatitis B. That's a serious deal! It's not just about perking you up—coffee's literally fighting off fibrosis, cirrhosis, and cancer." (Pace Palitti et al., 2022)

### Decaf vs. Regular: The Great Coffee Debate
As the conversation picked up, more café regulars gathered around. Someone asked the burning question, "So, which is better? Decaf or regular?"

Joe was ready for this one. "Good question! Turns out, both decaf and regular coffee offer benefits. Sure, caffeine has its own perks—it's great at blocking liver fibrosis—but chlorogenic acids are present in both types, and they're the real game-changer when it comes to liver health. Studies show that even if you're drinking decaf, you're still getting most of the benefits, especially when it comes to fighting inflammation and oxidative stress." (Hamden et al., 2021)

Old Man Frank, now feeling quite smug about his decaf, raised his mug. "So, no matter what, I'm still giving my liver a workout?"

"You bet," Joe said, tipping his own cup in a mock toast. "Whether you're drinking full caffeine or decaf, you're still giving your liver a fighting chance. Just don't go crazy—more than six cups a day might start to mess with your heart, so keep it balanced." (Pace Palitti et al., 2022)

### The Liver's Ultimate Sidekick
As the café patrons soaked in their newfound knowledge, Sue asked, "So, three to four cups a day keeps the liver in check? Is that the magic number?"

Joe nodded. "Pretty much. Three to four cups a day is the sweet spot. Studies show that people who hit that range have a 30-40% lower risk of liver fibrosis and liver cancer. But if you really want to get the best out of your coffee, stick with filtered coffee. None of that Turkish or espresso stuff—turns out the brewing process matters. Filtering helps keep all the good stuff in without the extra cholesterol-raising compounds." (Di Pietrantonio et al., 2020)

## The Town That Loved Coffee

By now, the whole café was on board. Liverton had officially declared coffee not just a morning necessity but the town's unofficial liver supplement. Even Old Man Frank, who had once been a staunch believer in cutting back on caffeine, was now sipping his decaf with newfound respect.

"Here's to coffee," Joe said, raising his cup high. "The liver's best friend and the world's greatest beverage."

Sue rolled her eyes but smiled. "Alright, Joe, you've convinced me. I'll start thinking of every latte I pour as a little liver boost."

And so, in Liverton, coffee wasn't just keeping people awake—it was saving their livers one cup at a time. The town's residents kept sipping, knowing that with every gulp, they were giving their livers a well-deserved spa day.

As the coffee chatter reached new heights in Liverton, Joe Brewster decided to share one final nugget of wisdom with the café crowd, leaning in with a conspiratorial tone.

"Now, folks, if you really want to take your coffee—and your liver—up a notch, there's one more thing you need to know: not all coffee is created equal. The best brew for your liver? It's got to be single-origin, non-GMO, organic black pour-over coffee."

Sue, halfway through pouring another cup, looked up. "What, like the fancy stuff?"

"You bet," Joe said, nodding. "Single-origin coffee comes from one location, usually a small farm, meaning it's grown with fewer pesticides and chemicals. And when you choose organic and non-GMO, you're making sure that your coffee is free from any nasty additives that could mess with your liver's detox process. Plus, when you go for black pour-over, you're preserving all the chlorogenic acids and antioxidants that work their magic on liver health. It's basically the purest form of coffee, and studies show that it packs the most punch when it comes to protecting against fatty liver and other chronic liver diseases." (Di Pietrantonio et al., 2020;Hamden et al., 2021)

Old Man Frank raised an eyebrow. "So, no cream, no sugar, just black?"

Joe grinned. "Exactly. You want to keep it pure to get all those bioactive compounds straight into your system without any interruptions."
But Joe wasn't done yet. "And if you're dealing with fatty liver or want to go the extra mile, you can even add a bit of MCT oil to your coffee.
Studies suggest that medium-chain triglycerides (MCTs) can help reduce liver fat and improve liver function by promoting fat metabolism and reducing lipid accumulation in the liver.

It's like giving your coffee an extra boost in the fight against fatty liver disease." (St-Onge & Bosarge, 2021)

Sue raised her cup, now fully convinced. "So, single-origin, organic, non-GMO black pour-over with a splash of MCT oil?"

Joe lifted his mug in a celebratory toast. "The ultimate liver-loving brew!" And with that, Liverton's residents knew they weren't just sipping coffee anymore— they were crafting liver-saving potions, one perfect pour-over at a time.

Made in United States
North Haven, CT
01 December 2024

61306675R00202